# Immune Thrombocytopenia (ITP)

UNI-MED

UNI-MED Verlag AG
Bremen - London - Boston

**Kühne, Thomas:**
Immune Thrombocytopenia (ITP)/Thomas Kühne.-
3rd edition - Bremen: UNI-MED, 2022
(UNI-MED SCIENCE)
ISBN 978-3-8374-1624-4



Printed in Europe

# MEDICINE - STATE OF THE ART

UNI-MED Verlag AG, one of the leading medical publishing companies in Germany, presents its highly successful series of scientific textbooks, covering all medical subjects. The authors are specialists in their fields and present the topics precisely, comprehensively, and with the facility of quick reference in mind. The books will be most useful for all doctors who wish to keep up to date with the latest developments in medicine.

The publisher would like to thank the company Swedish Orphan Biovitrum for supporting the production of this edition. The publisher assures that the industry partner could not influence the content of the book in any way, especially not therapy recommendations.

# Preface to the 3rd edition

In recent years there was much movement in the area of immune thrombocytopenia (ITP). There is increasing knowledge in the understanding how platelets function and what is wrong with them under pathological conditions. It has been realized that platelets are not only cells involved in hemostatic processes, but also act in innate and adaptive immune responses and exert inflammatory functions. ITP occurs as a result of dysregulated immune responses based on probably many different mechanisms, which may cause thrombocytopenia as a result of an increased and premature destructive process of platelets and a disturbed mega- and thrombopoiesis. This destructive process may evolve into therapy-refractoriness ("autoimmune expansion") in certain patients that is not predictable. Our clinical observations and assessments of platelet counts however do not tell us clearly neither the bleeding risk of a given patient, nor his or her disease course. This may be due to the fact that there is usually absence of individual information of ITP pathomechanisms and that bleeding is a complex process influenced by intrinsic and extrinsic factors affecting platelet production and function. This complexity is the reason why ITP exhibits a strong clinical inter- and intra-patient variability with unpredictable response to therapies and thus demands for individual solutions. Moreover, there is increasing knowledge of symptoms other than bleeding, such as fatigue and reduced health-related quality of life, which may represent treatment endpoints and reflect patients' needs. Based on this knowledge new diagnostic and therapeutic strategies will be developed from which patients hopefully will benefit.

Elucidation of molecular pathways and targets and their disturbances are the basis for the development of new therapies, similarly to other areas in medicine. This process will probably continue with the aim for treating so-called targets reflecting the desire for tolerable, efficient and curative treatments for all patients without side effects and complications and development of strict patient selection criteria. We are far away from this ideal concept, but we may increasingly be aware of the way how to approach this ideal.

The third edition of this book attempts to reflect this departure into future time without omitting current scientific knowledge and clinical practice of children and adults with ITP. The material of ITP became so complex and substantial in recent years, that a comprehensive book would need much more time and volume. The current edition was written in a difficult time reflected by the COVID-19 pandemic with many obstacles and adversities. I would like to express my deep gratitude to all co-authors who worked hard on this edition and who contributed to the successful completion of this book. It was a real and great pleasure to collaborate with them and to see the book growing. I would like to thank the publisher UNI-MED Verlag Bremen, who always supported me, never lost patience and always demonstrated interest in this book project. I hope that this new edition contributes to optimal patient care and management.

*Basel, January 2022* *Thomas Kühne*

# Authors

Carlo L. Balduini
Ferrata-Storti Foundation
Pavia
Italy

*Chapter 6.*

Carolyn E Beck, MD, MSc, FRCPC
Associate Professor
Faculty of Medicine
University of Toronto
Division of Paediatric Medicine, Department of Paediatrics
The Hospital for Sick Children
Toronto
Ontario, Canada

*Chapter 9.*

George R. Buchanan, MD
Division of Hematology-Oncology
Center for Cancer and Blood Disorders
Children's Medical Center and
University of Texas Southwestern Medical Center
Dallas, Texas
USA

*Chapter 20.*

James B. Bussel, MD
Department of Pediatrics
Weill Medical College
525 East 68th Street P-695
New York NY 10021
USA

*Chapter 13.*

Andrew R. Crow, BRT
Transfusion Medicine Research
St. Michael's Hospital
30 Bond Street
Toronto, Ontario
Canada, M5B 1W8

*Chapter 15.*

Yoelys Cruz-Leal
Centre for Innovation
Canadian Blood Services
Ottawa, ON
Canada

Keenan Research Centre for Biomedical Science
St. Michael's Hospital
Unity Health Toronto
Toronto ON
Canada

Toronto Platelet Immunobiology Group
Toronto, ON
Canada

*Chapter 16.*

Samuel Deshayes
Service de médecine interne
CHU de Caen Normandie
Avenue de la Côte de Nacre
14033 Caen Cedex
France

*Chapter 11.*

Terry B. Gernsheimer, MD
Professor of Medicine and Hematology
University of Washington
Puget Sound Blood Center
Seattle
USA

*Chapter 14.*

Waleed Ghanima
Consultant Hematologist
Professor, Institute of Clinical Medicine
Østfold Hospital
University of Oslo, Norway

*Chapter 12.*

Lazaro Gil
Keenan Research Centre for Biomedical Science
St. Michael's Hospital
Unity Health Toronto
Toronto ON
Canada

Toronto Platelet Immunobiology Group
Toronto, ON
Canada

*Chapter 16.*

Bertrand Godeau, MD
Service de médecine interne
Centre labellisé de référence pour la prise en charge et la recherche sur les cytopénies auto-immunes de l'adulte
Centre Hospitalier Universitaire Henri-Mondor
Assistance Publique-Hôpitaux de Paris
Université Paris Est Créteil
51, avenue du Maréchal-de-Lattre-de-Tassigny
94010 Créteil cedex
France

*Chapter 11.*

Paul Imbach, MD
Division of Oncology/Haematology
University Children's Hospital
Postfach
Römergasse 8
CH-4005 Basel
Switzerland

*Chapter 2., 21.*

Robert Klaassen, MD, FRCP(C)
Professor, Department of Pediatrics
Division of Hematology/Oncology
Department of Pediatrics
University of Ottawa
Children's Hospital of Eastern Ontario
Ottawa
Ontario, Canada

*Chapter 9., 18.*

Thomas Kühne, MD
Division of Oncology/Haematology
University Children's Hospital
Postfach
Römergasse 8
CH-4005 Basel
Switzerland

*Chapter 1., 10.*

Michele P. Lambert, MD, MSTR
The Children's Hospital of Philadelphia
Division of Hematology, Philadelphia, PA
Perelman School of Medicine
University of Pennsylvania
Department of Pediatrics
Philadelphia, PA

*Chapter 4.*

Alan H. Lazarus
Centre for Innovation
Canadian Blood Services
Ottawa, ON
Canada

Department of Laboratory Medicine and Pathobiology
University of Toronto
Toronto, ON
Canada

Keenan Research Centre for Biomedical Science
St. Michael's Hospital
Unity Health Toronto
Toronto ON
Canada

Toronto Platelet Immunobiology Group
Toronto, ON
Canada

Department of Medicine
University of Toronto
Toronto, ON
Canada

*Chapter 15., 16.*

Joel Livingston MSc, MD, FRCPC
Clinical Fellow
Division of Haematology/Oncology
Department of Paediatrics
University of Toronto
The Hospital for Sick Children, Toronto
Ontario
Canada

*Chapter 18.*

Axel C. Matzdorff, MD, PhD
Director Dpt. of Hematology, Oncology, Hemostasis
Caritasklinikum Saarbruecken St. Theresia
Rheinstrasse 2
66113 Saarbrücken
Germany

*Chapter 17.*

Adrian Newland, CBE
Professor of Haematology
Barts and The London School of Medicine and Dentistry
Queen Mary University of London
London, UK
Email: a.c.newland@qmul.ac.uk

*Chapter 19.*

Peter A.A. Norris
Centre for Innovation
Canadian Blood Services
Ottawa, ON
Canada

Department of Laboratory Medicine and Pathobiology
University of Toronto
Toronto, ON
Canada

Keenan Research Centre for Biomedical Science
St. Michael's Hospital
Unity Health Toronto
Toronto ON
Canada

Toronto Platelet Immunobiology Group
Toronto, ON
Canada

*Chapter 16.*

Alessandro Pecci
University of Pavia
IRCCS Policlinico San Matteo Foundation
Pavia
Italy

*Chapter 6.*

Francesco Rodeghiero, MD
Department of Cell Therapy and Haematology
San Bortolo Hospital
Vicenza
Italy

*Chapter 8.*

Alexandra Schifferli
Department of Oncology/Hematology
University Children's Hospital Basel
Spitalstrasse 33
CH-4031 Basel, Switzerland

*Chapter 7.*

John W. Semple, PhD
Professor of Transfusion Medicine
Division of Hematology and Transfusion Medicine
Lund University
Clinical Immunology and Transfusion Medicine
Office of Medical Services
Region Skåne
Lund
Sweden

*Chapter 3.*

Zoya Tawhidi
Department of Laboratory Medicine and Pathobiology
University of Toronto
Toronto, ON
Canada

Keenan Research Centre for Biomedical Science
St. Michael's Hospital
Unity Health Toronto
Toronto ON
Canada

Toronto Platelet Immunobiology Group
Toronto, ON
Canada

*Chapter 16.*

Kevin D. Won
Department of Laboratory Medicine and Pathobiology
University of Toronto
Toronto, ON
Canada

Keenan Research Centre for Biomedical Science
St. Michael's Hospital
Unity Health Toronto
Toronto ON
Canada

Toronto Platelet Immunobiology Group
Toronto, ON
Canada

*Chapter 16.*

James L. Zehnder, MD
Professor of Pathology and Medicine (Hematology)
Director of Clinical Pathology, Department of Pathology
Stanford University School of Medicine
Director, Coagulation and Molecular Genetic Pathology Laboratories
Stanford Health Care
USA

*Chapter 5.*

# Contents

# 1. Introduction

"Immune thrombocytopenia" (ITP) was proposed by an international working group at the Vicenza Consensus Conference to be more appropriate than "idiopathic thrombocytopenic purpura" or "immune thrombocytopenic purpura", because of the immune-mediated mechanisms and because not all patients with ITP present with a purpura [1]. Furthermore, ITP was proposed by the same group to be classified as primary and secondary ITP. Primary ITP, formerly called idiopathic thrombocytopenic purpura, indicates absence of the knowledge of any initiating or underlying causes for thrombocytopenia and is the main topic of this book. Secondary ITP reflects immune mediated thrombocytopenia with a known cause, such as an infectious disease, lymphoproliferation, systemic lupus erythematosus, immune deficiency and other disorders, and is described elsewhere [2-5]. There is growing knowledge of secondary ITP both in children and adults [6, 7], particularly demonstrated by the SARS-CoV-2 pandemic.

Thrombocytopenia (platelet count <100 x $10^9$/L) is caused by premature platelet and megakaryocyte destruction by the monocytic-phagocytic system, which results in reduced survival of platelets, structural changes of platelets and their function, and in potential bleeding with a wide range of unpredictable clinical variability, from no or oligosymptomatic patients to severe fatal bleeding.

Mild and moderate bleeding, defined differently in the literature, is frequent, whereas severe fatal bleeding, such as intracranial haemorrhage, is rare in childhood and increases with age. Several reasons may be responsible for the variability and severity of bleeding, such as age of the patient, acquired and congenital co-morbidities, i.e. environmental and predisposing genetic factors, and drugs. Thrombocytopenia reflecting the key feature of ITP is the result of complex and not well-characterized various mechanisms involving the innate and adaptive immune system, the hematopoiesis, inflammatory system, and various regulatory systems. The classical pathophysiology with autoantibodies opsonizing platelets with their subsequent Fc-mediated phagocytosis is not always present. It is estimated that approximately one third of adult patients with ITP lack autoantibodies. Furthermore, autoimmunity represents a dynamic process with the potential of autoimmune expansion and epitope spreading, which may explain at least in part that chronic ITP may become therapy-refractory. Thus, an etiological background remains often unknown, which defines primary ITP. This unknown background of primary ITP must be taken into consideration when evaluating results of clinical trials. Despite rigorous inclusion and exclusion criteria, trial populations consist of individuals with a potentially highly heterogeneous pathophysiological background. This can be demonstrated when evaluating early cohort studies, which included patients with malignancies or patients treated with acetylsalicylic acid. Since the description of a patient with suspected "ITP" by Paul Gottlieb Werlhof in 1735 [8], basic science and clinical research have revealed many different acquired and inherited causes for thrombocytopenia, which cannot be classified as ITP based on modern definitions. Thus, the group of patients with primary ITP becomes steadily smaller during time. Primary ITP remains still a mystery and clinicians and researchers should be encouraged to critically use the diagnosis "primary ITP" and to continuously consider the large list of differential diagnoses. ITP may be simply considered as a symptom, rather than a "disease" ("Werlhof's disease"). The heterogeneity of ITP is a basis for controversies regarding pathophysiology and management of patients with ITP, and this unclear background is further fuelled by a substantial lack of knowledge of basic science and clinical research.

Lack of evidence and controversial management resulted in the establishment of various groups who developed national and international practice guidelines, which initially were based mainly on expert opinion and consensus conferences, rather than on evidence [9-13]. Although guidelines are appropriate and important tools to manage patients with ITP, there are also limitations, as critical questions have been asked, and as it has been shown that guidelines are not consistently followed [14-17]. Why is that? First of all, as it has been mentioned above, primary ITP is still a diagnosis of exclusion with the consequence, that the population of patients diagnosed with primary ITP represents a heterogeneous group causing difficulties in analyzing study results and drawing conclusions. Guidelines are not based solely on clinical evidence, demonstrated by George et al. [10], rather they reflect expert and consensus opinions based on relatively few clinical randomized trials, which are furthermore characterized by short follow-up time and frequently designed for objectives, which differ from objectives and their interpretations made in guidelines. These are reasons why there are various guidelines and why they are not consistent and even contradict each other in certain statements. Furthermore, they may not reflect the opinion of doctors working at "the front", because of different local circumstances, differences in availability of drugs and last but not least the complexity of such guidelines [11]. However, the development of guidelines stimulated a systematic and coordinated approach to the problems associated with ITP. With the development of thrombopoietin-receptor agonists, evidence-based medicine with strict criteria was introduced. Comprehensive and critical appraisal of the literature became the basis for an appropriate approach to and management of the patient with ITP, and optimization of research coordination including economical use of resources became goals of international activities.

Despite the difficulties associated with primary ITP many achievements have been made in recent years and will be discussed in this book, including growing knowledge in immunology, hemato- and megakaryopoiesis, platelet physiology, genetic aspects of autoimmune diseases, and pharmacology. Clinical achievements include a harmonization of terminology, definitions and outcome criteria [1], international activity in developing guidelines [11] and in coordinating research and communication, such as the Pediatric and Adult Registry on Chronic ITP (PARC-ITP) of the Intercontinental Cooperative ITP Study Group (ICIS, www.itpbasel.ch) and many other groups, and clearly the development of new drugs in recent years, such as monoclonal anti-CD20 antibodies, e.g., rituximab, and thrombopoietin receptor agonists, e.g., romiplostim, eltrombopag, avatrombopag, as well as fostamatinib, and drugs under development, such as FcRn-antagonists, BTK inhibitors, complement inhibitors and others. These new drugs created a new and fresh wind, which blows into algorithms and guidelines, resulting in new strategies of the management of patients with ITP. However, although the armamentarium of therapeutic interventions for such patients has been enriched with powerful new drugs, many scientific questions need to be answered and the exact clinical

| Problems in ITP |
|---|
| • Unknown etiology of primary ITP |
| • Primary ITP as a diagnosis of exclusion |
| • Difficulties in combining basic science and clinical research |
| • Predictability of chronic symptomatic ITP and of therapy refractory ITP |
| • Difficulty in estimation of individual bleeding risk |
| • Poorly defined endpoints and the use of the platelet count as treatment endpoint in the management of patients with ITP and in clinical trials |
| • Lack of validation of alternative treatment endpoints, such as bleeding, fatigue, health-related quality of life, adverse effects of platelet-enhancing drugs, and economical aspects |
| • Poorly defined prevention and treatment interventions of bleeding resulting in confusing assessments of their clinical benefit |
| • Substantial lack of investigator-driven clinical randomized trials and of real world data |
| • Substantial lack of knowledge of long-term natural history of ITP and long-term aspects after medical intervention, such as drugs and splenectomy |
| • Strategy of the management with novel drugs |
| • Integration of patients' needs and requirements and their voice in developing management strategies |

***Table 1.1:*** Problems in ITP (incomplete list).

strategical position of these drugs continues to await clarification. Furthermore, in developing new therapies and new management tools including practice guidelines it is important to integrate the patients' voice, in order to balance medical desires and treatment endpoints, as well as the patient's perspective and their needs [18].

As the world is becoming smaller and obstacles to collaborate are encountered less frequently, international activities become more feasible with the potential to overcome problems associated with rare diseases. Large numbers of patients can be approached better and faster, coordination of research may include many countries, and national borders may become conquerable with powerful communication tools to exchange study results within adequate time. There is, however, still a long list of substantial problems associated with ITP (☞ Table 1.1), which needs energy, courage, and investment for the realization of basic science and clinical research projects, but also for further improvement of international communication and coordination of resources and activities. Immune thrombocytopenia remains an attractive model disorder for autoimmunity and its treatment, in order to restore tolerance.

## References

1. Rodeghiero F, Stasi R, Gernsheimer T, et al. Standardization of terminology, definitions and outcome criteria in immune thrombocytopenic purpura (ITP) of adults and children. Report from an international working group. Blood 2009;113:2386-2393.

2. Liebman HA, Stasi R. Secondary immune thrombocytopenic purpura. Curr Opin Hematol. 2007;14:557-573.

3. Cines DB, Bussel JB, Liebman HA, Luning Prak ET. The ITP syndrome: pathogenic and clinical diversity. Blood. 2009;113:6511-6521.

4. Bussel JB. Therapeutic approaches to secondary immune thrombocytopenic purpura. Semin Hematol. 2009;46(Suppl 2):S44-58.

5. Kim TO, Despotovic JM. Primary and Secondary Immune Cytopenias Evaluation and Treatment Approach in Children. Hematol Oncol Clin N Am. 2019;33:489-506.

6. Schifferli A, Heiri A, Imbach P, et al. Misdiagnosed thrombocytopenia in children and adolescents: analysis of the Pediatric and Adult Registry on Chronic ITP. Blood Adv. 2021;5(6):1617-1626.

7. Michel M, Lega J-C, Terriou L. [Secondary ITP in adults] [Article in French]. Rev Med Interne. 2021;42(1): 50-57

8. Werlhof PG. De Variolis et Anthracibus. Hannover, 1735

9. Eden OB, Lilleyman JS Guidelines for management of idiopathic thrombocytopenic purpura. The British Paediatric Haematology Group. Arch Dis Child. 1992;67: 1056-1058.

10. George JN, Woolf SH, Raskob GE, et al. Idiopathic thrombocytopenic purpura: a practice guideline developed by explicit methods for The American Society of Hematology. Blood. 1996;88:3-40.

11. Provan D, Arnold DM, Bussel JB, et al. Updated international consensus report on the investigation and management of primary immune thrombocytopenia. Blood Adv. 2019;3(22):3780-3817.

12. Neunert C, Terrell DR, Arnold DM, et al. American Society of Hematology 2019 guidelines for immune thrombocytopenia [published correction appears in Blood Adv. 2020;4(2):252]. Blood Adv. 2019;3(23): 3829-3866.

13. Matzdorff A, Meyer O, Ostermann H, et al. Immune Thrombocytopenia – Current Diagnostics and Therapy: Recommendations of a Joint Working Group of DGHO, ÖGHO, SGH, GPOH, and DGTI. Oncol Res Treat 2018;(41 Suppl 5):1-30

14. Buchanan GR, de Alarcon PA, Feig SA, et al. Acute idiopathic thrombocytopenic purpura – management in childhood. Blood. 1997;89:1464-1465

15. Bolton-Maggs PHB, Moon I. Assessment of UK practice for management of acute childhood idiopathic thrombocytopenic purpura against published guidelines. Lancet 1997;350:620-623

16. Vesely S, Buchanan GR, Cohen A, et al. Self-reported diagnostic and management strategies in childhood idiopathic thrombocytopenic purpura: results of a survey of practicing pediatric hematology/oncology specialists. J Pediatr Hematol Oncol 2000;22:55-61

17. Matzdorff A, Arnold G. Treatment of chronic immune thrombocytopenic purpura: the patients' perspective. Eur J Haematol 2007;78:381-388

18. Terrell DR, Neunert CE, Cooper N, et al. Immune Thrombocytopenia (ITP): Current Limitations in Patient Management. Medicina 2020;56(12), 667

# 2. History of ITP

## 2.1. Introduction: What is thrombocytopenic bleeding?

Immune thrombocytopenia (ITP) is characterized by isolated destruction of platelets. Susceptible individuals are recognized with a low platelet count. Some of them demonstrate easy bruising, petechiae, suffusions, nose bleedings and rarely severe bleeding including hematuria, gastrointestinal bleeding, prolonged menstruation, and central nervous bleeding [1, 2] (☞ Table 2.1).

| Bleeding Grade Classification [20] | Bolton-Maggs & Moon % (n=427) | ICIS Registry II % (n=863) |
|---|---|---|
| None/mild | 76% (324) | 77% (665) |
| Moderate | 21% (90) | 20% (173) |
| Severe | 3% (13) | 3% (25)* |

***Table 2.1:*** Comparison of bleeding severity based on strict definitions of bleeding and bleeding scores by different authors. *Sites of bleeding (some with more than one site): epistaxis (15 cases), mouth (8 cases), gastrointestinal tract (8 cases), urinary tract (2 cases), multiple sites (12 cases), other (1 case), and menorrhagia and nervous system (1 case each).

For example, in the Intercontinental Cooperative ITP Study Group (ICIS) Registry II, 665 of 883 (70%) children with newly diagnosed ITP and a platelet count below 20 x $10^9$/L had no or mild bleeding at presentation, 173 (20%) had moderate bleeding, and 25 (3%) had severe bleeding. Bleeding was categorized as

(1) *none or mild*: no bleeding at all or bruising, petechiae, occasional mild epistaxis causing very little or no interference with daily living;

(2) *moderate*: more severe skin manifestations with some mucosal lesions and more troublesome epistaxis or menorrhagia; or

3) *severe*: bleeding episodes (epistaxis, melena, menorrhagia, and/or intracranial hemorrhage) requiring hospital admission and/or blood transfusions, i.e., symptoms interfering seriously with quality of life [3, 4].

The susceptibility of ITP is unknown. ITP often occurs as a para- or postinfectious event, which may indicate disturbed recovery of the subject's immune system. Most of these patients have a transient form of ITP. In other patients ITP is ongoing for 3 to 12 months (persistent ITP) or more than 12 months (chronic ITP). In persistent or chronic, secondary ITP may be present and a differential diagnosis must be performed (☞ Table 2.2).

| | |
|---|---|
| Primary ITP | 80 % |
| Para-/postinfectous (children) | (70 %) |
| Postvaccinal (children) | (1.2%) |
| Secondary ITP | 20 % |
| Systemic Lupus Erythematosus (SLE) | 5 % |
| Hepatitis C | 3 % |
| *Helicobacter pylori* | 2 % |
| Systemic infections | 2 % |
| Antiphospholipid Syndrome (APS) | 2 % |
| Evans Syndrome | 2 % |
| Chronic Lymphocytic Leukemia (CLL) | 2 % |
| Common Variable Immune Deficiency (CVID) | 1 % |
| Human Immunodeficiency Virus Infection | 1 % |

***Table 2.2:*** Short list of the differential diagnosis of primary and secondary ITP.

Pathophysiologically the severity of bleeding in patients with ITP reflects the balance between platelet production by megakaryocytes and the accelerated clearance of antibody-sensitized platelets. The antibodies are directed against specific epitopes on platelet glycoproteins (specific autoantibodies) or may be crossreactive, unspecific antibodies or immune complexes. The latter are mainly discussed in transient, postinfectious ITP.

The largest group of patients with thrombocytopenia are patients with cancer or autoimmune disorders under immunosuppressive treatment (chemotherapy, radiotherapy) leading to transient megakaryocyte suppression resulting in low platelet production as adverse effect. The group of patients is not included in this chapter.

## 2.2. History of bleeding

Bleeding signs are fearful for the patient and may disturb the quality of life of an individual. Since more than 2500 years bleeding was described and attempts made for resolvement.

During the Greek and Roman period beginning 700 years BCE spontaneous cutaneous bleeding has been named purpura, deduced from the greek porphyra which signifies the purple dye, secreted by the purple snail, used as status symbol during antiquity and the Middle Age. There was no knowledge of the different blood components and functions at that time.

In 1557 the Portuguese Amatus Lusitanus mentioned a condition *Morbus pulicaris absque fibre* (without fever). In his work *Curationum medicinalum* he describes "… a boy with dark macules, resembling flea bites, had no fever and for several days had bloody discharges, eventually recovering". His description could have been thrombocytopenic bleeding.

In the early seventeenth century, Riverius (Lazarus de la Rivière) in his *Praxis medica* mentioned "the spots arisen from the over thinness of the blood … does sprout forth of the capillary veins into the skin … where being retained, it looseth its own colour, and becomes either blewish or black, or light red, and causes great variety of spots…" [5].

In 1775 Paul Werlhof [6] (☞ Figure 2.1a) a poet, composer, linguist and physician described the disorder under the name of *Morbus Maculosus Haemorhhagicus.* He became physician to King George II of England, at the same time elector of Hannover. In his book *De Variolis et Anthracibus* (☞ Figure 2.1b) [7] he mentioned in a footnote a 16-year-old girl with cutaneous and mucosal bleeding which occurred after an infectious disease and recovered after Elixirium acidum Halleri (citric acid). The name of the elixir refers to Albrecht von Haller, famous Swiss physician, botanist and poet, who was professor at the University of Göttingen, where he contacted Werlhof.

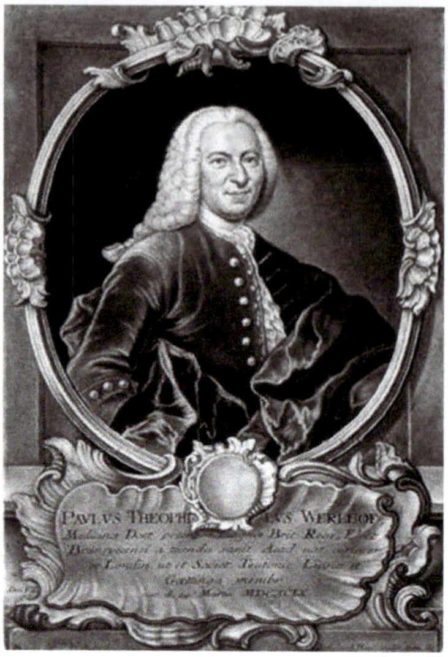

a

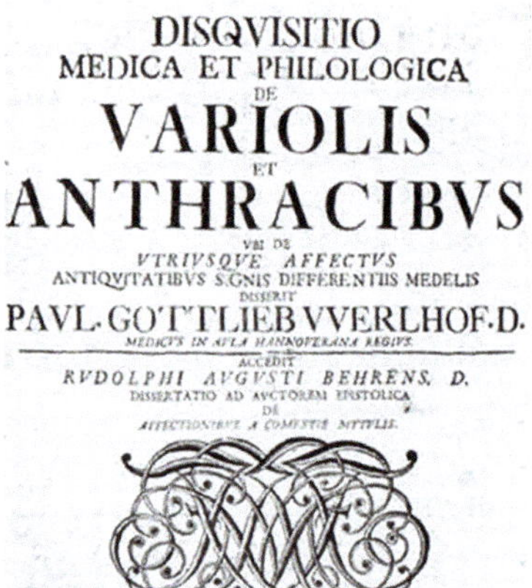
DISQVISITIO
MEDICA ET PHILOLOGICA
DE
VARIOLIS
ET
ANTHRACIBVS
VBI DE
VTRIVSQVE AFFECTVS
ANTIQVITATIBVS SIGNIS DIFFERENTIIS MEDELIS
DISSERIT
PAVL. GOTTLIEB VVERLHOF. D.
MEDICVS IN AVLA HANNOVERANA REGIVS.
ACCEDIT
RVDOLPHI AVGVSTI BEHRENS. D.
DISSERTATIO AD AVCTOREM EPISTOLICA
DE
AFFECTIONIBVS A COMESTIS MYTVLIS.

BOERHAAVE.
HANNOVERAE
SVMTIBVS HAEREDVM NICOLAI FOERSTERI ET FILII
clↄ Iↄcc xxxv.

b

***Figure 2.1a+b:*** **a**: Paul Gottlieb Werlhof. **b**: First page of his book *De Variolis et Anthracibus* (1735; with acknowledgement to Professor G. Gaedicke, Berlin, 1990).

The next milestone was the observation of a similar disorder by Dohrn in 1873 in a neonate and his mother. The term "platelets" was first used by Kraus 1883 [8] and Deny 1897 [9], who observed that platelets were diminished during the height of the purpura and increased when hemorrhage ceased. These findings were confirmed by Hayem [10] in 1895 who performed more accurate platelet counts.

## 2.3. History of the pathogenesis of ITP

In 1938, Troland and Lee [11] described a substance extracted from the spleens of patients with chronic ITP and named it "thrombocytopen". This substance produced transient thrombocytopenia when injected into rabbits. In 1951 in St. Louis, USA, Harrington et al [12] observed a child with purpura born to a mother with chronic ITP, a condition already described by Dohrn 1883 (☞ above). The child's purpura resolved spontaneously within three weeks, while the mother remained thrombocytopenic. Harrington then administered plasma from a patient with chronic ITP to himself and to nine volunteers with normal platelet counts. Eight of the recipients immediately developed transient thrombocytopenia. One of the volunteers, in spite of an earlier splenectomy, also responded, indicating that the spleen plays a secondary role. In his work, Harrington suggested an antiplatelet factor in the plasma as the cause of ITP (☞ Figure 2.3a).

With the development of plasmapheresis, Shulman et al. [13] in Boston in 1965 showed that the causative factor in the plasma of patients with ITP was associated with the IgG fraction. This factor bound to autologous and homologous platelets, as documented by Dixon [14] in 1975. Van Leeuven et al., in 1982 provided the first evidence for specific autoantibodies in chronic ITP: 32 of 42 eluates from ITP platelets bound to normal, but not to thrombasthenic (Glanzmann) platelets. As the latter are deficient in glycoprotein GP IIb-IIIa, the authors postulated that ITP patients have autoantibodies against one of these glycoproteins. Tests to measure platelet-associated antibodies (PAIgG) were established in 1987. These tests are characterized by high specificity (78-92%) and low sensitivity (49-66%) [15]. Recently, a new assessment of glycoprotein antibodies testing has been developed [16].

New insights into the pathogenesis of ITP have provided evidence of dysregulation of the immune response at the level of T-cells [17], of B-cells, of phagocytosis [18], and of dendritic cells/antigen presenting cells [17, 20]. Thus, immune dysregulation and suppression of platelets and megakaryocytes may play a primary role in the pathogenesis and the management of ITP, which is also true for many other inflammatory and autoimmune disorders (☞ Chapter 16.3.). In addition, not just peripheral platelets are involved in the pathogenesis of ITP, but megakaryocyte production and impaired maturation as well (☞ Chapter 2.6.).

Figure 2.2 roughly outlines the pathogenesis of ITP.

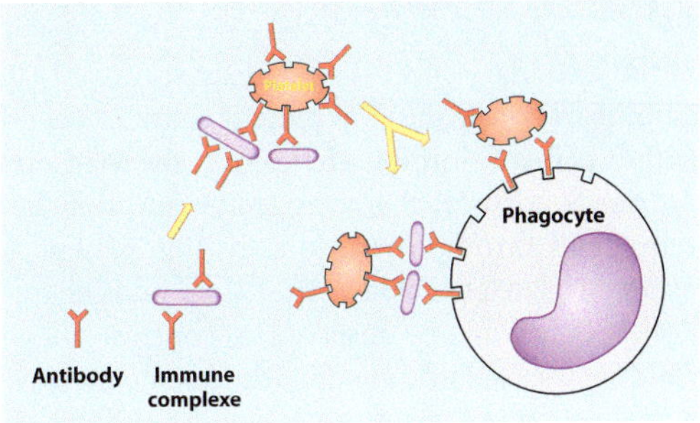


***Figure 2.2:*** Summary figure of pathogenesis in patients with ITP.

## 2.4. History of management of patients with ITP

In his 1808 book *On Cutaneous Diseases*, Willan [21] prescribed for Morbus Maculosus Haemorrhagicus "moderate exercise in the open air, a generous diet, and free use of wine."

In Prague 1916, the medical student Kaznelson hypothesized that ITP was analogous with hemolytic anemia based on the observation that excessive destruction of platelets occurs in the spleen [22]. He persuaded one of his tutors, Professor Schloffer, to perform a splenectomy in a woman with ITP. A dramatic platelet increase followed surgery. Since then, splenectomy has become a standard treatment for patients with severe bleeding in ITP.

Corticosteroids or other immunosuppressive agents increasing platelets have been used since 1951. The first controlled multicenter study, a randomized double-blind study of corticosteroids versus placebo for 21 days in children with newly diagnosed ITP was carried out by the Swiss J. Sartorius in Basel when he returned from Detroit, USA, in 1972. Detroit was a center for ITP under the leadership of W.W. Zuelzer [23]. Owing to the early death of Sartorius, the study was published posthumously [24]. The results showed a faster increase of platelet counts in the group randomized for corticosteroid treatment, but the outcome after one year was similar between treatment groups, and the side effects associated with long-term corticosteroid treatment prevented their liberal use in children.

In 1980, the impetus for the first immunomodulatory treatment in ITP was

1) the newly available intravenous immunoglobulin (IVIg) concentrates from healthy blood donors and

2) the secondary effect shown of substitutive IVIg administration against low platelet count in a child with a primary immunodeficiency, the Wiskott-Aldrich Syndrome, characterized by infection, eczema, and thrombocytopenia. In this patient, a minimal platelet increase after each administration of IVIg could be observed, in contrast to two children with aplastic anemia who had no increase in platelets after IVIg [25]. We wondered if this effect would translate to a patient with severe chronic ITP, and indeed, a 12-year-old boy with severe, refractory ITP lasting for 8 years, with a previous splenectomy and an intracranial bleeding episode, who needed long term immunosuppressants resulting in secondary immunodeficiency, dramatically responded to IVIg: after the first IVIg administration he immediately began a rapid platelet increase which was continued by administration of four further doses of 0.4 g IVIg/kg body weight, resulting in normal platelet counts (☞ Figure 2.3a). Immediately following this observation, a pilot study in 12 consecutive children with newly diagnosed or chronic ITP and without hypogammaglobulinemia showed similar dramatic effects in response to IVIg [26] (☞ Figure 2.3b). Of note, each child had a different, heterogenous pattern of platelet upon follow-up. Consequently, a controlled randomized multicenter study comparing corticosteroids with IVIg administration was performed, confirming this new treatment option [27] (☞ Figure 2.3c). In 1986 the FDA approved the IVIg indication of ITP; today the requirements of an approval of a new remedy by governmental authorities are much higher (e.g. for TPO-RAs with evidence based clinical studies, ☞ Chapter 2.6.).

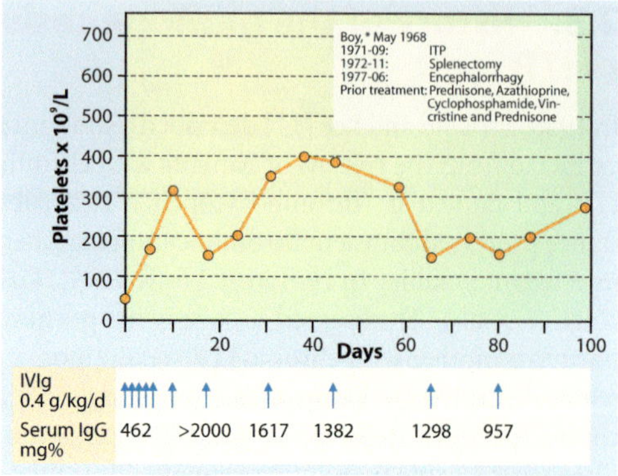


a

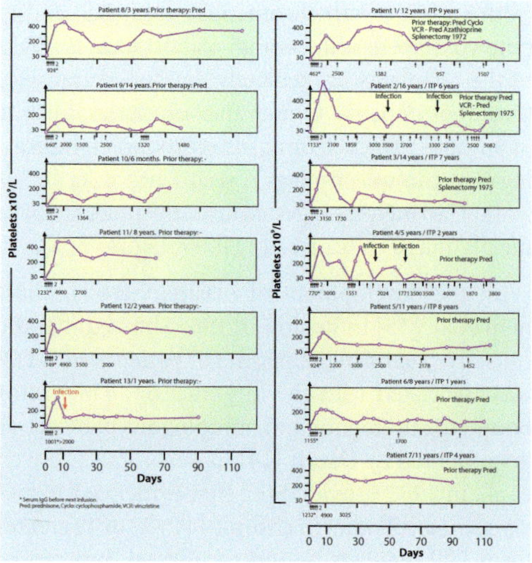


b

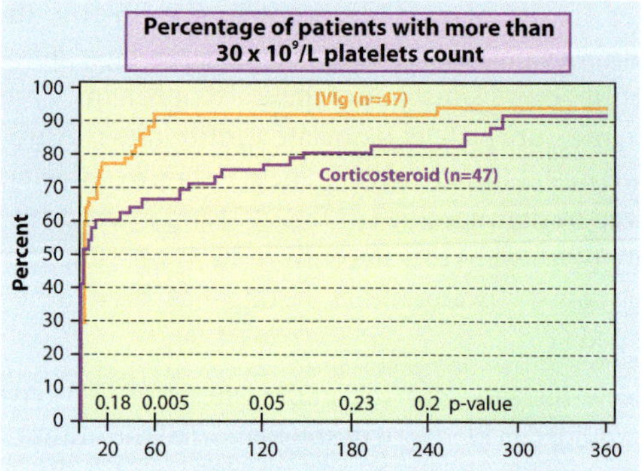


c

***Figure 2.3a-c:*** The first observation and translation from IVIg substitution to immunomodulation in children with ITP. **a**: Key patient. **b**: Pilotstudy of 6 children with newly diagnosed ITP and 7 children with chronic ITP [26]. **c**: Controlled randomized multicenter study comparing IVIg- versus steroid-treatment [27].

Thus, there are two opposite, not well-explained phenomena associated with circulating antibodies:

- Targeted platelet-associated antibodies from patients with ITP destroys platelets of healthy volunteers, and
- Antibody concentrates from healthy blood donors can rapidly increase platelet counts in patients with ITP [28] (☞ Figure 2.4a+b)

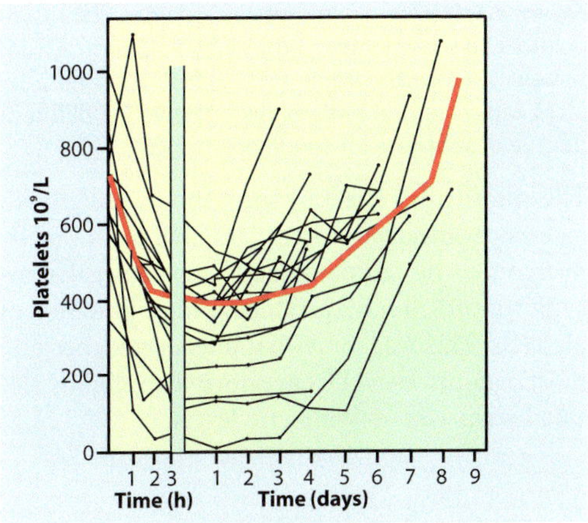


a

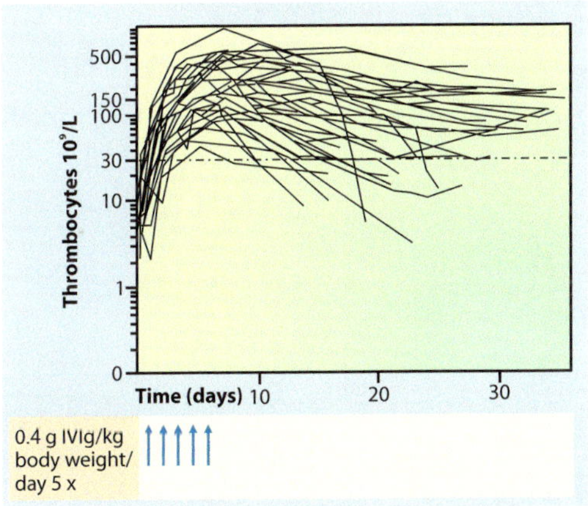


b

***Figure 2.4a+b:*** The effect of autoantibodies of patients with chronic ITP administered to healthy subjects with normal platelet counts representing Harrington's experiment (**a**), and the effect of antibody concentrate from healthy blood donors administered as intravenous immunoglobulins on patients with ITP (**b**).

## 2.5. The therapeutic translation of IVIg to other autoimmune disorders with similar pathophysiology as in ITP

☞ also Chapter 16.3.

Similar destructive pathogeneses and mechanisms of actions of IVIg are understood to be responsible for other chronic inflammatory and autoimmune disorders (reviewed in [29-31]). Clinical and laboratory studies document that IVIg is clinically beneficial and that its mechanism of action interacts with many different levels of the immune response (☞ Chapter 16., Figure 16.3). Over the 30 years since the first observation in 1980, PubMed counted over 78,800 publications on IVIg (☞ Table 2.3). ITP can be considered as a model disorder of autoimmunity. Today, the high demand for IVIg results in limitations on its availability. The worldwide use of the product increased from 300 kg in 1980 to over 90,000 kg per year today.

| Pub Med registered IVIg publications 1981-2010 | |
|---|---|
| Treatment | 33,731 |
| Mechanisms | 8,215 |
| Adverse/Effects | 6,437 |
| ITP | 2,503 |
| Kawasaki disease | 1,972 |
| Blood disorders (excl. ITP) | 1,374 |
| Neurology | 5,628 |
| Dermatology | 1,983 |
| Infection, toxic shock | 1,877 |
| Transplantation | 4,328 |
| Pregnancy | 257 |
| Reviews | 5,999 |
| Others | 3,896 |
| Primary immunodeficieny | 1,699 |

***Table 2.3:*** Pub Med registered publications 1981-2010 of IVIg mechanisms of actions and possible treatment indications.

Furthermore, the new immunomodulatory options provided by polyclonal antibody concentrates stimulated the translation and development of monoclonal, targeted antibodies and other targeted agents for the treatment of autoimmune and oncological disorders (☞ Chapter 16.3. and 16.5.).

In the early 1990s, a monoclonal anti-CD20 (B-cell) antibody, rituximab, became an established treatment option for ITP. More recently, a Syk-inhibitor, which blocks platelet clearance, was approved, and neonatal FCR-antagonists, which reduce the production of antibodies, entered phase II/III evaluation.

## 2.6. Stimulation of platelet production by megakaryocytes

A second development was the clinical research into megakaryocyte-stimulation by thrombopoietic growth factors in 1994. The basic immune pathophysiology experiment – similar to that by Harrington 1951, but in vitro rather than *in vivo* – demonstrated growth suppression of megakaryocyte cultures after incubation with plasma from patient with chronic ITP by Chang and McMillan [32-34] (☞ Figure 2.5).

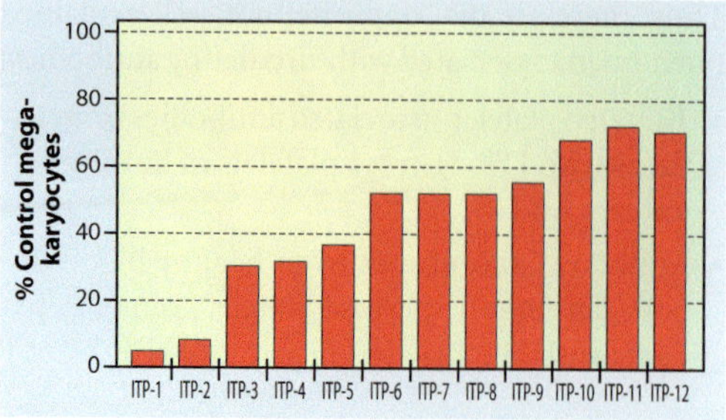


***Figure 2.5:*** Growth suppression of megakaryocyte cultures after incubation with individual plasma from patient 1-12 with chronic ITP. In this experiment by McMillan, each patient's plasma showed a different degree of suppression. Modified after [34].

The stimulatory effect by thrombopoietic growth factors on megakaryocytes was able to indirectly overcome the autoantibody-based megakaryocytic suppression by producing high numbers of platelets. This was somewhat unexpected, because most patients with ITP have normal or slightly elevated serum thrombopoietin levels.

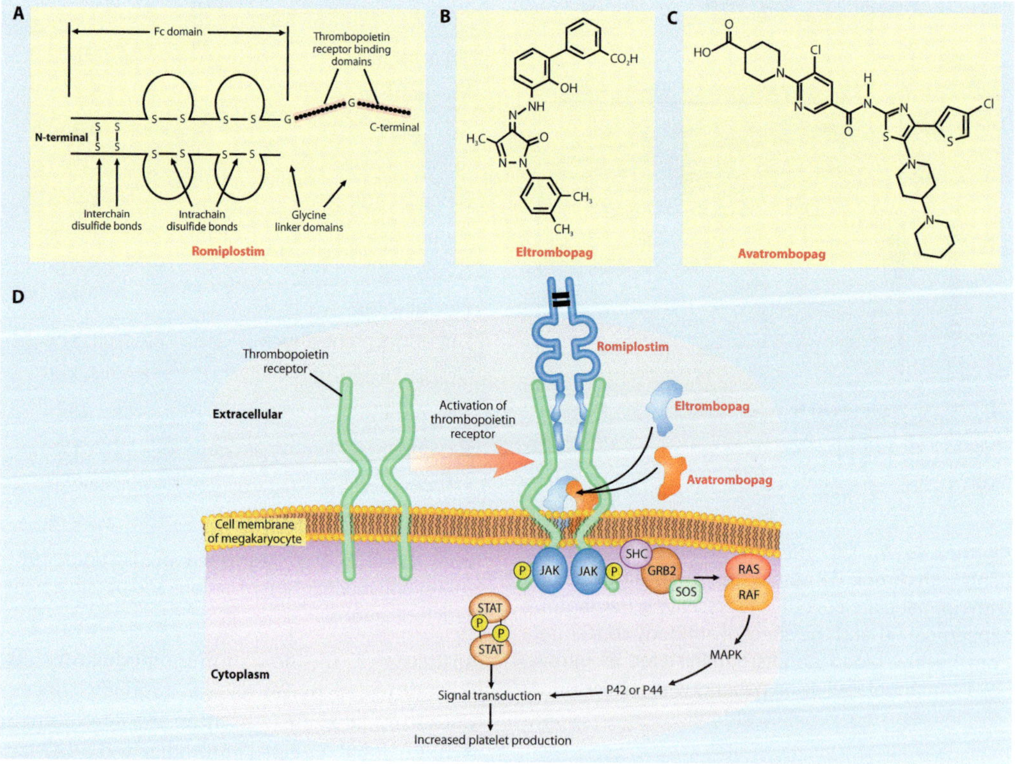


***Figure 2.6:*** Stimulation of platelet production on megakaryopoiesis. First thrombopoietin receptor agonists (TPO-RA, **A-C**) and their potential activation of the intracellular cascade of platelets production (**D**). Modified after [36].

The first generation of thrombopoietic growth factors, recombinant human thrombopoietin (rhTPO) and pegylated human recombinant megakaryocyte growth and development factor (PEG rHu MGDF) increases platelet counts in volunteers, efficiently (for review see [35]). However, the administration had to be stopped in clinical trials when autoantibodies against the factor (PEG rHu MGDF) were detected in healthy human subjects.

A second generation of thrombopoietin receptor agonists TPO-RAs (originally romiplostim and eltrombopag, and more recently avatrombopag and lusutrombopag) efficiently increase platelet counts (☞ details in Chapter 16.4.). Romiplostim is a large molecule administered subcutaneously or intravenously, also named pepti-body, and eltrombopag as well as avatrombopag are small molecules administrated orally (☞ Figure 2.6A-C).

The agonists have a high affinity for the thrombopoietin receptor and activate the intracellular cascade, which stimulates platelet production (☞ Figure 2.6C). These generation of TPO-RAs were clinically evaluated by standardized phase I-III studies. They demonstrated safety, tolerability, and efficacy in patients with ITP [36]. Thus, the stimulatory effect of TPO-RAs on megakaryocytes may indirectly overcome the autoantibody-based megakaryocytic suppression by a high production of platelets. In 2011 the Food and Drug Administration FDA approved romiplostim and eltrombopag and in 2019 avatrombopag for adults with refractory, chronic ITP with or without splenectomy (for reviews ☞ [36, 52]).

## 2.7. Recent development of clinical research of ITP and new aspects of platelets themselves

Since 1992 guidelines based on extensive reviews and followed by many national or local guidelines have been published [37-41]. These efforts on defining the natural history and management of ITP, on harmonization of terminology [42] and guidelines [43-45] have been published. These studies and reports are not evidence-based; they serve as arguments of adequate management recommendations. As a result of the large heterogeneities in individuals with ITP emerging in various controversies, current practice does not always follow these recommendations.

Since 1994 research of ITP evoked the initiative of the International Cooperative ITP Study (ICIS) group. Prospective registries of large numbers of patients with ITP, an international network of physicians and scientists collaborating into detailed analyses and publications and regular international expert meetings has been established stimulating the progress in ITP and autoimmunity (www.itpbasel. ch).

On the basis of such registry analyses evidenced based studies might be done in rare disorders such as ITP [51]. The ongoing Pediatric and Adult Registry on Chronic ITP (PARC ITP) database has the objective of defining subgroups within ITP concerning natural history, genetics, comorbidity, management, treatments and adverse effects and other criteria. This way algorithms of diagnostic procedures and of practical management [46] will steadily improve the care of patients with ITP.

A new area of research is the immune nature of the platelets themselves: Beside mediator of hemostasis the platelets interact as immunoregulatory agents against viruses including the recent Covid19 virus [47, 48] and various bacteria, together with endothelial and other components of the immune system [49, 50].

### References

1. Mithoowani S, Cervi A, Shah N, Ejaz R, Sirotich E, Barty R, Li N, Nazy I, Arnold DM. Management of major bleeds in patients with immune thrombocytopenia. J Thromb Haemost. 2020;18:1783-1790.

2. Neunert C, Noroozi N, Norman G, Buchanan GR, Goy J, Nazi I, Kelton JG, Arnold DM. Severe bleeding events in adults and children with primary immune thrombocytopenia: a systematic review. J Thromb Haemost. 2015;13:457-464.

3. Neunert CE, Buchanan GR, Imbach P, et al. Intercontinental Childhood ITP Study Group Registry II Participants. Severe hemorrhage in children with newly diagnosed immune thrombocytopenic purpura. Blood. 2008;112(10):4003-4008.

4. Neunert CE, Buchanan GR, Imbach P, et al. Intercontinental Cooperative ITP Study Group Registry II Participants. Bleeding manifestations and management of children with persistent and chronic immune thrombocytopenia: data from the Intercontinental Cooperative ITP Study Group (ICIS). Blood. 2013;121(22):4457-4462.

5. Rivierius L. Praxis medica or the Compleat Pratice of Physick. London 1658:618.

6. Werlhof PG. Opera omnia. Hannover 1775. Helwing, 748, In Major RH, (ed.): Classic Descriptions of Disease, 3rd ed. Springfield, IL, CC Thomas 1965.

7. Werlhof PG. De Variolis et Anthracibus. Hannover 1735.

8. Krauss E. Ueber Purpura. Inaugural dissertation, Heidelberg 1883.

9. Denys H. Etudes sur la coagulation du sang dans un cas de purpura avec diminution considérable des plaquettes. La Cellule 1887;3:445-462.

10. Hayem G. Du purpura. Presse Medical 1895;233-235.

11. Troland CE, Lee FC. Thrombocytopenia: A substance in the extract from the spleen of patients with idiopathic thrombocytopenic purpura that reduces the number of blood platelets. J Am Assoc. 1938;111:221-226.

12. Harrington WJ, Minnich V, Hollingsworth JW, Moore CV. Demonstration of a thrombocytopenic factor in the blood of patients with thrombocytopenic purpura. J Lab Clin Med. 1951;38:1-10.

13. Shulman NR, Marder VJ, Weinrach RS. Similarities between known antiplatelet antibodies and the factor responsible for thrombocytopenia in idiopathic purpura: physiologic, serologic and isotopic studies. Ann NY Acad Sci. 1965;124:499-542.

14. Dixon R, Rosse W, Ebbert L. Quantitative determination of antibody in idiopathic thrombocytopenic purpura. N Engl J Med. 1975;292:230-236.

15. Warner MN, Moore JC, Warkentin TE, et al. A prospective study of protein-specific assays used to investigate idiopathic thrombocytopenic pupura. Br J Haematol. 1999;104:442-447.

16. Al-Samkari H, Rosovsky RP, Karp Leaf RS, Smith DB, Goodarzi K, Fogerty AE, Sykes DB, Kuter DJ. A modern reassessment of glycoprotein-specific direct platelet autoantibody testing in immune thrombocytopenia. Blood Adv. 2020;4:9-18.

17. Semple JW, Milev Y, Cosgrave D, et al. Differences in serum cytokine levels in acute and chronic autoimmune thrombocytopenic purpura: Relationship to platelet phenotype and antiplatelet T-Cell reactivity. Blood 1996; 87:4245-4254.

18. Samuelsson A, Towers T, Ravetch J. Anti-inflammatory activity of IVIg mediated through the inhibitory Fc receptor. Science. 2001;291:484-486.

19. Siragam V, Crow AR, Brine D, et al. Intravenous immunoglobulin ameliorates ITP via activating Fcgamma receptors on dendritic cells. Nat Med. 2006;12:688-692.

20. Imbach P, Lazarus AH, Kühne T. Intravenous immunoglobulins induce potentially synergistic immunomodulations in autoimmune disorders. Vox Sang. 2010; 98:385-394.

21. Willan R. On Cutaneous Diseases, London, Barnard JG 1808;452-471.

22. Kaznelson P. Verschwinden der hämorrhagischen Diathese bei einem Falle von essentieller Thrombopenie (Frank) nach Milzexstirpation. Wien Klin Wochenschr. 1916;29:1451-1454.

23. Lusher JM, Zuelzer WW. Idiopathic thrombocytopenic purpura in childhood. J Pediatr. 1966;68:971-979.

24. Sartorius JA. Steroid treatment of idiopathic thrombocytopenic purpura in children. Preliminary results of a randomized cooperative study. Am J Pediatr Hematol Oncol. 1984;6:165-169.

25. Imbach P, Barandun S, Baumgartner C, et al. High-dose intravenous gammaglobulin therapy of refractory, in particular idiopathic thrombocytopenia in childhood. Helv Paediat Acta. 1981;46:81-86.

26. Imbach P, Barandun S, d'Apuzzo V, et al. High-dose intravenous gammaglobulin for idiopathic thrombocytopenic purpura in childhood. Lancet. 1981;1:1228-1231.

27. Imbach P, Berchtold W, Hirt A, et al. Intravenous immunoglobulin versus oral corticosteroids in acute immune thrombocytopenic purpura in childhood. Lancet. 1985;2:464-468.

28. Imbach P. Treatment of immune thrombocytopenia with intravenous immunoglobulin and insights for other diseases. A historical review. Swiss Med Wkly. 2012:142.

29. Negi VS, Elluru S, Sibéril S, et al. Intravenous immunoglobulin: an update on the clinical use and mechanisms of action. J Clin Immunol. 2007;27:233-245.

30. Gold R, Stangel M, Dalakas MC. Drug Insight: the use of intravenous immunoglobulin in neurology – therapeutic considerations and practical issues. Nat Clin Pract Neurol. 2007;3:36-44.

31. Jolles S, Hughes J. Use of IGIV in the treatment of atopic dermatitis, urticaria, scleromyxedema, pyoderma gangrenosum, psoriasis, and pretibial myxedema. Int Immunopharmacol. 2006;6:579-591.

32. McMillan R, Luiken GA, Levy R, Yelenosky R, Longmire RL. Antibody against megakaryocytes in idiopathic thrombocytopenic purpura. JAMA. 1978;239: 2460-24635.

33. Chang M, Nakagawa PA, Williams SA, Schwartz MR, Imfeld KL, Buzby JS, Nugent DJ. Immune thrombocytopenic purpura (ITP) plasma and purified ITP monoclonal autoantibodies inhibit megakaryocytopoiesis in vitro. Blood. 2003;102:887-895.

34. McMillan R, Wang L, Tomer A, Nichol J, Pistillo J. Suppression of in vitro megakaryocyte production by

antiplatelet autoantibodies from adult patients with chronic ITP. Blood. 2004;103:1364-1369.

35. Kuter DJ. New thrombopoietic growth factors. Blood. 2007;109:4607-4616.

36. Imbach P, Crowther M. Thrombopoietin-receptor agonists for primary immune thrombocytopenia. N Engl J Med. 2011;365:734-741.

37. Eden OB, Lilleyman JS. Guidelines for management of idiopathic thrombocytopenic purpura. The British Paediatric Haematology Group. Arch Dis Child. 1992; 67:1056-1058.

38. Shirahata A, Ishii E, Eguchi H, et al. ITP Committee of the Japanese Society of Pediatric Hematology. Consensus guideline for diagnosis and treatment of childhood idiopathic thrombocytopenic purpura. Int J Hematol. 2006;83:29-38.

39. Guidelines for the investigation and management of idiopathic thrombocytopenic purpura in adults, children and in pregnancy. Br J Haematol. 2003;120:574-596.

40. George JN, Woolf SH, Raskob GE, et al. Idiopathic thrombocytopenic purpura: a practice guideline developed by explicit methods for The American Society of Hematology. Blood. 1996;88:3-40.

41. Provan D, Stasi R, Newland AC, et al. International consensus report on the investigation and management of primary immune thrombocytopenia. Blood. 2010; 115:168-186.

42. Rodeghiero F, Stasi R, Gernsheimer T, et al. Standardization of terminology, definitions and outcome criteria in immune thrombocytopenic purpura of adults and children: report from an international working group. Blood. 2009;113:2386-2393.

43. Neunert C, Terrell DR, Arnold DM, Buchanan G, Cines DB, Cooper N, Cuker A, Despotovic JM, George JN, Grace RF, et al. American Society of Hematology 2019 guidelines for immune thrombocytopenia. Blood Adv. 2019;3:3829-3866.

44. Provan D, Arnold DM, Bussel JB, Chong BH, Cooper N, Gernsheimer T, Ghanima W, Godeau B, González-López TJ, Grainger J et al. Updated international consensus report on the investigation and management of primary immune thrombocytopenia. Blood Adv. 2019;3: 3780-3817.

45. Matzdorff A, Meyer O, Ostermann H, Kiefel V, Eberl W, Kühne T, Pabinger I, Rummel M. Immune Thrombocytopenia — Current Diagnostics and Therapy: Recommendations of a Joint Working Group of DGHO, ÖGHO, SGH, GPOH, and DGTI. Oncol Res Treat. 2018; 41 (Suppl. 5):1-30.

46. Schifferli A, Heiri A, Imbach P, Holzhauer S, Seidel MG, Nugent D, Michel M, Kühne T. Misdiagnosed thrombocytopenia in children and adolescents: analysis of the Pediatric and Adult Registry on Chronic ITP. Blood Adv. 2021;5(6):1617-1626.

47. Pavord S, Thachil J, Hunt BJ, Murphy M, Lowe G, Laffan M, Makris M, Newland AC, Provan D, Grainger JD, et al. Practical guidance for the management of adults with immune thrombocytopenia during the COVID-19 pandemic. Br J Haematol. 2020;189:1038-1043.

48. Mahévas M, Moulis G, Andres E, Riviere E, Garzaro M, Crickx E, Guillotin V, Malphettes M, Galicier L, Noel N, et al. Clinical characteristics, management and outcome of COVID-19-associated immune thrombocytopenia: a French multicentre series. Br J Haematol. 2020; 190:e224-e229.

49. Maouia A, Rebetz J, Kapur R, Semple J. W. The Immune Nature of Platelets Revisited. Transfus Med Rev. 2020;34(4):209-220.

50. Semple JW, Rebetz J, Maouia A, Kapur R. An update on the pathophysiology of immune thrombocytopenia. Curr Opin Hematol. 2020;27(6):423-429.

51. Imbach P, Kühne T, Müller D, Berchtold W, Zimmerman S, Elalfy M, Buchanan GR. Childhood ITP: 12 months follow-up data from the prospective registry I of the Intercontinental Childhood ITP Study Group (ICIS). Pediatr Blood Cancer. 2006;46:351-356.

52. Virk ZM, Kuter DJ, Al-Samkari H. An evaluation of avatrombopag for the treatment of thrombocytopenia. Expert Opin Pharmacother. 2021;22(3):273-280.

# 3. Basic immunology of ITP

Immune thrombocytopenia (ITP) is an organ-specific autoimmune bleeding disorder characterized by the production of autoreactive antibodies against one's own platelets, resulting in increased platelet destruction by phagocytic macrophages in the reticuloendothelial system (RES) [1-4]. In addition, the autoimmunity also affects the bone marrow leading to megakaryocyte destruction and/or inhibition and impaired platelet production [3-5]. Patients with ITP suffer from petechiae, purpura, mucocutaneous bleeding, and in rare cases intracranial hemorrhage which can be fatal [1, 6, 7]. Approximately 14,000 to 16,000 cases are diagnosed each year and the incidence of childhood ITP is about 2 to 5 per 100,000 [8-10]. Persistent ITP lasts between 3 to 12 months from diagnosis, in comparison to chronic ITP which lasts for more than 12 months [6, 7]. ITP often manifests following viral or bacterial infections, and these forms are referred to as secondary ITP, while primary ITP includes all cases without any underlying causes [6, 7]. Patients with ITP mainly produce IgG autoantibodies against glycoproteins (GP) GPIIb/IIIa, GPIb/IX or GPIa on the platelet surface and most patients display multiple specificities [11, 12]. Of interest, however, it is known that about 20-30 % of patients with ITP have no detectable platelet autoantibodies suggesting that alternative mechanisms of platelet destruction may exist [11, 12].

Newly diagnosed and persistent ITP in children often occurs after a viral or bacterial infection and usually spontaneously resolves within 6 months of diagnosis, however, in approximately 10 % of children, the disease progresses to the chronic form [5]. In contrast to childhood ITP, chronic ITP is predominantly found in adults, with more females being affected than males [1-6]. Although both childhood and adult ITP are immune-mediated, it is possible that the pathophysiological mechanisms may be different [16]. This chapter will give an overview of the abnormalities associated with T cell and B cells in ITP and how genetic and environmental factors may also relate to the disorder. It now appears that all of them may have a profound effect on the autoimmunity associated with ITP.

## 3.1. T cell and cytokine abnormalities in ITP

The majority of organ specific autoimmune diseases like ITP are correlated with a predominant T helper 1 (Th1)/Th17 activation pattern whereas anti-inflammatory Th2 responses are generally associated with remissions [13, 14]. Th1 responses are characterized by the production of cytokines which include interleukin (IL)-2, interferon (INF)-γ, and tumor necrosis factor (TNF)-α whereas Th17 respones are primarily identified by secretion of IL-17 [15]. These T cell responses are primarily responsible for the initiation of pro-inflammatory reactions. On the other hand, Th2 cytokine responses consists mainly of IL4, IL5, IL6, and IL10 and these cytokines are primarily associated with anti-inflammatory responses [15]. The vast majority of studies to date have shown that patients with chronic ITP in active disease have increased serum levels of IL2 and IFN-γ and there is a suppression of IL-4 and IL-6 [3, 16, 17]. These data suggest that there is a strong link between the pro-inflammatory cytokine milieu and active chronic ITP. Furthermore, early studies have shown that increased transforming growth factor (TGF)-β1 is found associated with remission of ITP whereas low levels of TGF-β1 were found in patients with active disease [18, 19]. TGF-β1 is an extremely immunosuppressive cytokine that is associated with the development of T regulatory (Treg) cells and has the ability to potently suppress B-cell proliferation and antibody production [20, 21].

Regulatory T cells (Tregs) are a small subgroup of $CD4^+$ T cells that play a vital role in establishing and maintaining self tolerance [22, 23]. They are marked by surface expression of CD25, CD62L, specific CD45 isoforms [22, 23] and they specifically express the transcription factor Foxp3 [22, 23]. Aberrant development of these cells is currently thought to be the main underlying defect in most organ-specific autoimmune diseases and these defects are now well known to occur in patients with chronic ITP [3, 17, 24]. Patients with active chronic ITP have a lower proportion of peripheral Treg cells in comparison to patients in remission or healthy controls [3, 17, 24]. It is quite possible that the lower proportion of Treg cells in combination with their lower suppressive activity cannot efficiently inhibit autoreactive Th cells, thereby the induction of autoreactive platelet antibodies proceeds and ITP occurs. Of interest, it now appears that in those patients with ITP that respond to treatments including prednisone, dexamethasone, IVIg, rituximab or thrombopoietin receptor agonists (TPO-RA) show a corresponding increase in Treg cell numbers and restoration of their suppressive function [2, 3]. Since these different therapies have very different mechanisms of actions, it is doubtful that they are all responsible for directly affecting the Treg levels in ITP. More specifically, it may be the rise in platelet counts (the increased platelet mass) is responsible for the normalization of Tregs in ITP. Platelets are known to be immune cells and, for example, contain the highest amounts of the Treg molecular switch TGF in the peripheral blood [25, 26]. Pre-clinical studies suggest that this may be the case with TPO-RA therapy for ITP [27]. Outlining all of the T cell abnormalities in ITP is beyond the scope of this chapter, but the reader is referred to several recent comprehensive reviews on the subject [17, 25, 28].

Taken together, however, it is clear that the balance of proinflammatory and anti-inflammatory T cells are the major driving factors in development and resolution of platelet autoimmunity in ITP.

## 3.2. B cell abnormalities

Autoantibodies in patients with ITP usually target GPIIb/IIIa or GPIb/IX, but also react with GPIa/IIa, GPIV, and GPV [11, 12]. It appears that the majority of patients with ITP have autoantibodies against multiple platelet antigens and few (approximately 5 %) have only single specificites [11, 12, 29]. The different epitopes recognized by platelet autoantibodies are of great interest because data has suggested that while some anti-platelet antibodies may be responsible for platelet destruction e.g. phagocytosis, others may have a platelet inhibitory role [30-34]. It may be that the balance of these events have a role to play in why some patients with ITP bleed and others do not. In addition, as many as 20-30 % of patients with ITP have no detectible antibodies [12]. Whether the lack of antibody detection is due to robustness of the antibody tests used or perhaps due to a purely T cell-mediated mechanisms of platelet destruction is still unknown.

Like Tregs, there is a subset of CD19+CD41hi CD38hi B-regulatory cells (Bregs) which also maintain peripheral tolerance and it appears that these cells are also impaired in patients with ITP, are also impaired in ITP [35]. These defective cells cannot limit CD4+ T cell activation or recruit Tregs. It appears that these types of Bregs are significantly elevated in the spleens of patients with ITP suggesting that their peripheral deficiency could be due to a sequestration process within lymphoid compartments [36]. Analogous mechanisms have been found for Tregs as well [37]. These data suggest that lymphocyte movements and sequestration patterns in ITP may play a profound role in tolerance mechanisms and lead to the development of platelet autoimmunity.

## 3.3. Dendritic Cells (DC) in ITP

DCs are the most efficient cells for antigen presentation and several studies have now shown their involvement in ITP [3, 24, 38]. For example, Li et al [39] have recently shown that an imbalance of plasmacytoid dendritic cells (pDC)/myeloid dendritic cells (mDC) together with an increase of IL-6, IL-12, and IL-23 leads to the increased differentiation of CD4+ T cells into Th1 and Th17 cells. This may explain the defects in Th1 and Th17 cells seen in the disorder. Perhaps related to ITP is the ability of platelets to affect DC and indirectly, T cells. Saris et al [40] examined the ability of platelets to immunomodulate monocyte-derived dendritic cells (moDC) as well as primary dendritic cells and their effects on T cell responses. It was shown that a secreted platelet factor could inhibit pro-inflammatory (IL-12, IL-6, TNF-α) and increase anti-inflammatory (IL-10) cytokine production by moDCs. Tis in turn, led to an inhibition of T cell priming. Taken toether, these results may explain a potential mechanism of how increasing platelet numbers in ITP may affect T cells and reduce the autoimmune pathogenesis. Moreover, it was also shown that silencing DC through the CD27/CD70 co-stimulatory axis may be important in DC 'licensing', which could initiate a series of anti-platelet autoreactive immune responses [41]. Silencing the CD70 genes on DC from patients with ITP decreased $CD4^+$ $CD25^-$ Tcell proliferation and Treg differentiation, while inducing higher IL-10 and lower IFN-$\gamma$ levels. It may be that interference with the CD27-CD70 costimulatory pathway might lead to the alleviation of the autoimmune reactions and polarization of Th2 response and induction of immune tolerance. It is now quite clear that eamining DC in ITP may be a fruitful avenue of designing specific therpaies for this autoimmune disorder.

## 3.4. Environmental factors in ITP

Environmental factors play a role in many immune diseases, particularly autoimmunity [42]. This is no better seen than in children with newly diagnosed ITP. Most children with ITP have a history of infections before the onset of ITP and a majority will resolve spontaneously without any need for therapy [6, 7]. It appears that in children with ITP, anti-platelet antibodies are predominantly due to a cross reaction with infectious agents. This was best demonstrated by Wright et al [43] who showed that anti-viral antibodies could cross react with platelet antigens e.g. molecular mimicry or by autoreactive B cells being directly stimulated by the infectious agents. One fascinating aspect of environmental factors causing ITP is that completely different antigenic structures e.g. HIV, Hepatitis C and the drug quinine can all lead to development of the same antibody specificity that targets GPIIbIIIa on the platelet surface. For example, patients with secondary ITP (either HIV-associated or Hep C-associated) or patients treated with quinine can generate an IgG autoantibody that reacts with a

| Antibodies | Effector Function |
|---|---|
| IgG Anti-GPIIbIIIa | • FcR-mediated phagocytosis<br>• Platelet function inhibition<br>• Complement mediated lysis<br>• Megakaryocyte destruction/inhibition |
| IgG Anti-GPIIbIIIa (HIV/HCV ITP) | • Platelet suicide by ROS |
| IgG Anti-GPIbIX | • FcR independent platelet destruction<br>• Platelet desialytion (Liver destruction)<br>• Platelet inhibition<br>• ROS<br>• Megakaryocyte destruction/inhibition (?) |
| IgM Anti-GPIIbIIIa | • FcR-mediated phagocytosis<br>• Platelet function inhibition<br>• Complement mediated lysis<br>• Megakaryocyte destruction/inhibition |
| IgA Anti-platelet antibodies | • FcR-mediated phagocytosis<br>• Platelet function inhibition<br>• Complement mediated lysis<br>• Megakaryocyte destruction/inhibition |
| T cells | |
| CD4+T cells | • Immune regulation |
| CD8+ T cells | • Platelet and megakaryocyte cytotoxicity |
| γ/δ T cells | ? |
| B cells | • Immune regulation/plasma cell source |
| Dendritic cells | • APC/T and B cell regulation/phagocytosis |
| Platelets/Megakaryocytes | • Immune regulation/APC |
| NK cells/Macrophages/Granulocytes | • ADCC/Phagocytosis (APC)/ROS |

***Table 3.1:*** Potential Effector Mechanisms in ITP [2, 25, 28, 48-52]. **APC**: antigen presenting cell, **ADCC**: antibody dependent cellular cytotoxicity, **FcR** : Fc receptor, **ROS**: reactive oxygen species.

GPIIIa epitope composed of amino acid residues 49-66 [44-47]. When the HIV-associated autoantibody bound to platelets, it stimulated platelet 12-lipoxygenase system to initiate production of reactive oxygen species that mediated platelet fragmentation [45].

Taken together, these results suggest that completely different antigenic challenges (either viruses or drugs) have the ability to generate autoantibodies that are reactive against the same platelet epitope.

This strongly supports the concept that infectious agents via molecular mimicry play a critical role in either initiating or deregulating platelet autoantibody production.

## 3.5. Alternative modes of thrombocytopenia in ITP

In recent years there have been several lines of evidence to suggest that in addition to the classical antibody-mediated platelet destruction by FcR-dependent phagocytosis in the spleen, there are other forms of platelet/megakaryocyte destruction or thrombocytopenia. Table 3.1 summarizes these various effector mechanisms and shows that there are alternative methods of thrombocytopenia in ITP. These studies support the concept that ITP is an extremely heterogeneous disorder with various immune effector mechanisms leading to thrombocytopenia.

## 3.6. Conclusions

ITP is a heterogeneous autoimmune disorder with multiple immune factors that contribute to the cause and severity of the disease. As suggested above, T and B cell abnormalities along with DC and environmental factors contribute to the pathogenesis of ITP. These factors are not mutually exclusive but are superimposed on each other and can intimately affect one another and the pathogenesis of ITP. With such a diverse and complex underlying cause to ITP, it is not surprising that the exact mechanism of immune dysfunction is still unclear. However, what is clear is that more research is required to gain a better understanding of this multifaceted disorder.

## References

1. Cines DB, Bussel JB, Liebman HA, Luning Prak ET. The ITP syndrome: pathogenic and clinical diversity. Blood. 2009;113(26):6511-21.

2. McKenzie CG, Guo L, Freedman J, Semple JW. Cellular immune dysfunction in immune thrombocytopenia (ITP). British journal of haematology. 2013;163(1):10-23.

3. Zufferey A, Kapur R, Semple JW. Pathogenesis and Therapeutic Mechanisms in Immune Thrombocytopenia (ITP). Journal of clinical medicine. 2017;6(2).

4. Semple JW, Rebetz J, Maouia A, Kapur R. An update on the pathophysiology of immune thrombocytopenia. Current opinion in hematology. 2020;27(6):423-9.

5. Singh A, Uzun G, Bakchoul T. Primary Immune Thrombocytopenia: Novel Insights into Pathophysiology and Disease Management. Journal of clinical medicine. 2021;10(4).

6. Provan D, Arnold DM, Bussel JB, Chong BH, Cooper N, Gernsheimer T, et al. Updated international consensus report on the investigation and management of primary immune thrombocytopenia. Blood advances. 2019;3(22):3780-817.

7. Neunert C, Terrell DR, Arnold DM, Buchanan G, Cines DB, Cooper N, et al. American Society of Hematology 2019 guidelines for immune thrombocytopenia. Blood advances. 2019;3(23):3829-66.

8. Rodeghiero F, Marranconi E. Management of immune thrombocytopenia in women: current standards and special considerations. Expert review of hematology. 2020;13(2):175-85.

9. Michel M. Immune thrombocytopenic purpura: epidemiology and implications for patients. Eur J Haematol Suppl. 2009(71):3-7.

10. Terrell DR, Beebe LA, Vesely SK, Neas BR, Segal JB, George JN. The incidence of immune thrombocytopenic purpura in children and adults: A critical review of published reports. American journal of hematology. 2010; 85(3):174-80.

11. Al-Samkari H, Rosovsky RP, Karp Leaf RS, Smith DB, Goodarzi K, Fogerty AE, et al. A modern reassessment of glycoprotein-specific direct platelet autoantibody testing in immune thrombocytopenia. Blood Adv. 2020;4 (1):9-18.

12. Porcelijn L, Huiskes E, Oldert G, Schipperus M, Zwaginga JJ, de Haas M. Detection of platelet autoantibodies to identify immune thrombocytopenia: state of the art. British journal of haematology. 2018;182(3): 423-6.

13. Geenen V. The thymus and the science of self. Seminars in Immunopathology. 2021;43(1):5-14.

14. Bluestone JA, Bour-Jordan H, Cheng M, Anderson M. T cells in the control of organ-specific autoimmunity. The Journal of clinical investigation. 2015;125(6):2250-60.

15. Pawlak M, Ho AW, Kuchroo VK. Cytokines and transcription factors in the differentiation of CD4 + T helper cell subsets and induction of tissue inflammation and autoimmunity. Current opinion in immunology. 2020;67:57-67.

16. LeVine DN, Brooks MB. Immune thrombocytopenia (ITP): Pathophysiology update and diagnostic dilemmas. Veterinary clinical pathology. 2019;48 Suppl 1:17-28.

17. Kostic M, Zivkovic N, Cvetanovic A, Marjanović G. CD4 + T cell phenotypes in the pathogenesis of immune thrombocytopenia. Cellular immunology. 2020;351: 104096.

18. Andersson PO, Stockelberg D, Jacobsson S, Wadenvik H. A transforming growth factor-beta1-mediated bystander immune suppression could be associated with remission of chronic idiopathic thrombocytopenic purpura. Annals of hematology. 2000;79(9):507-13.

19. Andersson PO, Olsson A, Wadenvik H. Reduced transforming growth factor-beta1 production by mononuclear cells from patients with active chronic idiopathic thrombocytopenic purpura. British journal of haematology. 2002;116(4):862-7.

20. Zhang S. The role of transforming growth factor β in T helper 17 differentiation. Immunology. 2018;155(1): 24-35.

21. Sheng J, Chen W, Zhu H-J. The immune suppressive function of transforming growth factor-β (TGF-β) in human diseases. Growth factors (Chur, Switzerland). 2015;33(2):92-101.

22. Zhang R, Miao J, Zhu P. Regulatory T cell heterogeneity and therapy in autoimmune diseases. Autoimmunity reviews. 2021;20(5):102715.

23. Tang Q, Bluestone JA. The Foxp3+ regulatory T cell: a jack of all trades, master of regulation. Nat Immunol. 2008;9(3):239-44.

24. Swinkels M, Rijkers M, Voorberg J, Vidarsson G, Leebeek FWG, Jansen AJG. Emerging Concepts in Immune Thrombocytopenia. Frontiers in immunology. 2018;9:880.

25. Maouia A, Rebetz J, Kapur R, Semple JW. The Immune Nature of Platelets Revisited. Transfus Med Rev. 2020;34(4):209-220.

26. Bertolini TB, Biswas M, Terhorst C, Daniell H, Herzog RW, Piñeros AR. Role of orally induced regulatory T cells in immunotherapy and tolerance. Cellular immunology. 2021;359:104251.

27. Kapur R, Aslam R, Speck ER, Rebetz JM, Semple JW. Thrombopoietin receptor agonist (TPO-RA) treatment raises platelet counts and reduces anti-platelet antibody levels in mice with immune thrombocytopenia (ITP). Platelets. 2020;31(3):399-402.

28. Semple JW, Rebetz J, Maouia A, Kapur R. An update on the pathophysiology of immune thrombocytopenia. Current opinion in hematology. 2020;27(6):423-9.

29. Porcelijn L, Schmidt DE, Oldert G, Hofstede-van Egmond S, Kapur R, Zwaginga JJ, et al. Evolution and Utility of Antiplatelet Autoantibody Testing in Patients with Immune Thrombocytopenia. Transfusion medicine reviews. 2020;34(4):258-69.

30. Webster ML, Sayeh E, Crow M, Chen P, Nieswandt B, Freedman J, et al. Relative efficacy of intravenous immunoglobulin G in ameliorating thrombocytopenia induced by antiplatelet GPIIbIIIa versus GPIbalpha antibodies. Blood. 2006;108(3):943-6.

31. Iraqi M, Perdomo J, Yan F, Choi PY, Chong BH. Immune thrombocytopenia: antiplatelet autoantibodies inhibit proplatelet formation by megakaryocytes and impair platelet production in vitro. Haematologica. 2015;100(5):623-32.

32. Audia S, Bonnotte B. Emerging Therapies in Immune Thrombocytopenia. Journal of clinical medicine. 2021; 10(5).

33. McMillan R. The pathogenesis of chronic immune thrombocytopenic purpura. Seminars in hematology. 2007;44(4 Suppl 5):S3-S11.

34. Leytin V, Mykhaylov S, Starkey AF, Allen DJ, Lau H, Ni H, et al. Intravenous immunoglobulin inhibits antiglycoprotein IIb-induced platelet apoptosis in a murine model of immune thrombocytopenia. British journal of haematology. 2006;133(1):78-82.

35. Li X, Zhong H, Bao W, Boulad N, Evangelista J, Haider MA, et al. Defective regulatory B-cell compartment in patients with immune thrombocytopenia. Blood. 2012;120(16):3318-25.

36. Aslam R, Segel GB, Burack R, Spence SA, Speck ER, Guo L, et al. Splenic lymphocyte subtypes in immune thrombocytopenia: increased presence of a subtype of B-regulatory cells. British journal of haematology. 2016; 173(1):159-60.

37. Aslam R, Hu Y, Gebremeskel S, Segel GB, Speck ER, Guo L, et al. Thymic retention of CD4+CD25+FoxP3+ T regulatory cells is associated with their peripheral deficiency and thrombocytopenia in a murine model of immune thrombocytopenia. Blood. 2012;120(10):2127-32.

38. Wen R, Wang Y, Hong Y, Yang Z. Cellular immune dysregulation in the pathogenesis of immune thrombocytopenia. Blood coagulation & fibrinolysis : an interna-

tional journal in haemostasis and thrombosis. 2020;31 (2):113-20.

39. Li Q, Liu Y, Wang X, Sun M, Wang L, Wang X, et al. Regulation of Th1/Th2 and Th17/Treg by pDC/mDC imbalance in primary immune thrombocytopenia. Experimental biology and medicine (Maywood, NJ). 2021: 15353702211009787.

40. Saris A, Steuten J, Schrijver DP, van Schijndel G, Zwaginga JJ, van Ham SM, et al. Inhibition of Dendritic Cell Activation and Modulation of T Cell Polarization by the Platelet Secretome. Frontiers in immunology. 2021; 12:631285.

41. Zhang X, Wang Y, Zhang D, Li H, Zhou Z, Yang R. CD70-silenced dendritic cells induce immune tolerance in immune thrombocytopenia patients. British journal of haematology. 2020;191(3):466-75.

42. Molina V, Shoenfeld Y. Infection, vaccines and other environmental triggers of autoimmunity. Autoimmunity. 2005;38(3):235-45.

43. Wright JF, Blanchette VS, Wang H, Arya N, Petric M, Semple JW, et al. Characterization of platelet-reactive antibodies in children with varicella-associated acute immune thrombocytopenic purpura (ITP). British journal of haematology. 1996;95(1):145-52.

44. Nardi MA, Liu LX, Karpatkin S. GPIIIa-(49-66) is a major pathophysiologically relevant antigenic determinant for anti-platelet GPIIIa of HIV-1-related immunologic thrombocytopenia. Proceedings of the National Academy of Sciences of the United States of America. 1997;94(14):7589-94.

45. Nardi M, Tomlinson S, Greco MA, Karpatkin S. Complement-independent, peroxide-induced antibody lysis of platelets in HIV-1-related immune thrombocytopenia. Cell. 2001;106(5):551-61.

46. Zhang W, Nardi MA, Borkowsky W, Li Z, Karpatkin S. Role of molecular mimicry of hepatitis C virus protein with platelet GPIIIa in hepatitis C-related immunologic thrombocytopenia. Blood. 2009;113(17):4086-93.

47. Peterson JA, Nelson TN, Kanack AJ, Aster RH. Fine specificity of drug-dependent antibodies reactive with a restricted domain of platelet GPIIIA. Blood. 2008;111 (3):1234-9.

48. Coopamah MD, Garvey MB, Freedman J, Semple JW. Cellular immune mechanisms in autoimmune thrombocytopenic purpura: An update. Transfusion medicine reviews. 2003;17(1):69-80.

49. Semple JW, Lazarus AH, Freedman J. The cellular immunology associated with autoimmune thrombocytopenic purpura: an update. Transfusion science. 1998; 19(3):245-51.

50. Panzer S, Szamait S, Bödeker RH, Haas OA, Haubenstock A, Mueller-Eckhardt C. Platelet-associated immunoglobulins IgG, IgM, IgA and complement C3 in immune and nonimmune thrombocytopenic disorders. American journal of hematology. 1986;23(2):89-99.

51. Kapur R, Zufferey A, Boilard E, Semple JW. Nouvelle Cuisine: Platelets Served with Inflammation. The Journal of Immunology. 2015;194(12):5579-87.

52. McMillan R, Nugent D. The effect of antiplatelet autoantibodies on megakaryocytopoiesis. Int J Hematol. 2005;81(2):94-9.

# 4. Megakaryopoiesis in ITP

## 4.1. Overview of normal thrombopoiesis

Platelets, like all circulating blood cells, derive from the hematopoietic stem cell (HSC; reviewed [1]). During hematopoietic differentiation, the HSC gives rise to progressively committed progenitors, including the common myeloid progenitor and the megakaryocyte-erythrocyte progenitor. The latter, bi-potential cell gives rise to both cells of the megakaryocytic and erythroid lineages, although increasing evidence also supports the existence of primary megakaryocyte "primed" hematopoietic progenitor cells capable of quickly repopulating the megakaryocyte pool and making platelets [1]. As megakaryocytic cells become progressively differentiated, they lose their proliferative ability and become polyploid. All megakaryocytic precursors express the integrin GPIIb (CD41), but the earliest precursors may be morphologically indistinguishable from lymphocytes. The first morphologically recognizable megakaryocytic cells are promegakaryoblasts, which give rise to tetraploid megakaryoblasts and the successively larger and more polyploid promegakaryocytes and megakaryocytes. Mature megakaryocytes can be 150 μM or more in diameter and are the largest hematopoietic cells in the bone marrow (☞ Figure 4.1).

Polyploidy is a defining feature of the mature megakaryocyte, but the purpose for acquiring multiple chromosome complements is unknown. It is theorized that polyploidization facilitates the massive protein and membrane synthesis required for later platelet production through functional gene amplification [2]]. There is some correlation between the degree of megakaryocyte ploidy and platelet production; for example, neonatal megakaryocytes are typically of low ploidy and may have reduced capacity to produce platelets relative to their adult counterpart, but increased proliferative capacity [3-5]. These differences may come down to differences in mTOR signaling [6, 7]. However, examination of different mouse strains in which the modal megakaryocyte ploidy varies does not uphold a correlation between ploidy and steady state platelet counts [8], suggesting that either this relationship is not as simple, or mice and human megakaryocyte biology differ with respect to this relationship. The mechanism of polyploidization, or endomitosis, is also an enigma. During endomitosis, megakaryocytes enter anaphase, separate their chromosomes, and even go so far as to initiate cleavage furrow formation [9, 10]. At that point, furrows regress and the nuclei fail to separate, resulting in the formation of a multilobulated, polyploid nucleus [10]. Furrow regression may be due

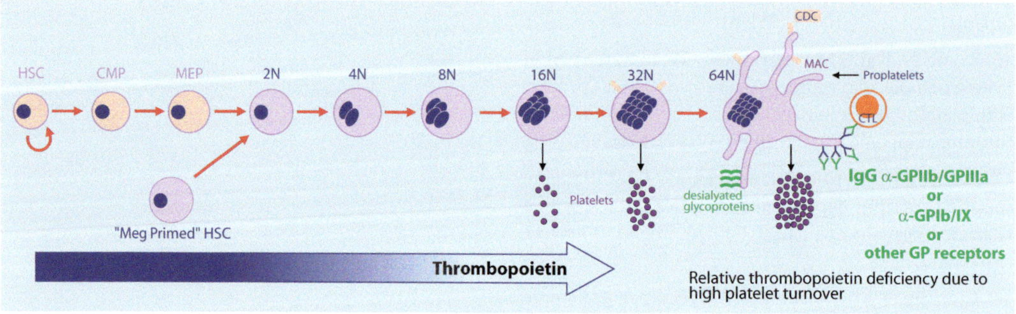


***Figure 4.1:*** Impact of the immune response on thrombopoiesis. Megakaryocytes develop from hematopoietic stem cells under the influence of thrombopoietin. Anti-platelet antibodies (IgG) promote platelet destruction and inhibit megakaryopoiesis and platelet production. Complement dependent cytotoxicity may directly mediate megakaryocyte toxicity and apoptosis, contributing to ineffective thrombopoiesis through formation of membrane attack complex on megakaryocytes. Direct cytotoxic T cell mediated cytotoxicity has been demonstrated in some patients with ITP and may also target megakaryocytes. Finally, changes in sialylation on megakaryocyte glycoproteins may also alter platelet release. **HSC**: hematopoietic stem cell, **CMP**: common myeloid progenitor, **MEP**: megakaryocyte erythroid progenitor, **MK**: megakaryocyte, **CTL**: cytotoxic lymphocyte, **MAC**: membrane attack complex, **CDC**: complement dependent toxicity.

the failure to properly localize or regulate active RhoA at the contractile ring [11], and endomitosis has been established as a defect in late cytokinesis [10, 12] and karyokinesis [13, 14]. Interestingly, despite significant gains in our understanding of this process, the precise mechanism by which megakaryocytes escape the tetraploid checkpoint [15, 16].

In addition to polyploidization, maturation of the megakaryocyte is marked by the formation of an extensive demarcation membrane system (DMS) and the accumulation of alpha and dense granules (reviewed [1]). The DMS is an elaborate membrane network that ultimately fills the megakaryocyte cytoplasm except for a narrow band at the periphery of the cell. This membrane system is continuous with the plasma membrane of the cell and is in contact with the external environment and has been proposed to serve as a reservoir of membrane to support proplatelet formation [17]. Alpha granules are formed in the Golgi complex and contain both endogenously produced proteins (e.g. platelet factor 4, von Willebrand factor) and proteins derived from the extracellular environment through receptor-mediated endocytosis and pinocytosis (e.g. fibrinogen, factor V). These granules and other megakaryocyte organelles are essential components that will be transferred into the forming platelets. Megakaryocyte cytoplasmic maturation and polyploidization are separately regulated, and even low ploidy megakaryocytes can be fully mature, giving rise to platelets[18].

Two models have been proposed to explain platelet formation from mature megakaryocytes. In the **proplatelet model**, megakaryocytes in the bone marrow develop multiple proplatelet processes that extend into the marrow sinusoids to release platelets into the circulation. Using live cell microscopy, Italiano and colleagues elegantly documented the elaboration of a network of branching proplatelets by cultured megakaryocytes [19]. Junt and colleagues extended these results by imaging the bone marrow compartment in a living mouse, demonstrating that fluorescently-labeled megakaryocytes release platelet-like particles into marrow sinusoids [20]. In the **fragmentation model**, megakaryocytes travel from the bone marrow to the lung where they are fragmented into platelets in the microvasculature [21]. Multiple studies have now confirmed megakaryocyte presence in the lungs, and recent use of intravital 2-photon microscopy was able to demonstrate immobile MKs residing in lung interstitium and de novo platelet production [22-25], confirming the lung as a site of thrombopoiesis and a contributor to overall circulating platelet mass. Recently, Yeung and colleagues used single cell RNA sequencing to profile bone marrow and lung megakaryocytes and demonstrated that there are significant differences in the expression profiles of megakaryocytes from lung and bone marrow, suggesting a more immune modulatory role for lung megakaryocytes and a hemostatic role for bone marrow megakaryocytes [26].

The process of by which proplatelet are formed (whether in bone marrow or lung) is only partially understood. New evidence suggests that that control of cytoplasmic maturity is under the control of RhoA and Cdc42 [27] and that endomitosis and cytoplasmic maturation are separately regulated processes with different controls. Loss of Cdc42 in murine knockout models results in decreased proplatelet formation and macrothrombocytopenia [28, 29] due to alternations in demarcation membrane formation/polarization and mice that lacked both RhoA and Cdc42 demonstrated markedly decreased proplatelet formation through aberrant MKL/SRF signaling resulting in abnormal microtubule organization [27]. Proplatelet formation is preceded by a reorganization of the actin-tubulin cytoskeleton in the megakaryocyte, with tubulin adopting a peripheral localization within the cell. Pseudopodia then bulge from the megakaryocyte surface and elongate into processes that branch distally; the microtubules within these processes are arranged in opposing directions and form coiled loops at the tips of the processes [19]. These loops correspond to the marginal band that gives the platelet its disc-like shape [30]. Granules and other megakaryocyte organelles traffic along the microtubules out to the tips of the processes where they accumulate in the nascent platelet [31]. Interactions with the extracellular matrix are also important in regulating platelet formation and may help to restrict it to the vascular niche [32]. In particular, the von Willebrand factor receptor GPIb on megakaryocytes is an important regulator of proplatelet formation, as the autosomal recessive inheritance of mutations involving GPIb (Bernard Soulier syndrome) results in abnormal megakaryocyte maturation and macrothrombocytopenia [33, 34] and antibodies to GPIb inhibit megakaryopoiesis and platelet production *in vitro* [35], perhaps contributing to the thrombocytopenia of ITP.

Proplatelet formation is a terminal process, leaving nothing of the megakaryocyte but a nuclear remnant that is engulfed by macrophages [19, 36]. Apoptosis plays a complex role in both platelet survival [37-39] and megakaryopoeisis [40]. Inhibition of apoptosis is required however for megakaryocytes to survive during polyploidization and proplatelet formation as loss of BclxL results in megakaryocyte apoptosis and failure of platelet shedding [41]. Conversely, in humans, several variants in cytochrome c that enhances apoptosis have been described with autosomal dominant thrombocytopenia [42-44]. Although platelet lifespan and megakaryocyte frequency were unaffected, megakaryocytes forming proplatelets could be seen within the marrow space, suggesting that premature and ineffective proplatelet formation is the mechanism of peripheral thrombocytopenia in this disorder. Thus, apoptosis is an important regulator of thrombopoiesis, but its role is incompletely understood.

Multiple factors regulate megakaryopoiesis, the most important of which is **thrombopoietin (TPO)**. TPO is critical for megakaryocyte growth and development [45-50]. Its receptor c-Mpl is expressed primarily on platelets, megakaryocytes and megakaryocyte precursors, and without TPO c-Mpl platelet numbers are reduced to approximately 10 % of normal values [51, 52]. In addition, hematopoietic stem cells and progenitors of erythroid and myeloid lineages are also reduced, speaking to the importance of TPO for all hematopoiesis [53, 54]. TPO is produced by the liver, although small amounts are also produced by the kidney and marrow stromal cells [55]. Unlike erythropoietin, whose production is modulated by tissue oxygen requirements, TPO is produced by the liver at a constant rate. Circulating TPO levels are regulated by platelet mass through receptor-mediated uptake and degradation [56, 57]. When platelet production is high, TPO is bound by platelet-expressed c-Mpl and removed from the circulation, resulting in less free TPO available to stimulate megakaryopoiesis. When platelet production is low, more TPO is free to stimulate megakaryopoiesis. Circulating TPO levels are highest when megakaryopoiesis itself is impaired, such as in patients with aplastic anemia or congenital amegakaryocytic thrombocytopenia [58]. The development of recombinant TPO and now peptide and non-peptide TPO receptor agonists have provided valuable tools not only for the study of megakaryopoiesis in cell line and animal models but also for treatment of clinical states of thrombocytopenia (☞ below).

## 4.2. Thrombopoiesis in ITP: evidence for accelerated platelet destruction

ITP is a disease of accelerated platelet destruction, mediated by anti-platelet antibodies that bind platelets and lead to their uptake and destruction in the reticuloendothelial system (reviewed [59]). T-cells also play an important role in the immune attack on platelets. Current therapies such as corticosteroids, IVIg, anti-D, splenectomy, and the spleen tyrosine kinase inhibitor, fostamatinib, target platelet destruction either by suppressing the immune response or reducing the uptake of antibody-coated platelets and are generally effective.

The effects of anti-platelet antibodies have been studied in animal models. When animals are injected with an anti-platelet antibody, there is a rapid onset of thrombocytopenia, and in response to the decrease in platelet count TPO levels increase and promote an increase in bone marrow megakaryocyte number and ploidy, harbingers of platelet recovery. The bold experiment of Harrington demonstrated analogous results in humans, when he infused plasma from patients with ITP to healthy volunteers including himself and caused a rapid onset of severe thrombocytopenia [60]. Clinically, assays employing direct monoclonal antibody immobilization of platelet antigens (MAIPA) detect antiplatelet antibodies in up to 85 % of ITP patients [61].

Previous studies have suggested heterogenous effects on platelet production, but early studies with $^{51}$Cr-labelled donor platelets in ITP patients indicated that compared to controls, platelet turnover was significantly increased in ITP, due to both reduced platelet survival and compensatory platelet production [62, 63]. Although this type of labelling study cannot be routinely performed in the clinic, it is possible to measure the immature platelet fraction (IPF). The immature platelet fraction is analogous to the reticulocyte count, and it is usually increased in patients with ITP [64]. Studies of patients with ITP show that while the absolute IPF is reduced, the IPF as a percentage of total platelets is increased in many patients with ITP. Furthermore, IVIg and anti-D therapies tended to have little effect on the absolute IPF, suggesting that they work by reducing platelet destruction [65]. These findings fit a model in which ITP is a disease of platelet destruction, although the fact that the absolute IPF is not higher in ITP suggests that platelet production is suboptimal.

Most recently, studies have suggested that platelet clearance by hepatocyte Ashwell-Morell receptors recognizing abnormally desialylated platelets contributes to decreased platelet survival [66] supported by the clinical observation of case reports of improved platelet counts with oseltamivir [67, 68]. Finally, platelet (not megakaryocyte) apoptosis due to antibody-dependent cytotoxicity may also contribute to impaired platelet survival/accelerated destruction.

Additional work has also demonstrated a role for peripheral platelet destruction by antibody dependent cellular phagocytosis by macrophages expressing Fc Gamma receptors [69, 70], supported by clinical responses to both splenectomy and fostamatinib. Finally, more recent attention has focused on a role for antibody dependent cellular cytotoxicity [71] as well as a role for complement activation through macrophage complement receptor 1[72, 73]. These mechanisms are covered in more detail elsewhere.

## 4.3. Thrombopoiesis in ITP: evidence for impaired platelet production

Although not diminishing the importance of platelet destruction, additional evidence suggests that ITP is also a disorder of impaired platelet production. Further thrombokinetic studies concluded that, when $^{111}$In-labelled autologous platelets were infused into patients with ITP, platelet turnover was equal or less than that in normal subjects, indicating reduced platelet production. The discrepant results may be due in part to shortened survival of allogeneic relative to autologous platelets and *in vivo* elution of the $^{51}$Cr label, falsely elevating estimates of platelet destruction [73, 74]. The authors hypothesized that impaired platelet production was due to antibody-mediated damage to megakaryocytes and megakaryocyte precursors.

In fact, *in vitro* studies demonstrate that antibodies in ITP can impair megakaryopoiesis and proplatelet production. When CD34+ cells were differentiated in culture in the presence of plasma from patients with ITP or healthy controls, the ITP plasma inhibited the development of megakaryocytic cells. Similar inhibitory effects were seen when purified antibodies to GPIbα, GPIIb or GPIIIa were used, and pre-incubation of patient plasma with platelets to adsorb the anti-platelet antibodies eliminated its negative effects on megakaryopoiesis [30]. Anti-platelet antibodies in ITP also blocked proplatelet formation *in vitro* and these effects were particularly prominent with anti-GPIbα antibodies [29, 30, 75]. A recent study found that ITP patients who were non-responders to thrombopoietin receptor agonists had ineffective platelet production, with no rise in the absolute IPF despite increased numbers of marrow megakaryocytes, suggesting that in these patients anti-platelet antibodies are inhibiting proplatelet formation or platelet release [72]. Although the mechanisms by which antibodies inhibit megakaryopoiesis are not clear, apoptosis may play a role. Early light microscopy studies of bone marrow from patients with ITP revealed that a large number of the megakaryocytes appeared damaged [74, 75]. Further studies with electron microscopy showed that despite increased numbers of marrow megakaryocytes, up to 78 % of megakaryocytes in bone marrow specimens from adults with ITP had ultrastructural findings consistent with para-apoptosis or apoptosis; in addition, electron microscopy of CD34+ cells cultured with plasma from patients with ITP demonstrated similar evidence of megakaryocyte damage [76-78]. Less mature megakaryocytes also demonstrate morphologic changes. This last observation has led to the alternative hypothesis that ineffective thrombopoiesis, rather than absolute loss of total megakaryocyte mass results in relative TPO deficiency (see below), normal or increased megakaryocytes in bone marrow and overall thrombocytopenia [79]. The accelerated megakaryocyte maturation and proplatelet formation, which is characterized by physiologic apoptosis [80], results in ineffective platelet production, an elevated IPF and overall low platelet count.

In addition to the ineffective thrombopoiesis, platelet production may be reduced in ITP because circulating TPO levels are inappropriately low relative to the degree of thrombocytopenia. Although in animal models of acute immune thrombocytopenia TPO levels rise within 24 hr of antibody administration [81], in humans with chronic ITP TPO levels were only modestly increased over healthy controls [58, 82]. This is in stark contrast to patients with thrombocytopenia due to aplastic anemia. These findings were confirmed in the clinic by the development of the TPO-receptor agonists as therapeutic strategies for the treatment of ITP and the approval of several molecules now for the treatment of ITP (both oral and subcutaneous) in both pediatric and adult ITP, and current recommendations for their use as preferred second line treatment [83, 84].

## 4.4. Megakaryopoiesis in ITP: evidence for direct roles of megakaryocytes

Recent studies have implicated megakaryocytes in a much more direct role in the pathobiology of ITP. More recent evidence suggest aberrant micro (mi)RNA expression directing megakaryocyte differentiation, proliferation and platelet production as well as defective apoptosis and abnormal proliferation and differentiation of mesenchymal stromal cells supporting megakaryopoiesis [85]. An elegant study examined the role of the bone marrow niche in the pathophysiology of ITP, looking at the contribution of mesenchymal stromal cells, as well as the distribution of megakaryocytes within the bone marrow, and demonstrated that megakaryocyte distribution was abnormal with significant increase in apoptosis of nestin$^{+}$ mesenchymal stromal cells [86]. Further, investigators have also detected anti-GPIIb/IIIa and anti-Ib/IX antibodies in bone marrow aspirates and directly on megakaryocytes from bone marrow aspirates of patients with chronic ITP, demonstrating that megakaryocytes are at least a target cell [87] for the immune response, and may be actively contributing to the pathophysiology of the immune process of ITP.

## References


1. Noetzli LJ, French SL, Machlus KR. New Insights Into the Differentiation of Megakaryocytes From Hematopoietic Progenitors. Arterioscler Thromb Vasc Biol. 2019;39:1288-300.

2. Raslova H, Roy L, Vourc'h C, Le Couedic JP, Brison O, Metivier D, Feunteun J, Kroemer G, Debili N, Vainchenker W. Megakaryocyte polyploidization is associated with a functional gene amplification. Blood. 2003; 101:541-4.

3. Davenport P, Liu ZJ, Sola-Visner M. Changes in megakaryopoiesis over ontogeny and their implications in health and disease. Platelets. 2020;31:692-9.

4. Bornstein R, Garcia-Vela J, Gilsanz F, Auray C, Cales C. Cord blood megakaryocytes do not complete maturation, as indicated by impaired establishment of endomitosis and low expression of G1/S cyclins upon thrombopoietin-induced differentiation. Br J Haematol. 2001; 114:458-65.

5. Mattia G, Vulcano F, Milazzo L, Barca A, Macioce G, Giampaolo A, Hassan HJ. Different ploidy levels of megakaryocytes generated from peripheral or cord blood CD34+ cells are correlated with different levels of platelet release. Blood. 2002;99:888-97.

6. Raslova H, Baccini V, Loussaief L, Comba B, Larghero J, Debili N, Vainchenker W. Mammalian target of rapamycin (mTOR) regulates both proliferation of megakaryocyte progenitors and late stages of megakaryocyte differentiation. Blood. 2006;107:2303-10.

7. Liu ZJ, Italiano J, Jr., Ferrer-Marin F, Gutti R, Bailey M, Poterjoy B, Rimsza L, Sola-Visner M. Developmental differences in megakaryocytopoiesis are associated with up-regulated TPO signaling through mTOR and elevated GATA-1 levels in neonatal megakaryocytes. Blood. 2011;117:4106-17.

8. Corash L, Levin J. The relationship between megakaryocyte ploidy and platelet volume in normal and thrombocytopenic C3H mice. Exp Hematol. 1990;18: 985-9.

9. Vitrat N, Cohen-Solal K, Pique C, Le Couedic JP, Norol F, Larsen AK, Katz A, Vainchenker W, Debili N. Endomitosis of human megakaryocytes are due to abortive mitosis. Blood. 1998;91:3711-23.

10. Geddis AE, Fox NE, Tkachenko E, Kaushansky K. Endomitotic megakaryocytes that form a bipolar spindle exhibit cleavage furrow ingression followed by furrow regression. Cell Cycle. 2007;6:455-60.

11. Gao Y, Smith E, Ker E, Campbell P, Cheng EC, Zou S, Lin S, Wang L, Halene S, Krause DS. Role of RhoA-specific guanine exchange factors in regulation of endomitosis in megakaryocytes. Dev Cell. 2012;22:573-84.

12. Lordier L, Jalil A, Aurade F, Larbret F, Larghero J, Debili N, Vainchenker W, Chang Y. Megakaryocyte endomitosis is a failure of late cytokinesis related to defects in the contractile ring and Rho/Rock signaling. Blood. 2008;112:3164-74.

13. Lordier L, Chang Y, Jalil A, Aurade F, Garcon L, Lecluse Y, Larbret F, Kawashima T, Kitamura T, Larghero J, Debili N, Vainchenker W. Aurora B is dispensable for megakaryocyte polyploidization, but contributes to the endomitotic process. Blood. 2010;116:2345-55.

14. Geddis AE, Kaushansky K. Endomitotic megakaryocytes form a midzone in anaphase but have a deficiency in cleavage furrow formation. Cell Cycle. 2006;5:538-45.

15. Ganem NJ, Cornils H, Chiu SY, O'Rourke KP, Arnaud J, Yimlamai D, Thery M, Camargo FD, Pellman D. Cytokinesis failure triggers hippo tumor suppressor pathway activation. Cell. 2014;158:833-48.

16. Andreassen PR, Lohez OD, Lacroix FB, Margolis RL. Tetraploid state induces p53-dependent arrest of nontransformed mammalian cells in G1. Mol Biol Cell. 2001; 12:1315-28.

17. Schulze H, Korpal M, Hurov J, Kim SW, Zhang J, Cantley LC, Graf T, Shivdasani RA. Characterization of the megakaryocyte demarcation membrane system and its role in thrombopoiesis. Blood. 2006;107:3868-75.

18. Mazzi S, Lordier L, Debili N, Raslova H, Vainchenker W. Megakaryocyte and polyploidization. Exp Hematol. 2018;57:1-13.

19. Italiano JE, Jr., Lecine P, Shivdasani RA, Hartwig JH. Blood platelets are assembled principally at the ends of proplatelet processes produced by differentiated megakaryocytes. J Cell Biol. 1999;147:1299-312.

20. Junt T, Schulze H, Chen Z, Massberg S, Goerge T, Krueger A, Wagner DD, Graf T, Italiano JE, Jr., Shivdasani RA, von Andrian UH. Dynamic visualization of thrombopoiesis within bone marrow. Science. 2007; 317:1767-70.

21. Sharnoff JG, Scardino V. Platelet-count differences in blood of the rabbit right and left heart ventricles. Nature. 1960;187:334-5.

22. Levine RF, Eldor A, Shoff PK, Kirwin S, Tenza D, Cramer EM. Circulating megakaryocytes: delivery of large numbers of intact, mature megakaryocytes to the lungs. Eur J Haematol. 1993;51:233-46.

23. Slater DN, Trowbridge EA, Martin JF. The megakaryocyte in thrombocytopenia: a microscopic study which supports the theory that platelets are produced in the pulmonary circulation. Thromb Res. 1983;31:163-76.

24. Lefrancais E, Looney MR. Platelet Biogenesis in the Lung Circulation. Physiology (Bethesda). 2019;34:392-401.

25. Lefrancais E, Ortiz-Munoz G, Caudrillier A, Mallavia B, Liu F, Sayah DM, Thornton EE, Headley MB, David T, Coughlin SR, Krummel MF, Leavitt AD, Passegue E, Looney MR. The lung is a site of platelet biogenesis and a reservoir for haematopoietic progenitors. Nature. 2017; 544:105-9.

26. Yeung AK, Villacorta-Martin C, Hon S, Rock JR, Murphy GJ. Lung megakaryocytes display distinct transcriptional and phenotypic properties. Blood Adv. 2020; 4:6204-17.

27. Heib T, Hermanns HM, Manukjan G, Englert M, Kusch C, Becker IC, Gerber A, Wackerbarth LM, Burkard P, Dandekar T, Balkenhol J, Jahn D, Beck S, Meub M, Dutting S, Stigloher C, Sauer M, Cherpokova D, Schulze H, Brakebusch C, Nieswandt B, Nagy Z, Pleines I. RhoA/Cdc42 signaling drives cytoplasmic maturation but not endomitosis in megakaryocytes. Cell Rep. 2021;35:109102.

28. Aslan JE, McCarty OJ. Rho GTPases in platelet function. J Thromb Haemost. 2013;11:35-46.

29. Pleines I, Cherpokova D, Bender M. Rho GTPases and their downstream effectors in megakaryocyte biology. Platelets. 2019;30:9-16.

30. Italiano JE, Jr., Bergmeier W, Tiwari S, Falet H, Hartwig JH, Hoffmeister KM, Andre P, Wagner DD, Shivdasani RA. Mechanisms and implications of platelet discoid shape. Blood. 2003;101:4789-96.

31. Richardson JL, Shivdasani RA, Boers C, Hartwig JH, Italiano JE, Jr. Mechanisms of organelle transport and capture along proplatelets during platelet production. Blood. 2005;106:4066-75.

32. Avecilla ST, Hattori K, Heissig B, Tejada R, Liao F, Shido K, Jin DK, Dias S, Zhang F, Hartman TE, Hackett NR, Crystal RG, Witte L, Hicklin DJ, Bohlen P, Eaton D, Lyden D, de Sauvage F, Rafii S. Chemokine-mediated interaction of hematopoietic progenitors with the bone marrow vascular niche is required for thrombopoiesis. Nat Med. 2004;10:64-71.

33. Nurden AT, Didry D, Rosa JP. Molecular defects of platelets in Bernard-Soulier syndrome. Blood Cells. 1983;9:333-58.

34. Ware J, Russell S, Ruggeri ZM. Generation and rescue of a murine model of platelet dysfunction: the Bernard-Soulier syndrome. Proc Natl Acad Sci U S A. 2000;97: 2803-8.

35. Alimardani G, Guichard J, Fichelson S, Cramer EM. Pathogenic effects of anti-glycoprotein Ib antibodies on megakaryocytes and platelets. Thromb Haemost. 2002; 88:1039-46.

36. Radley JM, Haller CJ. Fate of senescent megakaryocytes in the bone marrow. Br J Haematol. 1983;53:277-87.

37. Mason KD, Carpinelli MR, Fletcher JI, Collinge JE, Hilton AA, Ellis S, Kelly PN, Ekert PG, Metcalf D, Roberts AW, Huang DC, Kile BT. Programmed anuclear cell death delimits platelet life span. Cell. 2007;128:1173-86.

38. Zhang H, Nimmer PM, Tahir SK, Chen J, Fryer RM, Hahn KR, Iciek LA, Morgan SJ, Nasarre MC, Nelson R, Preusser LC, Reinhart GA, Smith ML, Rosenberg SH, Elmore SW, Tse C. Bcl-2 family proteins are essential for platelet survival. Cell Death Differ. 2007;14:943-51.

39. Lebois M, Josefsson EC. Regulation of platelet lifespan by apoptosis. Platelets. 2016;27:497-504.

40. Josefsson EC, Vainchenker W, James C. Regulation of Platelet Production and Life Span: Role of Bcl-xL and Potential Implications for Human Platelet Diseases. Int J Mol Sci. 2020;21:7591.

41. Josefsson EC, James C, Henley KJ, Debrincat MA, Rogers KL, Dowling MR, White MJ, Kruse EA, Lane RM, Ellis S, Nurden P, Mason KD, O'Reilly LA, Roberts AW, Metcalf D, Huang DC, Kile BT. Megakaryocytes possess a functional intrinsic apoptosis pathway that must be restrained to survive and produce platelets. J Exp Med. 2011;208:2017-31.

42. Morison IM, Cramer Borde EM, Cheesman EJ, Cheong PL, Holyoake AJ, Fichelson S, Weeks RJ, Lo A, Davies SM, Wilbanks SM, Fagerlund RD, Ludgate MW, da Silva Tatley FM, Coker MS, Bockett NA, Hughes G, Pippig DA, Smith MP, Capron C, Ledgerwood EC. A mutation of human cytochrome c enhances the intrinsic apoptotic pathway but causes only thrombocytopenia. Nat Genet. 2008;40:387-9.

43. De Rocco D, Cerqua C, Goffrini P, Russo G, Pastore A, Meloni F, Nicchia E, Moraes CT, Pecci A, Salviati L, Savoia A. Mutations of cytochrome c identified in patients with thrombocytopenia THC4 affect both apoptosis and cellular bioenergetics. Biochim Biophys Acta. 2014;1842:269-74.

44. Liptak MD, Fagerlund RD, Ledgerwood EC, Wilbanks SM, Bren KL. The proapoptotic G41S mutation to human cytochrome c alters the heme electronic structure and increases the electron self-exchange rate. J Am Chem Soc. 2011;133:1153-5.

45. Kaushansky K, Lok S, Holly RD, Broudy VC, Lin N, Bailey MC, Forstrom JW, Buddle MM, Oort PJ, Hagen FS, et al. Promotion of megakaryocyte progenitor expansion and differentiation by the c-Mpl ligand thrombopoietin. Nature. 1994;369:568-71.

46. Lok S, Kaushansky K, Holly RD, Kuijper JL, Lofton-Day CE, Oort PJ, Grant FJ, Heipel MD, Burkhead SK, Kramer JM, et al. Cloning and expression of murine thrombopoietin cDNA and stimulation of platelet production in vivo. Nature. 1994;369:565-8.

47. Wendling F, Maraskovsky E, Debili N, Florindo C, Teepe M, Titeux M, Methia N, Breton-Gorius J, Cosman D, Vainchenker W. cMpl ligand is a humoral regulator of megakaryocytopoiesis. Nature. 1994;369:571-4.

48. Bartley TD, Bogenberger J, Hunt P, Li YS, Lu HS, Martin F, Chang MS, Samal B, Nichol JL, Swift S, et al. Identification and cloning of a megakaryocyte growth and development factor that is a ligand for the cytokine receptor Mpl. Cell. 1994;77:1117-24.

49. Kuter DJ, Beeler DL, Rosenberg RD. The purification of megapoietin: a physiological regulator of megakaryocyte growth and platelet production. Proc Natl Acad Sci U S A. 1994;91:11104-8.

50. de Sauvage FJ, Hass PE, Spencer SD, Malloy BE, Gurney AL, Spencer SA, Darbonne WC, Henzel WJ, Wong SC, Kuang WJ, et al. Stimulation of megakaryocytopoiesis and thrombopoiesis by the c-Mpl ligand. Nature. 1994;369:533-8.

51. Gurney AL, Carver-Moore K, de Sauvage FJ, Moore MW. Thrombocytopenia in c-mpl-deficient mice. Science. 1994;265:1445-7.

52. Bunting S, Widmer R, Lipari T, Rangell L, Steinmetz H, Carver-Moore K, Moore MW, Keller GA, de Sauvage FJ. Normal platelets and megakaryocytes are produced in vivo in the absence of thrombopoietin. Blood. 1997; 90:3423-9.

53. Murone M, Carpenter DA, de Sauvage FJ. Hematopoietic deficiencies in c-mpl and TPO knockout mice. Stem Cells. 1998;16:1-6.

54. Carver-Moore K, Broxmeyer HE, Luoh SM, Cooper S, Peng J, Burstein SA, Moore MW, de Sauvage FJ. Low levels of erythroid and myeloid progenitors in thrombopoietin-and c-mpl-deficient mice. Blood. 1996;88: 803-8.

55. McCarty JM, Sprugel KH, Fox NE, Sabath DE, Kaushansky K. Murine thrombopoietin mRNA levels are modulated by platelet count. Blood. 1995;86:3668-75.

56. Kuter DJ, Rosenberg RD. The reciprocal relationship of thrombopoietin (c-Mpl ligand) to changes in the platelet mass during busulfan-induced thrombocytopenia in the rabbit. Blood. 1995;85:2720-30.

57. Nagata Y, Shozaki Y, Nagahisa H, Nagasawa T, Abe T, Todokoro K. Serum thrombopoietin level is not regulated by transcription but by the total counts of both megakaryocytes and platelets during thrombocytopenia and thrombocytosis. Thromb Haemost. 1997;77:808-14.

58. Mukai HY, Kojima H, Todokoro K, Tahara T, Kato T, Hasegawa Y, Kobayashi T, Ninomiya H, Nagasawa T, Abe T. Serum thrombopoietin (TPO) levels in patients with amegakaryocytic thrombocytopenia are much higher than those with immune thrombocytopenic purpura. Thromb Haemost. 1996;76:675-8.

59. Audia S, Mahevas M, Nivet M, Ouandji S, Ciudad M, Bonnotte B. Immune Thrombocytopenia: Recent Advances in Pathogenesis and Treatments. Hemasphere. 2021;5:e574.

60. Harrington WJ, Minnich V, Hollingsworth JW, Moore CV. Demonstration of a thrombocytopenic factor in the blood of patients with thrombocytopenic purpura. J Lab Clin Med. 1951;38:1-10.

61. Porcelijn L, Huiskes E, Oldert G, Schipperus M, Zwaginga JJ, de Haas M. Detection of platelet autoantibodies to identify immune thrombocytopenia: state of the art. Br J Haematol. 2018;182:423-6.

62. Harker LA, Finch CA. Thrombokinetics in man. J Clin Invest. 1969;48:963-74.

63. Branehog I. Platelet kinetics in idiopathic thrombocytopenic purpura (ITP) before and at different times after splenectomy. Br J Haematol. 1975;29:413-26.

64. Briggs C, Kunka S, Hart D, Oguni S, Machin SJ. Assessment of an immature platelet fraction (IPF) in peripheral thrombocytopenia. Br J Haematol. 2004;126: 93-9.

65. Barsam SJ, Psaila B, Forestier M, Page LK, Sloane PA, Geyer JT, Villarica GO, Ruisi MM, Gernsheimer TB, Beer JH, Bussel JB. Platelet production and platelet destruction: assessing mechanisms of treatment effect in immune thrombocytopenia. Blood. 2011;117:5723-32.

66. Li J, van der Wal DE, Zhu G, Xu M, Yougbare I, Ma L, Vadasz B, Carrim N, Grozovsky R, Ruan M, Zhu L, Zeng Q, Tao L, Zhai ZM, Peng J, Hou M, Leytin V, Freedman J, Hoffmeister KM, Ni H. Desialylation is a mechanism of Fc-independent platelet clearance and a therapeutic target in immune thrombocytopenia. Nat Commun. 2015; 6:7737.

67. Revilla N, Corral J, Minano A, Mingot-Castellano ME, Campos RM, Velasco F, Gonzalez N, Galvez E, Berrueco R, Fuentes I, Gonzalez-Lopez TJ, de la Morena-Barrio ME, Gonzalez-Porras JR, Vicente V, Lozano ML. Multirefractory primary immune thrombocytopenia targeting the decreased sialic acid content. Platelets. 2019;30:743-51.

68. Shaim H, McCaffrey P, Trieu JA, DeAnda A, Yates SG. Evaluating the effects of oseltamivir phosphate on platelet counts: a retrospective review. Platelets. 2020;31: 1080-4.

69. Norris PAA, Segel GB, Burack WR, Sachs UJ, Lissenberg-Thunnissen SN, Vidarsson G, Bayat B, Cserti-Gazdewich CM, Callum J, Lin Y, Branch D, Kapur R, Semple JW, Lazarus AH. FcgammaRI and FcgammaRIII on splenic macrophages mediate phagocytosis of anti-glycoprotein IIb/IIIa autoantibody-opsonized platelets in immune thrombocytopenia. Haematologica. 2021; 106:250-4.

70. Kuwana M, Okazaki Y, Ikeda Y. Splenic macrophages maintain the anti-platelet autoimmune response via uptake of opsonized platelets in patients with immune thrombocytopenic purpura. J Thromb Haemost. 2009;7: 322-9.

71. Olsson B, Andersson PO, Jernas M, Jacobsson S, Carlsson B, Carlsson LM, Wadenvik H. T-cell-mediated cytotoxicity toward platelets in chronic idiopathic thrombocytopenic purpura. Nat Med. 2003;9:1123-4.

72. Peerschke EI, Panicker S, Bussel J. Classical complement pathway activation in immune thrombocytopenia purpura: inhibition by a novel C1s inhibitor. Br J Haematol. 2016;173:942-5.

73. Castelli R, Lambertenghi Delilliers G, Gidaro A, Cicardi M, Bergamaschini L. Complement activation in patients with immune thrombocytopenic purpura according to phases of disease course. Clin Exp Immunol. 2020;201:258-65.

74. Pisciotta AV, Stefanini M, Dameshek W. Studies on platelets. X. Morphologic characteristics of megakaryocytes by phase contrast microscopy in normals and in patients with idiopathic thrombocytopenic purpura. Blood. 1953;8:703-23.

75. Dameshek W, Miller EB. The megakaryocytes in idiopathic thrombocytopenic purpura, a form of hypersplenism. Blood. 1946;1:27-50.

76. Houwerzijl EJ, Blom NR, van der Want JJ, Esselink MT, Koornstra JJ, Smit JW, Louwes H, Vellenga E, de Wolf JT. Ultrastructural study shows morphologic features of apoptosis and para-apoptosis in megakaryocytes from patients with idiopathic thrombocytopenic purpura. Blood. 2004;103:500-6.

77. Stahl CP, Zucker-Franklin D, McDonald TP. Incomplete antigenic cross-reactivity between platelets and megakaryocytes: relevance to ITP. Blood. 1986;67:421-8.

78. Houwerzijl EJ, Blom NR, van der Want JJ, Vellenga E, de Wolf JT. Megakaryocytic dysfunction in myelodysplastic syndromes and idiopathic thrombocytopenic purpura is in part due to different forms of cell death. Leukemia. 2006;20:1937-42.

79. von Gunten S, Wehrli M, Simon HU. Cell death in immune thrombocytopenia: novel insights and perspectives. Semin Hematol. 2013;50 Suppl 1:S109-15.

80. Ucar C, Oren H, Irken G, Ates H, Atabay B, Turker M, Vergin C, Yaprak I. Investigation of megakaryocyte apoptosis in children with acute and chronic idiopathic thrombocytopenic purpura. Eur J Haematol. 2003;70: 347-52.

81. Yang C, Li YC, Kuter DJ. The physiological response of thrombopoietin (c-Mpl ligand) to thrombocytopenia in the rat. Br J Haematol. 1999;105:478-85.

82. Kosugi S, Kurata Y, Tomiyama Y, Tahara T, Kato T, Tadokoro S, Shiraga M, Honda S, Kanakura Y, Matsuzawa Y. Circulating thrombopoietin level in chronic immune thrombocytopenic purpura. Br J Haematol. 1996; 93:704-6.

83. Neunert C, Terrell DR, Arnold DM, Buchanan G, Cines DB, Cooper N, Cuker A, Despotovic JM, George JN, Grace RF, Kuhne T, Kuter DJ, Lim W, McCrae KR, Pruitt B, Shimanek H, Vesely SK. American Society of Hematology 2019 guidelines for immune thrombocytopenia. Blood Adv. 2019;3:3829-66.

84. Al-Samkari H, Kuter DJ. Optimal use of thrombopoietin receptor agonists in immune thrombocytopenia. Ther Adv Hematol. 2019;10: 2040620719841735.

85. Khodadi E, Asnafi AA, Shahrabi S, Shahjahani M, Saki N. Bone marrow niche in immune thrombocytopenia: a focus on megakaryopoiesis. Ann Hematol. 2016; 95:1765-76.

86. Wang M, Feng R, Zhang JM, Xu LL, Feng FE, Wang CC, Wang QM, Zhu XL, He Y, Xue J, Fu HX, Lv M, Kong Y, Chang YJ, Xu LP, Liu KY, Huang XJ, Zhang XH. Dysregulated megakaryocyte distribution associated with nestin(+) mesenchymal stem cells in immune thrombocytopenia. Blood Adv. 2019;3:1416-28.

87. Shrestha S, Nazy I, Smith JW, Kelton JG, Arnold DM. Platelet autoantibodies in the bone marrow of patients with immune thrombocytopenia. Blood Adv. 2020;4: 2962-6.

# 5. Genetics of ITP

## 5.1. Challenges in defining a genetic etiology of ITP

Immune thrombocytopenia (ITP) is an autoimmune disease that is presently a diagnosis of exclusion, lacking a simple confirmatory diagnostic test. Many diseases can mimic ITP, including autoimmune lymphoproliferative syndrome (ALPS), common variable immunodeficiency (CVID), inherited disorders with thrombocytopenia (e.g., Bernard Soulier disease, RUNX1, ANKRD26, and ETV6 – associated thrombocytopenia). It is important to rigorously exclude these alternative diseases as the etiology. ITP also is frequently observed in association with other autoimmune diseases such as systemic lupus erythematosus, autoimmune hemolytic anemia and antiphospholipid antibody syndrome. Whether ITP occurring in the background of another autoimmune disease should be considered true ITP or secondary to the other autoimmune process is also uncertain, reflecting the lack of knowledge generally in the genetic basis of autoimmune disorders. While it is generally believed that these autoimmune diseases likely reflect a genetic predisposition plus an environmental provocation, this hypothesis has proven difficult to study.

Thrombotic thrombocytopenic purpura (TTP) can serve as a model for thinking about some of the challenges in defining a genetic basis for ITP. TTP can present as an inherited germline disorder or as an acquired autoimmune deficiency of ADAMTS13. However even in this case where the disease mechanism is well understood (inherited or acquired deficiency of ADAMTS13 with decreased processing of von Willebrand factor (VWF) leading to prothrombotic large VWF multimers), it is complicated by the fact that ADAMTS13 deficiency is necessary but not sufficient for the phenotype as the clinical presentations of patients with acute TTP are consistent with an environmental trigger on a background of ADAMTS13 deficiency. In inherited TTP, pregnancy, infection and age have been implicated but much remains to be known about the mechanism of triggering the TTP phenotype [5, 15]. Defining such environmental triggers and how they interact with an underlying genetic predisposition is a major unmet need in understanding the etiology of autoimmune disease generally. If disease risk is polygenic and/or multifactorial, as has been hypothesized for ITP, the challenge is greater.

## 5.2. Germline single-nucleotide variant (SNV) candidate gene approach

Candidate gene approach is based on prior knowledge or hypotheses about specific pathways and require rigorous validation using a multiple independent sample sets with large numbers of patients. Several reviews compiled candidate genes implicated in ITP [1, 2, 10, 16]. Polymorphism in Fcγ receptors, one of the most studied genes in this field, have been associated with the onset and pathogenesis of ITP as well as response to treatment. A long list of variants in cytokines (both proinflammatory and anti-inflammatory), transcription factors, redox regulators, phosphorylation regulators, DNA methyltransferase, and miRNAs have been studied. A limiting factor in many of these studies is sample size and diversity. The utility of this approach remains to be defined and will require larger confirmatory studies. At this time, there are no clinically actionable findings using this approach.

## 5.3. Familial ITP

If there is a genetic (hereditary) basis for ITP, then study of families is a promising avenue to pursue. Previous reports on familial ITPs are few. The generally incomplete family history information and the complexity in its diagnosis might have been limited and confounded its identification. In a literature review, Pujol-Moix et al. found total of 60 familial ITP cases from 20 families, with the first familial ITP case reported in 1953, which was decades later than the first report on ITP [4, 6, 9] However, Pujol-Moix et al. were able to identify 16 familial ITP cases from 8 families from their single center, the Platelet Pathology Unit of the Hospital de la Santa Creu I Sant Pau (Spain), in a period of 28 years. Similarly, Pediatric and Adult Registry on Chronic ITP (PARC-ITP) data revealed that 10 of 445 pediatric ITP patients had a positive family history [11]. These findings are consistent with a role of genetic predisposition in the etiology of ITP.

Most studies on familial ITPs have been focused on clinical characteristics, recently, with the availability of whole-exome sequencing and gene expression analysis, familial ITP studies began to provide genetic insights into the disease pathogenesis. Applying these methods on a familial cases, Peng et al. identified a potential pathogenic heterozygous mutation in *TNFRSF13B* (G76S) [8]. TNFRSF13B is a B-cell receptor belongs to TNF receptor superfamily. The authors demonstrated that, compared with healthy subjects or ITP patients with a wild type *TNFRSF13B,* the G76S mutation was associated with higher expression levels of *TNFRSF13B* mRNA and protein, enhanced binding capacity of APRIL ligand to B cells, and elevated serum T-cell activating markers, including IL-17a, TNF-α, IFN-γ and BAFF. Also, Epstein-Barr virus transformed B cells with the G76S mutation induced apoptosis of a human megakaryocytic cell line [8]. These data suggest a possible role of *TNFRSF13B* G76S in ITP. However, one family member harboring the same mutation appeared to be healthy. Similarly, this mutation was detected in healthy populations (2/233), albeit with a lower prevalence than in sporadic ITP patients (3/112). These findings are consistent with the notion that the etiology of ITP is multifactorial. And this study suggested that *TNFRSF13B* G76S mutation may contribute to genetic risk of ITP [8].

Of note, ITP could be secondary to CVID, and mutations in *TNFRSF13B* have been associated with CVID, although these mutations tend to be associated with compromised gene functions in CVID [3, 12], unlike the gain-of-function effects observed for the G76S mutation in familial ITP. By checking the IgG, IgM and IgA levels, Peng et al excluded the diagnosis of CVID in the familial and sporadic ITP cases with G76S mutation [8]. Yet, Ma et al screened 176 refractory pediatric ITP cases and identified 2 patients harboring the single G76S mutation in *TNFRSF13B* gene, and further evaluations on these cases suggested a suspicious CVID diagnosis [7]. In addition, Vandrovcova et al sequenced the *TNFRSF13B* gene in 130 ITP patients and did not observe any potential pathogenic mutations [18]. Taken together, the role and impact of *TNFRSF13B* G76S in ITP still need to be further evaluated.

One characteristic of familial ITP is that they are more often associated with other autoimmune diseases than sporadic ITP [9]. Interestingly, besides the potential linkages with ITP and/or CVID, the *TNFRSF13B* G76S mutation was also found to be associated with pulmonary artery hypertension [13]. Similarly, several other TNF receptor superfamily members have been shown to be involved in shared genetics among multiple autoimmune diseases [21].

## 5.4. Genome-wide association studies (GWAS)

GWAS is a powerful tool for identifying genetic loci associated with disease risk. A recent pooling GWAS study in Chinese Han population with 200 ITP patients and 200 controls identified 4 novel loci—GBE1/LINC02027 (rs117503120), TIMP3/SYN3 (rs5998634), TENM4 (rs4483616), and RBM45/OSBPL6 (rs16866133), to be strongly associated with ITP; three of these loci (rs117503120, rs5998634, and rs16866133) were also validated with a TaqMan assay in a separate cohort of 250 ITP cases and 250 controls [20]. The investigators also performed pathway analysis based on GWAS data and identified three candidate pathways potentially involved in the etiology of ITP: JAK-STAT signaling pathway, neuroactive ligand-receptor interaction, and pathways in cancer. The JAK-STAT pathway has been previously shown to be implicated in the pathogenesis of pediatric ITP by gene expression profiling studies [14].

Another recent study by Wang et al. [19] investigated the association between immune checkpoint related gene polymorphisms and the susceptibility as well as therapeutic effect of primary ITP in a cohort of 307 ITP patients and 295 age-matched healthy controls in the Chinese population. The investigators found that rs1980422 in CD28 was associated with an increased risk of ITP, and the CT genotype is associated with significantly higher CD28 expression at both the mRNA and protein levels the TT genotype. Furthermore, they identified the T allele of PD1 rs36084323 as a risk factor and the T allele of LAG3 rs870849 as a protective factor for ITP severity. In terms of corticosteroid-resistance, they identified the T allele of DNAM1 rs763361 as a risk factor and the T allele of ICOS rs6726035 as protective factor. These novel findings provide new candidate genetic factors as potential prognostic markers and therapeutic targets in ITP.

## 5.5. Future Directions

In the future, we hope to see more genetic insights obtained from familial ITP studies and more high quality GWAS studies of rigorously curated ITP patients. We believe that these two approaches are the most promising for delivering on the challenge of defining genetic risk of ITP, illuminating the underlying molecular mechanisms and identifying novel therapeutic targets. Moreover, somatic mutations have been emerging in the etiology of autoimmune diseases [17], and it will be interesting to see whether somatic mutations have contributed to ITP pathogenesis.

### References


1. Audia S, Mahévas M, Samson M, Godeau B, Bonnotte B. Pathogenesis of immune thrombocytopenia. Autoimmun Rev. 2017;16(6):620-632.

2. Bergmann AK, Grace RF, Neufeld EJ. Genetic studies in pediatric ITP: outlook, feasibility, and requirements. Ann Hematol. 2010;89 Suppl 1(Suppl 1):S95-S103.

3. Castigli E, Wilson SA, Garibyan L, et al. TACI is mutant in common variable immunodeficiency and IgA deficiency. Nat Genet. 2005;37(8):829-834.

4. De Spirito A. Thrombocytopenic purpura in twins. Clin Proc Child Hosp Dist Columbia. 1953;9(12):256-261.

5. Fujimura Y, Matsumoto M, Isonishi A, et al. Natural history of Upshaw-Schulman syndrome based on ADAMTS13 gene analysis in Japan. J Thromb Haemost. 2011;9 Suppl 1:283-301.

6. Lee RI, Robertson OH. The Effect of Antiplatelet Serum on Blood Platelets and the experimental Production of Purpura Hemorrhagica. J Med Res. 1916;33(3):323-336.

7. Ma J, Fu L, Gu H, et al. Screening for Genetic Mutations for the Early Diagnosis of Common Variable Immunodeficiency in Children With Refractory Immune Thrombocytopenia: A Retrospective Data Analysis From a Tertiary Children's Center. Front Pediatr. 2020; 8:595135.

8. Peng HL, Zhang Y, Sun NN, et al. A gain-of-function mutation in TNFRSF13B is a candidate for predisposition to familial or sporadic immune thrombocytopenia. J Thromb Haemost. 2017;15(11):2259-2269.

9. Pujol-Moix N, Jimenez B, Muñiz-Diaz E, Roca M, Souto JC. Familial Immune Thrombocytopenia. Report of 16 Cases and Literature Review. J Rare Dis Res Treat. 2018;4(1):52-60.

10. Rezaeeyan H, Jaseb K, Alghasi A, Asnafi AA, Saki N. Association between gene polymorphisms and clinical features in idiopathic thrombocytopenic purpura patients. Blood Coagul Fibrinolysis. 2017;28(8):617-622.

11. Rischewski JR, Imbach P, Paulussen M, Kühne T. Idiopathic thrombocytopenic purpura (ITP): is there a genetic predisposition? Pediatr Blood Cancer. 2006;47(5 Suppl):678-680.

12. Salzer U, Chapel HM, Webster AD, et al. Mutations in TNFRSF13B encoding TACI are associated with common variable immunodeficiency in humans. Nat Genet. 2005;37(8):820-828.

13. Shinya Y, Hiraide T, Momoi M, et al. TNFRSF13B c.226G>A (p.Gly76Ser) as a Novel Causative Mutation for Pulmonary Arterial Hypertension. J Am Heart Assoc. 2021;10(5):e019245.

14. Sood R, Wong W, Gotlib J, Jeng M, Zehnder JL. Gene expression and pathway analysis of immune thrombocytopenic purpura. Br J Haematol. 2008;140(1):99-103.

15. Sukumar S, Lämmle B, Cataland SR. Thrombotic Thrombocytopenic Purpura: Pathophysiology, Diagnosis, and Management. J Clin Med. 2021;10(3):536.

16. Swinkels M, Rijkers M, Voorberg J, Vidarsson G, Leebeek FWG, Jansen AJG. Emerging Concepts in Immune Thrombocytopenia. Front Immunol. 2018;9:880.

17. Van Horebeek L, Dubois B, Goris A. Somatic Variants: New Kids on the Block in Human Immunogenetics. Trends Genet. 2019;35(12):935-947.

18. Vandrovcova J, Salzer U, Grimbacher B, et al. FAS mutations are an uncommon cause of immune thrombocytopenia in children and adults without additional features of immunodeficiency. Br J Haematol. 2019;186 (6):e163-e165.

19. Wang S, Zhang X, Leng S, et al. Immune Checkpoint-Related Gene Polymorphisms Are Associated With Primary Immune Thrombocytopenia. Front Immunol. 2021;11:615941.

20. Xu Y, Li J, Yang W, Tang X, Huang B, Liu J, Lin J, Zhang J, Yang W, Li S, Sun F, Deng L, Wang X. A Pooling Genome-Wide Association Study Identifies Susceptibility Loci and Signaling Pathways of Immune Thrombocytopenia in Chinese Han Population. Int J Genomics. 2020 11;2020:7531876.

21. Zhernakova A, Withoff S, Wijmenga C. Clinical implications of shared genetics and pathogenesis in autoimmune diseases. Nat Rev Endocrinol. 2013;9(11):646-659.

# 6. Differential diagnosis of ITP: Inherited Thrombocytopenias

Diagnosis of immune thrombocytopenia (ITP) remains of exclusion because no tests can ascertain that a patient with a recently discovered thrombocytopenia of unknown origin is affected by this disorder. Inherited thrombocytopenias (ITs) are therefore one of the conditions that have to be excluded before making a diagnosis of ITP. Although this distinction might seem simple, several literature reports indicate that misdiagnosis of ITs with ITP is common. This is well illustrated by the finding that 57 of 181 consecutive women with ITs had a previous diagnosis of ITP and 44 of them had received treatments that are not only useless, but also potentially harmful, such as immunosuppressive agents and splenectomy [11]. Moreover, 289 patients with *MYH9*-related disease (*MYH9*-RD), monoallelic Bernard-Soulier syndrome (BSS) or *ANKRD26*-related thrombocytopenia (*ANKRD26*-RT) were correctly diagnosed at an average age of 30, 33 and 35 years, respectively, after most of them had been previously classified as having ITP and nearly 20 % had received futile treatments [8, 9, 12]. Misdiagnosis with ITP not only exposes patients with ITs to the risk of undue therapies, but also prevent them to be considered for treatments and follow-up strategies that can improve quality of life and/or radically ameliorate prognosis [15]. Thus, striving to rule out an IT before diagnosing ITP is mandatory.

## 6.1. Inherited Thrombocytopenias

ITs are genetic disorders characterized by the presence from birth of severe to clinically irrelevant thrombocytopenia. We presently know 45 forms of IT caused by mutations in 41 different genes, but just under 50 % of patients have forms whose genetic defects have not yet been discovered. In spite of this wide genetic heterogeneity, only 5 disorders affect almost 80 % of patients with known ITs in our series of over 600 patients from about 300 families. These diseases are, in decreasing order of frequency, *MYH9*-RD, monoallelic BSS, *ANKRD26*-RT, biallelic BSS, and *ACTN1*-related thrombocytopenia (*ACTN1*-RT). Of note, the frequency of monoallelic BSS is much higher in Italy than in all other countries because the most frequent causative variant (p.Ala172Val in *GP1BA*) is almost exclusive of the Italian population.

The estimated prevalence of 2.7 in 100,000 places ITs among the rare diseases [1]. According to the prevalence of rare diseases calculated in 2021 by Orphanet (http://www.orphanet-italia.it), ITs are about ten times rarer than ITP and have a prevalence similar to severe hemophilia A and myelofibrosis with myeloid metaplasia. These data suggest that physicians dealing with blood diseases should expect to examine at least some individuals with ITs during their professional life.

The most useful classification of ITs from a practical point of view distinguishes forms characterized by only thrombocytopenia, forms presenting with other associated congenital alterations, and forms that predispose to acquire additional diseases during life. Table 6.1 reports ITs classified according to these criteria, while Table 6.2 details the additional congenital defects and the acquired disorders that can associate with thrombocytopenia in specific ITs.

### 6.1.1. Clinical and laboratory peculiarities of inherited thrombocytopenias

ITs have some peculiarities that are not shared with ITP and must therefore be carefully researched for differentiating these conditions.

#### Family history of thrombocytopenia

The finding of other family members with thrombocytopenia must raise a strong suspicion that the thrombocytopenia of the patient under examination is inherited. On the other hand, the absence of affected relatives does not exclude an IT, because many forms have recessive or sex-linked transmission (☞ Table 6.1). Moreover, some forms with dominant transmission have variable penetrance and family members carrying the same mutation as the proband may have platelet counts at the lower limit of the normal range. Finally, *MYH9*-RD, the most frequent form of IT, is characterized by a high frequency of sporadic cases deriving from

| Disease (abbreviation, OMIM entry) | Freq.[1] | Gene | Inh.[2] | Degree of TCP[3] | Excessive bleeding[4] | Platelet size |
|---|---|---|---|---|---|---|
| Forms with only thrombocytopenia | | | | | | |
| Bernard-Soulier syndrome, biallelic form (bBSS, 231200) | ++++ | *GP1BA* *GP1BB* *GP9* | AR | ++/+++ | yes | giant |
| Bernard-Soulier syndrome, monoallelic form (mBSS, 153670) | +++ | *GP1BA* *GP1BB* | AD | +/++ | no | large |
| *ACTN1*-related thrombocytopenia (*ACTN1*-RT, 615193) | +++ | *ACTN1* | AD | +/++ | no | large |
| Gray platelet syndrome (GPS, 139090) | ++ | *NBEAL2* | AR | ++/+++ | yes | large |
| Platelet-type von Willebrand disease (PTvWD, 177820) | ++ | *GP1BA* | AD | +/+++ | no | normal |
| *GFI1b*-related thrombocytopenia, monoallelic form (*GFI1b*-RT, 187900) | ++ | *GFI1B* | AD | +/++ | no | large |
| *GFI1b*-related thrombocytopenia, biallelic form (*GFI1b*-RT, 187900) | + | | AR | +++ | no | large |
| *TUBB1*-related thrombocytopenia (*TUBB1*-RT, 613112) | + | *TUBB1* | AD | +/++ | no | large |
| *ITGA2B*/*ITGB3*-related thrombocytopenia (*ITGA2B*/*ITGB3*-RT, 187800) | + | *ITGA2B* *ITGB3* | AD | +/++ | yes | large |
| *CYCS*-related thrombocytopenia (*CYCS*-RT or THC4, 612004) | + | *CYCS* | AD | + | no | normal |
| *SLFN14*-related thrombocytopenia (*SLFN14*-RT, 616913) | + | *SLFN14* | AD | +/++ | yes | large |
| *FLI1*-related thrombocytopenia, mono-allelic form (*FLI1-RT*, 617443) | + | *FLI1* | AD | + | yes | large |
| *FLI1*-related thrombocytopenia, biallelic form (*FLI1-RT*, 617443) | + | | AR | ++ | yes | large |
| *IKZF5*-related thrombocytopenia (*IKZF5*-RT, na) | + | *IKZF5* | AD | +/++ | no | normal |
| Thrombocytopenia caused by monoallelic *THPO* mutation (*THPO*-RT, na) | + | *THPO* | AD | + | no | normal |
| *FYB*-related thrombocytopenia (*FYB*-RT or THC3, 273900) | + | *FYB* | AR | ++/+++ | no | small |
| *TRPM7*-related thrombocytopenia (*TRPM7*-RT, na) | + | *TPRM7* | AD | ++ | no | large |
| *TPM4*-related thrombocytopenia (*TPM4*-RT, na) | + | *TPM4* | AD | + | no | large |
| *PTPRJ*-related thrombocytopenia (*PTPRJ*-RT, na) | + | *PTPRJ* | AR | ++/+++ | no | small |
| *PRKACG*-related thrombocytopenia (*PRKACG*-RT, 616176) | + | *PRKACG* | AR | +++ | no | large |
| Syndromic forms (☞ also Table 6.2) | | | | | | |
| Wiskott-Aldrich syndrome (WAS, 301000) | ++++ | *WAS* | XL | +++ | no | small |
| X-linked thrombocytopenia (XLT or THC1, 313900) | | | | ++/+++ | no | small |
| Jacobsen syndrome (JBS, 147791), Paris-Trousseau thrombocytopenia (TCPT, 188025) | ++++ | Deletions in 11q23 | AD | ++/+++ | yes | normal/ large |
| Thrombocytopenia with absent radii (TAR, 274000) | +++ | *RBM8A* | AR | +++ | no | normal |
| *GATA1*-related disorders: X-linked thrombocytopenia with thalassemia (XLTT, 314050), X-linked thrombocytopenia with dyserythropoietic anemia (XLTDA, 300367) | ++ | *GATA1* | XL | +/+++ | no | normal |

| Disease (abbreviation, OMIM entry) | Freq.[1] | Gene | Inh.[2] | Degree of TCP[3] | Excessive bleeding[4] | Platelet size |
|---|---|---|---|---|---|---|
| Platelet abnormalities with eosinophilia and immune-mediated inflammatory disease (PLTEID, 617718) | ++ | *ARPC1B* | AR | ++/+++ | no | small |
| Stormorken syndrome (STRMK, 185070) | ++ | *STIM1* | AD | ++ | no | nr |
| York platelet syndrome (YPS, na) | + | | AD | +/++ | no | normal |
| Takenouchi-Kosaki syndrome with macrothrombocytopenia (TKS, 616737) | + | *CDC42* | AD | ++ | no | large |
| *KDSR*-related thrombocytopenia (*KDSR*-RT, na) | + | *KDSR* | AR | +++ | no | normal |
| *ACTB*-associated syndromic thrombocytopenia (*ACTB*-AST, na) | + | *ACTB* | AD | +/++ | no | large |
| *FLNA*-related thrombocytopenia (*FLNA*-RT, na) | + | *FLNA* | XL | ++ | no | large |
| Thrombocytopenia, anemia, and myelofibrosis (THAMY, 617441) | + | *MPIG6B* | AR | +/+++ | no | large |
| *GALE*-related thrombocytopenia (*GALE*-RT, na) | + | *GALE* | AR | +++ | no | large |
| Forms predisposing to additional diseases (☞ also Table 6.2) | | | | | | |
| *MYH9*-related disease (*MYH9*-RD, 155100) | ++++ | *MYH9* | AD | +/+++ | no | giant |
| *ANKRD26*-related thrombocytopenia (*ANKRD26*-RT or THC2, 188000) | +++ | *ANKRD26* | AD | ++/+++ | no | normal |
| Familial platelet disorder with propensity to acute myelogenous leukemia (FPD-AML, 601399) | +++ | *RUNX1* | AD | +/++ | yes | normal |
| *ETV6*-related thrombocytopenia (*ETV6*-RT or THC5, 616216) | ++ | *ETV6* | AD | +/++ | no | normal |
| Congenital amegakaryocytic thrombocytopenia (CAMT, 604498) | +++ | *MPL* | AR | +++ | no | normal |
| Congenital amegakaryocytic thrombocytopenia variant due to biallelic *THPO* mutation (CAMTv, na) | + | *THPO* | AR | +++ | no | normal |
| *MECOM*-associated syndrome (*MECOM*-AS), including radioulnar synostosis with amegakaryocytic thrombocytopenia 2 (RUSAT2, 616738) | ++ | *MECOM* | AD | +++ | no | normal |
| Radioulnar synostosis with amegakaryocytic thrombocytopenia 1 (RUSAT1, 605432) | + | *HOXA11* | AD | +++ | no | normal |
| *DIAPH1*-related disorder (*DIAPH1*-RD, na) | + | *DIAPH1* | AD | +/++ | no | large |
| *GNE*-related thrombocytopenia (*GNE*-RT, na) | + | *GNE* | AR | +++ | no | large |
| *SRC*-related thrombocytopenia (*SRC*-RT or THC6, 616937) | + | *SRC* | AD | +/+++ | no | large |

***Table 6.1:*** Inherited thrombocytopenias identified so far. na = not available

[1] Freq. = frequency; + less than 10 reported families, ++ more than 10 reported families, +++ more than 50 reported families, ++++ more than 200 reported families.

[2] Inh. = inheritance. AD: autosomal dominant, AR: autosomal recessive, XL: X-linked.

[3] Degree of thrombocytopenia (TCP) = degree of thrombocytopenia in the majority of the patients reported for each disorder; + platelet count > $100 \times 10^9$/L, ++ platelet count 50 to $100 \times 10^9$/L, +++ platelet count < $50 \times 10^9$/L.

[4] Bleeding tendency more severe than predicted by platelet count.

| Associate conditions | Inherited thrombocytopenias |
|---|---|
| **Congenital defects** | |
| Immunodeficiency, eczema | WAS, XLT |
| Physical growth delay, intellectual disability, craniofacial dysmorphisms, malformations of the heart, gastrointestinal tract, CNS, kidney, urinary tract, and/or skeleton, cryptorchidism, other malformations | JBS, TCPT |
| Bilateral radial aplasia ± other upper and lower limb bone abnormalities. Possible kidney, cardiac, and/or CNS malformations | TAR |
| Bilateral radioulnar synostosis. In *MECOM*-AS, other skeletal or organ malformations and sensorineural deafness may be present | RUSAT1, *MECOM*-AS |
| Abnormalities of the erythroid series consisting in dyserythropoietic or hemolytic anemia with laboratory abnormalities resembling beta-thalassemia. Splenomegaly. Congenital erythropoietic porphyria may be present | XLTT, XLTDA |
| Immunodeficiency. Systemic inflammation, with variable presence of leukocytoclastic vasculitis, inflammatory colitis, eosinophilia, eczema, lymphadenomegaly, hepato-splenomegaly. Growth failure | PLTEID |
| Myopathy with tubular aggregates. Possible asplenia or hyposplenia, congenital miosis, ichthyosis, short stature, mild cognitive impairment, migraines, and/or hypocalcaemia | STRMK |
| Myopathy with rimmed vacuoles | YPS |
| Defective growth and psychomotor development, facial abnormalities, brain malformation. Possible muscle tone abnormalities, immunodeficiency, eczema, hearing/visual disability, lymphedema, and cardiac, genitourinary, and/or skeletal malformations | TKS |
| Dermatologic involvement ranging from palmoplantar and anogenital hyperkeratosis/erythema to a more severe picture of Harlequin ichthyosis | *KDSR*-RT |
| Microcephaly, minor facial anomalies, mild intellectual disability, developmental delay. Other possible features include leukocytosis with eosinophilia, leukopenia and other malformations | *ACTB*-AST |
| Periventricular nodular heterotopia | *FLNA*-RT |
| Microcytic anemia, myelofibrosis, possible leukocytosis | THAMY |
| Anemia and recurrent neutropenia | *GALE*-RT |
| Facial dysmorphisms, intellectual disability, severe osteoporosis | *SRC*-RT |
| **Acquired disorders** | |
| Nephropathy and/or presenile sensorineural deafness and/or presenile cataracts and/or elevated liver enzymes | *MYH9*-RD |
| Acute leukemia, myelodysplastic syndrome, myeloproliferative neoplasms, or other hematological malignancies | *ANKRD26*-RT, FPD-AML, *ETV6*-RT |
| Bone marrow aplasia | CAMT, CAMTv, RUSAT1, *MECOM*-AS |
| Sensorineural deafness during infancy or childhood | *DIAPH1*-RD |
| Myopathy with rimmed vacuoles with onset in early adulthood | *GNE*-RT |
| Young-onset myelofibrosis and splenomegaly. Premature edentulism | *SRC*-RT |

***Table 6.2:*** Congenital or acquired conditions associated with inherited thrombocytopenias.

*de novo* mutational events (about 30 % of index cases) [14].

## History of additional manifestations of ist

As reported in Table 6.2, some of the genetic defects responsible for ITs can cause other congenital manifestations or expose to acquire additional illnesses during life. Thus, the collection of patient's personal and family history must include not only thrombocytopenia and bleeding diathesis, but also the congenital defects and acquired diseases that are associated with specific ITs.

## Bleeding tendency from infancy or childhood

The first ITs described at the end of the last century, such as biallelic BSS, gray platelet syndrome (GPS), congenital amegakaryocytic thrombocytopenia, and Wiskott-Aldrich syndrome (WAS), were all characterized by spontaneous and severe hemorrhagic manifestations from an early age and this has long been considered a constant feature of this group of diseases. However, the large number of new forms discovered since the beginning of this century and the analysis of large case series radically changed this view and showed that hemorrhagic diathesis is modest or even absent in most ITs patients. For instance, about 50 % of subjects with *MYH9*-RD [12], *ANKRD26*-RT [8] or monoallelic BSS [9] (the three most frequent ITs) do not have spontaneous bleeding at all. Similarly, only 35 % of patients with *ACTN1*-RT, the fourth disease in order of frequency [5], present spontaneous hemorrhages. For this reason, it is quite common that the reduced platelet count of subjects with ITs is discovered incidentally long after birth or even in adulthood. In summary, although bleeding diathesis from infancy or childhood is a distinctive feature of genetic thrombocytopenias that must be systematically sought, its absence does not rule out an IT.

## Stability of platelet count over time

The extent of thrombocytopenia varies greatly among different forms of IT (☞ Table 6.1). Moreover, it may vary also among different individuals affected by the same form, depending on the functional consequences of causative variants [13] and the individual genetic background, which affects the degree of thrombocytopenia in the same way it is responsible for the variability of platelet count in healthy subjects [4]. On the other hand, platelet count usually remains stable over time in the individual patients with IT. Only four forms of IT are exceptions to this rule. In thrombocytopenia with absent radii (TAR) and Jacobsen syndrome/Paris-Trousseau thrombocytopenia (JBS/TCPT), platelet count often increases over time, even up to normal values, while in GPS it tends to decrease with age. In Platelet-type von Willebrand disease, platelet count typically greatly decreases under stress conditions, such as infection, surgery or pregnancy. Finally, thrombopoietin, the natural hormone that stimulates platelet production, behaves like an acute phase protein and its elevation in acute, severe infections can transiently increase platelet count, sometimes up to normal values, in many forms of IT.

## Bleeding tendency disproportionate to the platelet count

A peculiar feature of some ITs is that bleeding tendency is more severe than expected based on platelet count. This is due to the fact that the genetic defect that hampers platelet production also results in defective platelet function. Paradigmatic in this respect is biallelic BSS, where the functional defect of platelets is clinically relevant and in itself puts the patient at risk of serious bleeding. The various causative mutations all hinder the expression of the GPIb-IX-V complex in the platelet membrane, which is essential for platelets to bind to the subendothelium exposed by a vascular lesion and start the hemostatic process. Thus, bleeding tendency is moderate to severe even when thrombocytopenia is mild. Other ITs in which thrombocytopenia may associate with clinically relevant defects of platelet function are GPS, Familial platelet disorder with propensity to acute myelogenous leukemia, *ITGA2B*/*ITGB3*-related thrombocytopenia, JBS/TCPT, *SLFN14*-related thrombocytopenia, and *FLI1*-related thrombocytopenia (*FLI1*-RT).

## Morphological abnormalities of blood cells

The genetic defects that cause thrombocytopenia are often responsible also for morphological abnormalities of platelets and, sometimes, of leukocytes and erythrocytes (☞ Table 6.3). A few of these defects are pathognomonic of specific ITs, as Döhle-like inclusions in neutrophils of *MYH9*-RD (☞ Figure 6.1) and single, giant platelet alpha

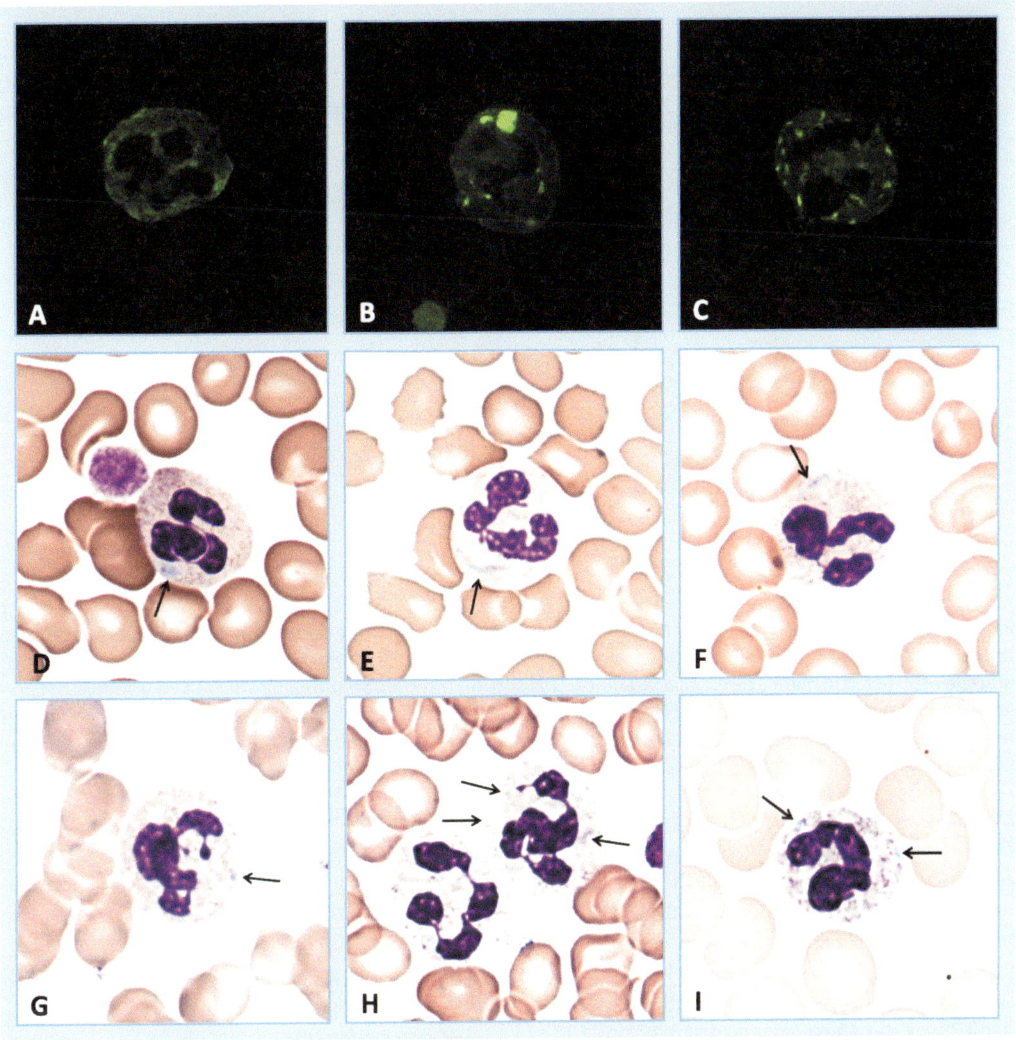


***Figure 6.1:*** **Leukocyte inclusions in *MYH9*-related disease.** A constant finding of *MYH9*-RD is the presence of clumps of the MYH9 protein in granulocytes cytoplasm. Immunofluorescence analysis recognizes these aggregates in all neutrophils of all patients, and this test has therefore very high sensitivity for making diagnosis. Specificity is also very good, since MYH9 is distributed homogeneously in healthy subjects as well as in patients with other forms of acquired or inherited thrombocytopenia (**A**). Mutations in the C-terminal tail domain of the MYH9 protein usually result in a single or few large aggregates possibly associated with small aggregates (**B**), while mutations in the N-terminal head domain result in many small aggregates (**C**). In May-Grünwald-Giemsa stained blood films, the MYH9 aggregates can be recognized as basophilic inclusions called Döhle-like bodies. Döhle-like inclusions are evident in a small percentage of neutrophils in 42-84 % % of *MYH9*-RD patients. The large aggregates due to mutations in the tail domain of MYH9 are easily identified as round or spindle shaped, light blue inclusions usually located at the cell periphery (**D-F**, arrows). The small aggregates associated with mutations in the head of MYH9 (**G-I**, arrows) are more difficult to identify. From: Balduini CL, Pecci A. Inherited thrombocytopenias. Haematologica. 2020; 105(Suppl 1):S237-247, with permission.

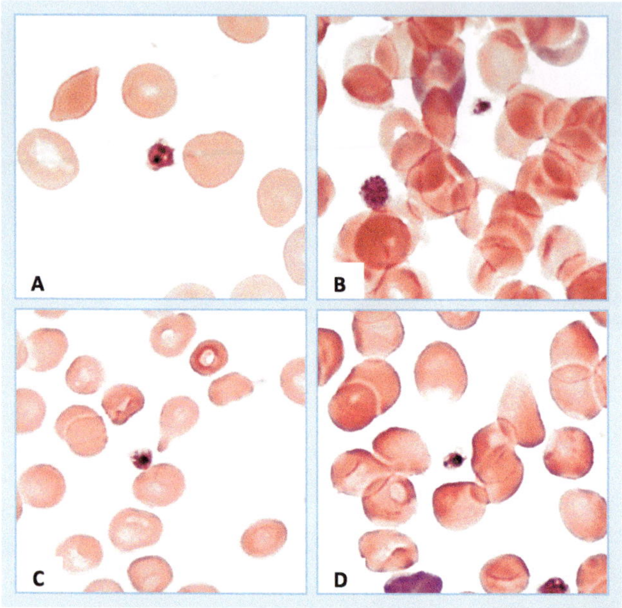


***Figure 6.2:*** **Giant platelet granules.** Mutations in FLI1 (FLI1-related thrombocytopenia, FLI1-RT) and large deletions in 11q23 including FLI1 (Jacobsen syndrome and Paris-Trousseau thrombocytopenia) cause the fusion of $\alpha$-granules and result in giant azurrophilic granules. This pathognomonic abnormality affects a very limited proportion of platelets (usually less than 2-3 %) and careful examination of blood films is required to identify it. Platelets may have one or two of these giant granules, sometimes with a few, residual, normal-sized granules. From: Balduini CL, Pecci A. Inherited thrombocytopenias. Haematologica. 2020; 105(Suppl 1):S237-247, with permission.

granules in subjects with *FLI1* alterations (TCPT/JBS and *FLI1*-RT, ☞ Figure 6.2), while others, as abnormalities of platelet size, defective alpha granule content, and platelet vacuolization, are common to different disorders (☞ Figure 6.3). Thus, in many cases, the examination of blood films can suggest that thrombocytopenia of the subject under investigation has a genetic origin or provide by itself the diagnosis of specific ist.

### 6.1.2. When to suspect inherited thrombocytopenias

The essential characteristic of ITs is that thrombocytopenia is present from birth. In clinical practice, this information is rarely available, but can sometimes be inferred from a history of bleeding episodes from an early age. However, as discussed above, most IT patients have no spontaneous hemorrhages and the absence of bleeding history does not exclude that thrombocytopenia is congenital. Thus, especially when thrombocytopenia has been identified incidentally by tests done for check-up or in preparation for surgery, the inability to ascertain that platelet count was normal at a previous blood count is in itself an element that must lead to suspect the genetic origin of thrombocytopenia. The identification of one or more of the peculiarities of ITs described above further strengthens the suspicion that the platelet deficiency is inherited.

The suspicion of IT must also arise when a patient diagnosed as ITP does not respond to therapy with immunosuppressants or intravenous immunoglobulins, as these drugs have no effects in ITs. Even an absent or a very short duration response to splenectomy could lead to the suspicion of an IT, because, except for WAS and its allelic variant X-linked thrombocytopenia (XLT), ITs do not respond to spleen removal. It is worth mentioning here that, in contrast, a response to thrombopoietin receptor agonists does not confirm a diagnosis of ITP, as these drugs proved to be effective in increasing platelet count in all the ITs in which they have been used so far [2]. A recent phase 2 clinical trial showed that the rise in platelet count is excellent, even up to the normalization, in *MYH9*-RD and in monoallelic BSS, and a clinically relevant response is observed in *ANKRD26*-RT and in WAS/XLT [16].

## 6.2. Differential diagnosis between ITP and inherited thrombocytopenias

The flow chart reported in Figure 6.4 shows the sequence of questions to answer in order to exclude that the patient with thrombocytopenia we are examining has an IT instead of ITP. The tools required for this purpose are available to everyone, because only medical history, physical examination and blood film evaluation are required.

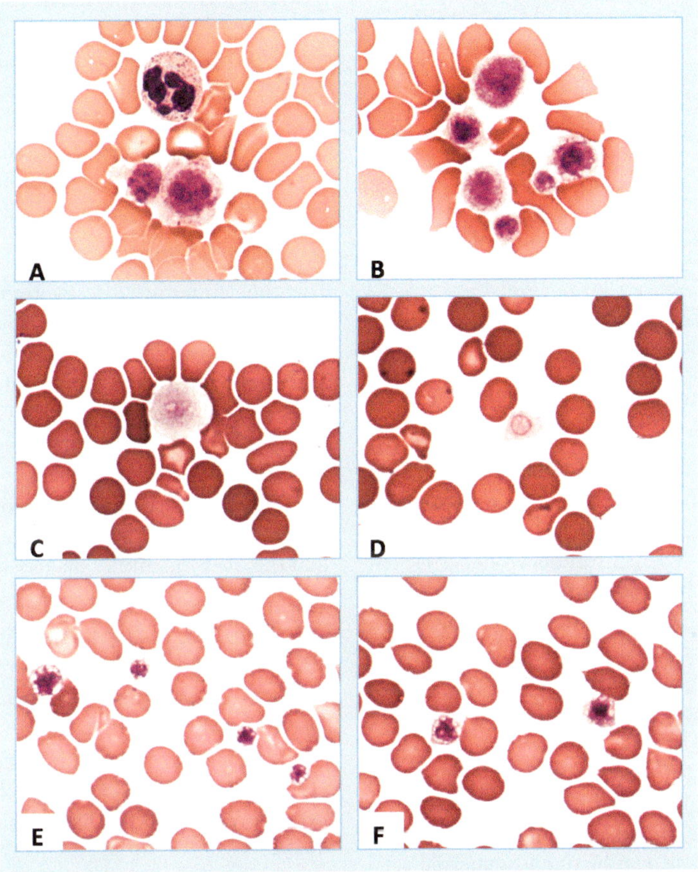


***Figure 6.3:*** **Giant, agranular and vacuolated platelets.** Many platelets larger than red cells or even neutrophils (**A, B**) are a distinguishing feature of *MYH9*-related disease (MYH9-RD), the most frequent form of inherited thrombocytopenia, and the classical, biallelic form of Bernard-Soulier syndrome (BSS), a rarer condition. Giant platelets can also be observed in myeloproliferative diseases, especially primary myelofibrosis, but the difference in the clinical picture does not pose problems of differential diagnosis. Large platelets that look 'pale' due to the complete (or nearly complete) absence of platelet azurrophilic $\alpha$-granules (**C, D**) are the distinguishing feature of gray platelet syndrome (GPS). The average diameter of platelets is slightly less than half of a red cell, but giant platelets are often observed (**C**). Circumferential bundles of microtubules are increased in GPS, and this is the reason why these structure may be sometimes recognized in a few platelets (**D**). Many enlarged platelets with abundant vacuoles (**E, F**) may be observed in *GATA1*-related disease (*GATA1*-RD). From: Balduini CL, Pecci A. Inherited thrombocytopenias. Haematologica. 2020; 105(Suppl 1):S237-247, with permission.

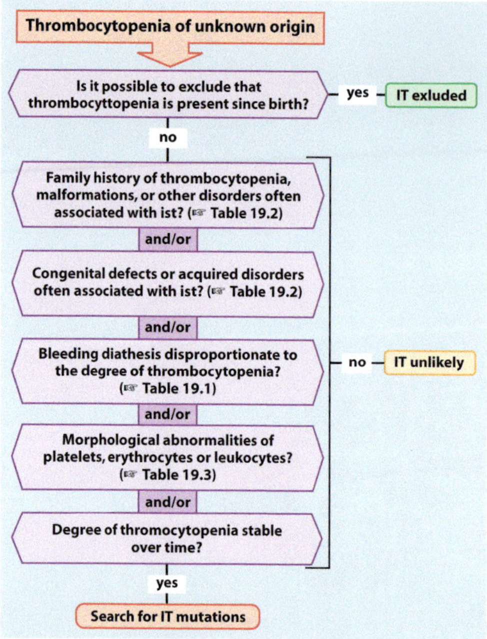


***Figure 6.4:*** Flow chart for suspecting that thrombocytopenia of unknown origin is inherited.

## Medical history

The most critical point of diagnostic reasoning is the emergence of the doubt that a genetic defect rather than an immune mechanism is responsible for thrombocytopenia. In fact, this suspicion might not arise when thrombocytopenia is first identified many years after birth or even in adulthood. We therefore suggest that trying to exclude with a very accurate medical history that thrombocytopenia is congenital rather than acquired is the first, essential step to avoid classifying an IT patient as having ITP. The only exception to this rule is represented by the clinical setting of neonatal thrombocytopenia. At birth, conditions other than ITs can underlie an isolated thrombocytopenia, which, for example, can be due to maternal-fetal incompatibility for human platelet antigens or the transmission of antibodies by a mother with ITP. In these conditions, however, thrombocytopenia tends to resolve spontaneously within a few days.

If it is not possible to exclude that thrombocytopenia is present since birth, the hypothesis of an IT becomes more and more probable the greater the number of affirmative answers to the next 5 questions of the flow chart in Figure 6.4. Again, medical history is required to ascertain whether one or more of the family members have thrombocytopenia or one of the congenital or acquired conditions frequently associated with ITs (☞ Table 6.2), the bleeding tendency is more severe than expected based on platelet count and/or the degree of thrombocytopenia is stable over time.

## Physical examination

The physical examination has an important role in the differential diagnosis between ITs and ITP because the finding of one of the congenital or acquired conditions reported in Table 6.2 must lead to the strong suspicion that thrombocytopenia derives from a genetic defect. Due to the heterogeneity of the defects to be sought, it is required that the examination is very accurate and does not neglect cognitive abilities. Physical examination, as well as medical history, may indicate the need for additional laboratory or instrumental investigations.

## Blood film evaluation

The only laboratory investigation always required by the diagnostic algorithm is microscope examination of blood films to identify the morphological alterations of platelets, erythrocytes and /or leukocytes that often characterize ITs. Of note, this diagnostic assessment is recommended not only by our algorithm, but by all guidelines for diagnosing ITP [6]. The assistance of a hematologist with experience in this type of analysis can increase the chance that this study identifies diagnostic anomalies.

The most frequent morphological abnormalities of ITs are those of platelet size. As shown in Table 6.1, most ITs have platelets that are larger than normal or even giant (i.e. larger than red cells), while in a few forms they are smaller than normal. Concerning platelet macrocytosis, also patients with ITP have large platelets, and this limits the usefulness of platelet size assessment for differential diagnostics. However, in *MYH9*-RD and biallelic BSS, the degree of platelet macrocytosis is significantly greater than in ITP, and evaluation of blood smears is therefore very useful for suspecting these conditions. In particular, a mean platelet diameter higher than 3.7 μm and/or the finding that more than 40 % of platelets are larger than 4 μm (i.e. half the diameter of red cells) have excellent sensitivity and specificity for differentiating these two conditions from ITP [11]. Conversely, some ITs have platelets with reduced size, and a mean platelet diameter smaller than 2.6 μm has 83 % sensitivity

| Blood cell abnormalities | Inherited thrombocytopenias |
|---|---|
| Platelets | |
| Giant platelets and >40 % of platelets larger than half a red blood cell | *MYH9*-RD, biallelic BSS |
| Small platelets and/or <10 % of platelets larger than half a red blood cell | WAS, XLT, CAMT, *CYCS*-RT |
| Agranular ('pale') platelets (with large platelets) | GPS, *GFI1b*-RT, *SRC*-RT |
| Hypo-granular platelets (with normal-sized platelets) | *ANKRD26*-RT |
| Some platelets with one single giant granule | TCPT/JBS, *FLI1*-RT |
| Vacuolated platelets | XLTT |
| Leukocytes | |
| "Döhle-like" inclusions in neutrophils | *MYH9*-RD |
| Red blood cells | |
| Anisopoikilocytosis or anisocytosis | *GATA1*-related disorders, *GFI1b*-RT |
| Anisopoikilocytosis with dacryocytosis | GPS |

***Table 6.3:*** Abnormal findings at blood film evaluation that are typical of inherited thrombocytopenias.

and 90 % specificity for distinguishing them from ITP. The most frequent ITs with small-sized platelets are WAS and XLT [10].

Measurement of platelet size by blood film evaluation is time consuming and operator-dependent, and the use of blood cell counters could therefore represent a convenient alternative. However, these instruments do not recognize very large platelets and therefore greatly underestimate mean platelet volume (and platelet count) in ITs with very large platelets. Anyway, it has been shown that mean platelet volumes higher than 51 % with respect to healthy subjects has 91 % specificity and 66 % sensitivity in distinguishing *MYH9*-RD and biallelic BSS from ITP [7].

The other morphological anomalies to be sought for are described in Table 6.3 and in Figures 6.1-6.3.

## 6.3. How to confirm the suspicion of inherited thrombocytopenia

The diagnostic flow-chart in Figure 6.4 can lead to a very strong suspicion of IT. For example, if the presence of thrombocytopenia in family members identifies a dominant transmission of the condition, an IT is almost certain and ITP can be excluded. Of note, the familiarity for ITP is so rare that the existence of inherited ITP is still only a hypothesis [3].

In some cases, very simple tests can definitively confirm specific IT and thus rule out ITP. For instance, the presence of giant platelets in blood films and the absence of platelet aggregation after stimulation with ristocetin are sufficient to make a diagnosis of certainty of biallelic BSS. The absence of the GPIb/IX/V complex on the platelet membrane ascertained with flow cytometry has the same diagnostic significance as the lack of platelet aggregation to ristocetin. Another disease that can be diagnosed with certainty with simple tests is *MYH9*-RD. The finding of very large platelets (☞ above) and of "Döhle-like" inclusions in neutrophils (☞ Figure 6.1) give certainty that the patient has this disease and not ITP.

In many cases, the strong suspicion of IT raised by the diagnostic flow chart cannot be confirmed by simple tests, and the only possibility to confirm the suspicion is the identification of gene variants responsible for IT. However, it is important to remind at this point that 50 % of IT patients have yet unknown forms and genetic analysis will therefore not identify their defects. In these cases, our clinical decisions will have to be based simply on the diagnostic hypothesis. To maximize the likelihood that the genetic analysis identifies the gene mutation causative of thrombocytopenia, we suggest referring the patient to a center experienced in inherited platelet disorders. In fact, the sequencing of panels of genes or of the exome or of the entire genome often identifies gene variants whose pathogenetic significance must be ascertained with phenotypic and functional analyses that require advanced skills. Furthermore, if the patient is affected by a still unknown form, the in-depth study of the case may lead to the identification of new genes responsible for IT and to the advancement of knowledge of these still insufficiently known diseases.

## References

1. Balduini CL, Pecci A, Noris P. Inherited thrombocytopenias: the evolving spectrum. Hämostaseologie 2012;32 (4):259-270.

2. Bastida JM, Gonzalez-Porras JR, Rivera J, Lozano ML. Role of thrombopoietin receptor agonists in Inherited thrombocytopenia. Int J Mol Sci. 2021;22(9):4330.

3. Bergmann AK, Grace RF, Neufeld EJ. Genetic studies in pediatric ITP: outlook, feasibility, and requirements. Ann Hematol. 2010;89(Suppl 1):S95-103.

4. Biino G, Santimone I, Minelli C, Sorice R, Frongia B, Traglia M, Ulivi S, Di Castelnuovo A, Gögele M, Nutile T, Francavilla M, Sala C, Pirastu N, Cerletti C, Iacoviello L, Gasparini P, Toniolo D, Ciullo M, Pramstaller P, Pirastu M, de Gaetano G, Balduini CL. Age- and sex-related variations in platelet count in Italy: a proposal of reference ranges based on 40987 subjects' data. PLoS One. 2013;8(1):e54289.

5. Bottega R, Marconi C, Faleschini M, Baj G, Cagioni C, Pecci A, Pippucci T, Ramenghi U, Pardini S, Ngu L, Baronci C, Kunishima S, Balduini CL, Seri M, Savoia A, Noris P. ACTN1-related thrombocytopenia: identification of novel families for phenotypic characterization. Blood 2015;125(5):869-872.

6. Lozano ML, Revilla N, Gonzalez-Lopez TJ, Novelli S, González-Porras JR, Sánchez-Gonzalez B, Bermejo N, Pérez S, Lucas FJ, Álvarez MT, Arilla MJ, Perera M, do Nascimento J, Campos RM, Casado LF, Vicente V. Real-life management of primary immune thrombocytopenia (ITP) in adult patients and adherence to practice guidelines. Ann Hematol. 2016;95(7):1089-98.

7. Noris P, Klersy C, Zecca M, Arcaini L, Pecci A, Melazzini F, Terulla V, Bozzi V, Ambaglio C, Passamonti F, Locatelli F, Balduini CL. Platelet size distinguishes between inherited macrothrombocytopenias and immune thrombocytopenia. J Thromb Haemost 2009;7(12): 2131-2136.

8. Noris P, Perrotta S, Seri M, Pecci A, Gnan C, Loffredo G, Pujol-Moix N, Zecca M, Scognamiglio F, De Rocco D, Punzo F, Melazzini F, Scianguetta S, Casale M, Marconi C, Pippucci T, Amendola G, Notarangelo LD, Klersy C, Civaschi E,et al. Mutations in ANKRD26 are responsible for a frequent form of inherited thrombocytopenia: analysis of 78 patients from 21 families. Blood 2011;117: 6673-80.

9. Noris P, Perrotta S, Bottega R, Pecci A, Melazzini F, Civaschi E, Russo S, Magrin S, Loffredo G, Di Salvo V, Russo G, Casale M, De Rocco D, Grignani C, Cattaneo M, Baronci C, Dragani A, Albano V, Jankovic M, Scianguetta S, et al. Clinical and laboratory features of 103 patients from 42 Italian families with inherited thrombocytopenia derived from the monoallelic Ala156Val mutation of GPIb{alpha} (Bolzano mutation). Haematologica 2012;97:82-8.

10. Noris P, Klersy C, Gresele P, Giona F, Giordano P, Minuz P, Loffredo G, Pecci A, Melazzini F, Civaschi E, Mezzasoma A, Piedimonte M, Semeraro F, Veneri D, Menna F, Ciardelli L, Balduini CL; Italian Gruppo di Studio delle Piastrine. Platelet size for distinguishing between inherited thrombocytopenias and immune thrombocytopenia: a multicentric, real life study. Br J Haematol. 2013;162(1):112-9.

11. Noris P, Biino G, Pecci A, et al. Platelet diameters in inherited thrombocytopenias: analysis of 376 patients with all known disorders. Blood. 2014;124(6):e4-e10.

12. Pecci A, Panza E, Pujol-Moix N, Klersy C, Di Bari F, Bozzi V, Gresele P, Lethagen S, Fabris F, Dufour C, Granata A, Doubek M, Pecoraro C, Koivisto PA, Heller PG, Iolascon A, Alvisi P, Schwabe D, De Candia E, Rocca B, et al. Position of nonmuscle myosin heavy chain IIA (NMMHC-IIA) mutations predicts the natural history of MYH9-related disease. Hum Mutat. 2008;29:409–17.

13. Pecci A, Klersy C, Gresele P, et al. MYH9-related disease: a novel prognostic model to predict the clinical evolution of the disease based on genotype-phenotype correlations. Hum Mutat. 2014;35(2):236-47.

14. Pecci A, Ma X, Savoia A, Adelstein RS. MYH9: Structure, functions and role of non-muscle myosin IIA in human disease. Gene. 2018 Jul 20;664:152-67.

15. Pecci A, Balduini CL. Inherited thrombocytopenias: an updated guide for clinicians. Blood Rev. 2020 Dec 1:100784. doi: 10.1016/j.blre.2020.100784. Epub ahead of print. PMID: 33317862.

16. Zaninetti C, Gresele P, Bertomoro A, Klersy C, De Candia E, Veneri D, Barozzi S, Fierro T, Alberelli MA, Musella V, Noris P, Fabris F, Balduini CL, Pecci A. Eltrombopag for the treatment of inherited thrombocytopenias: a phase II clinical trial. Haematologica. 2020; 105(3):820-8.

# 7. Secondary ITP

## 7.1. Definition and limitation

Immune thrombocytopenia (ITP) is an autoimmune disorder resulting from various etiologies, characterized by increased platelet destruction and impaired production. Thrombocytopenia can be linked to an underlying condition (secondary ITP) or no apparent cause can be found (primary ITP). In an attempt to standardize terminology and definitions, Rodeghiero et al. in 2009 proposed this definition on behalf of an international working group: "*Secondary ITP: All forms of immune-mediated thrombocytopenia except primary ITP.*" [1]. This is somewhat confusing and could suggest that the diagnosis of primary ITP is accurate, which unfortunately is not the case. To cite again this working group "*the diagnosis of primary ITP remains one of exclusion; no robust clinical or laboratory parameters are currently available to establish its diagnosis with accuracy.*" [1] In clinical practice we say: primary ITPs regroup all forms of suspected immune-mediated thrombocytopenia not related to another disease, even after a long period of observation. The diagnosis of primary ITP can only be performed retrospectively; therefore, differential diagnostic consideration should never stop completely.

In some cases, it is challenging to assess the immunological or non-immunological background of thrombocytopenia. Non-immune thrombocytopenia (non-IT) regroups other causes of thrombocytopenia, such as congenital thrombocytopenia and acquired bone marrow failure (e.g., aplastic anemia [AA], myelodysplastic syndrome [MDS]) or diseases of enhanced destruction (e.g., hypersplenism, microangiopathy, complement deficiency, inflammation, state of hypercoagulability). Immunological and non-immunological mechanisms may simultaneously induce thrombocytopenia in some cases – indeed, this is true for many forms of secondary ITP following viral infection (e.g., HCV, HIV, CMV) [2, 3], and oncological diseases combining immunological phenomena, impaired megakaryopoiesis and/or increased peripheral consumption [4,5]. Asymptomatic congenital platelet disorders (or carrier) may predispose to ITP or trigger its symptoms, and could explain patients recovering from a profound thrombocytopenia to longtime steady-state values $<100 \times 10^9$/L, patients with poor or moderate response to first-line treatment, and the spectrum of bleeding propensity.

The effective management of patients with ITP is therefore still limited by the lack of specific diagnostic tests and the uncertainty of individual bleeding risk. An underlying condition may influence both the prognosis and the management of ITP. Of course, the primary goal should be to treat the underlying cause of autoimmunity, even if the condition itself is incurable.

## 7.2. Etiology

In recent years, it has been possible to identify the pathogenesis and etiology of ITP more frequently, leading to a diagnostic shift from primary to secondary ITP or non-IT (☞ Table 7.1). Secondary ITP and misdiagnosed ITP is growing with knowledge [6-8].

Infectious diseases, especially acute infections (e.g., EBV, CMV, Parvovirus, VZV), are probably underestimated in all registries and cohorts because these patients may recover spontaneously and probably never see the hematologist, or only be discussed in an interdisciplinary consultation [9-12]. In many children, banal infections of the upper respiratory or gastrointestinal tract occur some weeks before the clinical manifestation of ITP, leading to the hypothesis that childhood ITP is due to the cross-reactivity of antiplatelet antibodies and viral antigens (i.e., antigenic mimicry) [10, 13, 14]. However pediatricians classify the disease in these cases as primary. The rate of chronic infection-associated ITP with HCV, HIV, and *Helicobacter pylori* is high worldwide but depends greatly on geographic and demographic, or social factors.

Other known causes of secondary ITP include systemic autoimmune disorders, primary or secondary immunodeficiency, paraneoplastic syndrome (e.g., lymphomas), and drug-dependent antibodies [10, 14-16] Autoimmune cytopenia is frequently the first manifestation of lymphoproliferation, systemic lupus erythematosus (SLE), or immunodeficiency. However, many of these con-

| Differential diagnosis of primary ITP | | |
|---|---|---|
| Secondary ITP | Non-immune thrombocytopenia | |
| | Congenital thrombocytopenia | Other |
| • Systemic autoimmune diseases (e.g. SLE, Evans syndrome)<br>• Immune deficiencies<br>- primary (CVID, ALPS, CTLA-4 deficiency))<br>- acquired (e.g. post HSCT)<br>• Lymphoproliferative disease (e.g. CLL, HL)<br>• Chronic infection (HCV, HIV, *Helicobacter pylori*)<br>• Acute Infection (nonspecific viral illness, EBV, CMV)<br>• Drug-induced | • Wiskott-Aldrich syndrome/ X-linked thrombocytopenia<br>• Myosin heavy chain 9-related disorders (MYHA-9)<br>• Bernard-Soulier syndrome<br>• Gray platelet syndrome<br>• Platelet-type von Willebrand disease<br>• Defects in megakaryocyte maturation (e.g Familial platelet disorder with propensity to acue myelogenous leukemia [RUNX1] mutation)/GATA1-related disease/ETV6-related thrombocytopenia/Paris-Trousseau thrombocytopenia/ and much more)<br>• Congenital amegakaryocytic thrombocytopenia<br>*and much more* | • Bone marrow failure<br>- inborn (e.g. Fanconi anemia)<br>- acquired (e.g. SAA, MDS)<br>• Bone marrow infiltration (Leukemia)<br>• Antiphospholipid antibody syndrome<br>• Consumptive thrombocytopenia (thrombotic microangiopathy, hypersplenism, M. Gaucher)<br>• Infection (e.g. malaria, EBV, CMV)<br>• Incidental thrombocytopenia of pregnancy<br>• Liver disease/alcohol-related thrombocytopenia<br>• EDTA-dependent pseudothrombocytopenia |

***Table 7.1:*** Differential diagnosis of primary ITP. **ALPS**: autoimmune lymphoproliferative syndrome, **CLL**: chronic lymphocytic leukemia, **CVID**: common variable immunodeficiency, **HL**: Hodgkin lymphoma, **HSCT**: hematopoietic stem-cell transplantation, **SLE**: systemic lupus erythematosus.

ditions are rare and require specific knowledge, as the clinical picture results in overlap syndromes combining immunodeficiency and autoimmunity (e.g., autoimmune lymphoproliferative syndrome [ALPS], common variable immunodeficiency [CVID]), or cancer and autoimmunity (e.g., Hodgkin lymphoma [HL], chronic lymphocytic leukemia [CLL]). Moreover, specific manifestations of the underlying disease may emerge only during the follow-up period [17-19]. It is therefore important to periodically re-examine for secondary causes. However, the diagnostic workflow may benefit from better definition and validation because the diagnosis is frequently identified with considerable delay.

## 7.3. Diagnostic workflow

Early discrimination between primary or secondary ITP and non-IT is important since clinical management protocols and prognosis may differ [14, 20, 21]. In the Canadian McMaster Registry, nearly 1 in 7 adults with ITP were reported to be initially misdiagnosed [22]. In children, secondary ITP is much rarer, but revision of the diagnosis is frequently delayed and 35 % of all misdiagnosed patients will be correctly diagnosed more than 6 months after initial diagnosis [23]. A clear algorithm might help shorten the delay or even improve the diagnosis upfront. Primary ITP is a diagnosis of exclusion, and there are no available laboratory tests to confirm ITP. According to international practice guidelines, medical and family history-taking, clinical examination, complete blood count assessment, and blood smear analysis are sufficient to diagnose the primary form [24, 25]. However, despite these recommendations, initial bone marrow puncture is frequently undertaken as seen in reports of the PARC registry (children > 40 %, and adults > 70 %) [23, 26], but this may not reflect the general approach, especially of smaller institutions. Other investigations that are frequently done in the daily routine comprise serologic tests for HIV, hepatitis C, antiphospholipid antibodies, antinuclear antibodies (ANA), and more rarely antiplatelet antibodies.

Diagnostic recommendations exist in the literature mostly in case of chronic or refractory ITP with the aim to describe, which analyses should be

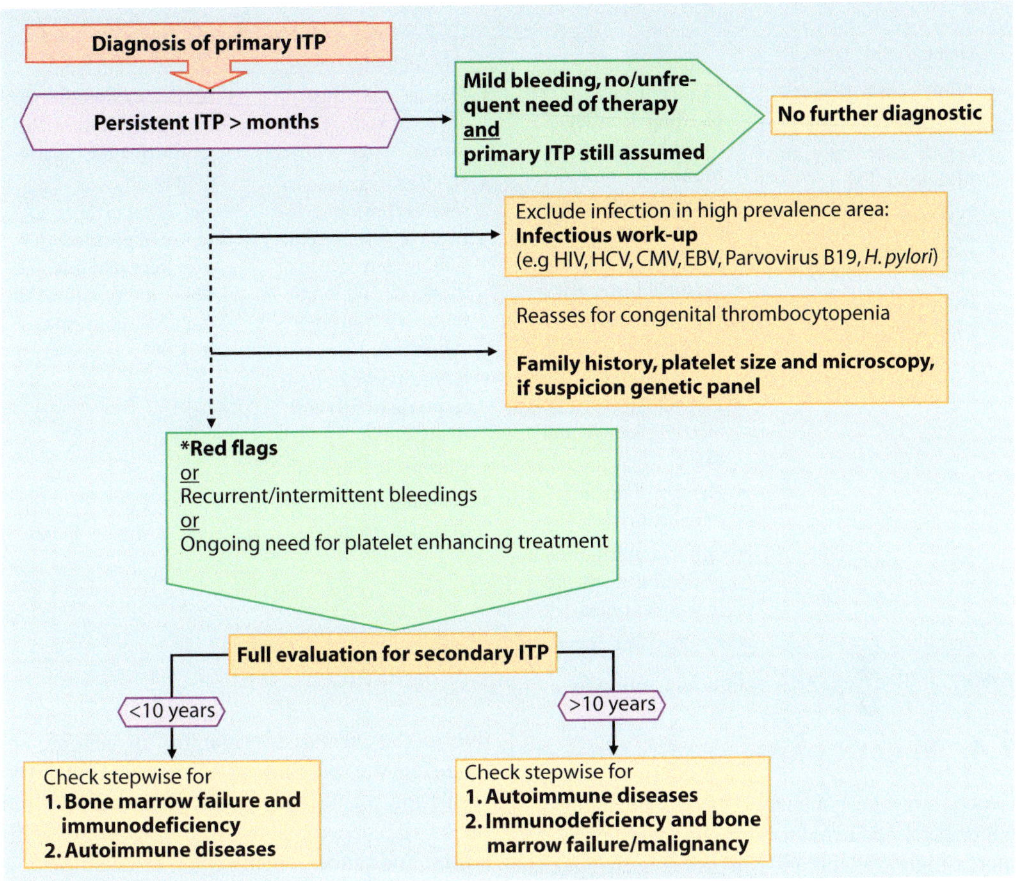


***Figure 7.1:*** Diagnostic workflow in children. Adapted from Schifferli A 2021 [23].
* *Red Flags for secondary ITP or non-IT:* female sex, age older than 10 years, moderate thrombocytopenia greater than 20 but less than $100 \times 10^9$/L, positive family history for ITP, comorbidities, and nonresponse to first-line treatment.
All patients with new symptoms or laboratory abnormalities during the disease course do not appear in the algorithm, since the diagnosis is guided by the new findings.

undertaken, but do not appear in a subsequent and informative order (e.g., international ITP guidelines [24], Italian guidelines [27]). Recently, Consolini et al. [15] suggested a progressive algorithm with further investigations to be performed in children with ITP. The algorithm is driven by the specific examination that should be undertaken in the course of the disease, without differentiating other clinical features (e.g., age, sex, level of platelet count). In a study on misdiagnosed ITP in children, the authors propose an algorithm based on the duration/evolution of the disease, specific red flags and the probability of possible differential diagnosis for different age groups (☞ Figure 7.1) [23]. The diagnosis can only be made after following patients over time, as the disease evolves and additional investigations are done to exclude other causes. Beside these different algorithms, the clinician should carefully search and recognize red flags or risk factors that raise the suspicion of secondary ITP and other non-immune causes of thrombocytopenia. These are summarized below (☞ Table 7.2) [8, 15, 22, 23, 28-34].

Despite the fact that patients diagnosed with secondary ITP or non-IT do not have a greater risk of bleeding [22, 34], except for HCV-associated ITP, many publications recommend conducting an expanded evaluation in patients with life-threatening and persistent bleeding requiring therapy.

| Red flags | | | |
|---|---|---|---|
| Demographic factors | Personal factors | ITP/platelet factors | Progression factors |
| • Adolescent > 10 years (over small children)<br>• Senior (over young and midlife adults)<br>• Women > men<br>• Population with increased risk of infection (e.g., *Helicobacter pylori*, HCV, HIV) | • Family history for ITP, bleeding disorders, thrombosis, autoimmunity, immunodeficiency, lymphoproliferative disease/ leukemia<br>• Personal history of recurrent infection (also upper airways: otitis, sinusitis), or diarrhea<br>• Personal history of bleeding (congenital cause)<br>• History of thrombosis or abortion<br>• Other comorbidities or physical abnormalities (e.g., splenomegaly)<br>• Drugs or vaccines | • Platelet size either above or below the normal range<br>• Moderate (instead of severe) thrombocytopenia at first presentation, or persistence of moderate and long-term stable thrombocytopenia<br>• Nonresponse or poor response to first-line treatments<br>• Chronic ITP in adults<br>• Persistent ITP in children (>6 months) | • All new symptoms or laboratory abnormalities during the disease course<br>• e.g., other cytopenia, repeated positive ANA titer, repeated infections, enteropathy, skin manifestations, splenomegaly |

***Table 7.2:*** Red flags. ANA: antinuclear antibody.

## 7.4. Genetic panel

Genetic screening panels for both congenital thrombocytopenia and hereditary immunodeficiencies are increasingly available and can probably change the landscape of thrombocytopenia. Rates of detection and new disorders will surely rise in the future and probably explain much of the clinical heterogenicity of ITP [7, 8, 24, 28, 31, 35-37] The frequency of positive analysis in chronic or refractory ITP is not clear, but arouse big interest [7, 38]. Detecting these conditions may have a considerable impact, because of associated conditions and increasing options of targeted therapy [8].

It is now clear that many congenital thrombocytopenias have much stronger consequences than a lifetime risk of hemorrhage. Particularly, RUNX1, ANKRD26, and ETV6 can be associated with the development of hematological malignancies, MPL and MECOM can evolve to bone marrow aplasia, SRC to juvenile myelofibrosis, and MYH9-related disorders with end-stage renal disease [39]. It is also clear that many inborn errors of immunity (IEIs) predispose patients to recurrent infections and to autoimmune disorders, allergy, lymphoproliferation, and malignancy. In the last decade, due to the increased availability of genome sequencing, the spectrum of IEIs with immune dysregulation phenotype rapidly expanded [40] and the overlap between autoimmunity, immunodeficiency, and cancer is being better understood. It is now clear that immunological activity can simultaneously be overactive and suppressed or defective.

As an example, diagnosis of multilineage cytopenia has shown considerable progress, and ALPS and CVID are now frequently detected [41-45].

## 7.5. Adult versus children

The rate of secondary ITP varies in the literature, mostly depending on the age group, sex, and on which disease state is being evaluated (newly diagnosed, persistent, and chronic). In adults, 18-38 % of patients diagnosed with ITP have an underlying disease, comorbid condition, and/or comedication, making the diagnosis of secondary ITP or non-immune thrombocytopenia more probable [10, 12, 22, 33, 46]. The frequency of secondary ITP increases with age [33]. Causes of secondary ITP depend also on demographical and socioeconomic factors (☞ Figure 7.2a-c). Especially, infection-associated secondary ITP (e.g., HCV, *Helicobacter pylori*) shows strong geographic disparities [10, 47, 48]. In the McMaster Registry, 93 of 362 ITP patients (26 %) were diagnosed with a secondary form, of them 42 were caused by systemic autoimmune disease (Evans syndrome n=14, SLE n=13, other autoimmune condition n=15), 9 were drug-induced, 6 with antiphospholipid antibody syndrome (APS), 20 with infection, 4 with immunodeficiency, and 4 secondary to lymphoproliferation. In total, 12 % of initial primary patients were reclassified as having non-immune or secondary ITP at follow-up [22] A nationwide French study including ITPs necessitating in-hospital care, reported secondary ITP in 19 % of cases. Malignancy was the main cause of secondary ITP (60 %), followed by systemic autoimmune disease (14 %) and immunodeficiency (9 %), and 7 % were due to hepatitis B/C and HIV. Surprisingly, drug-induced ITP was not reported [33].

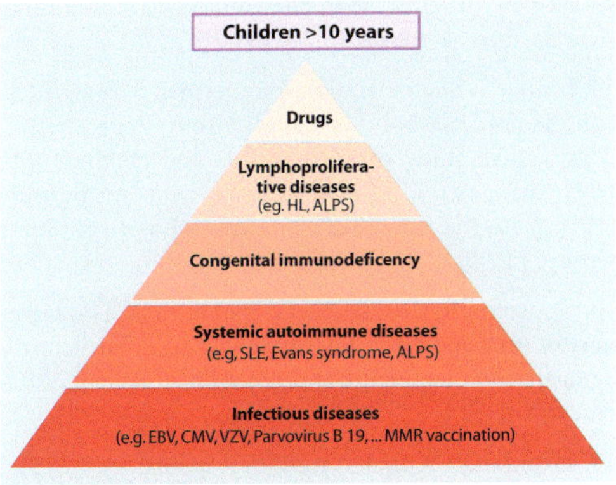


a

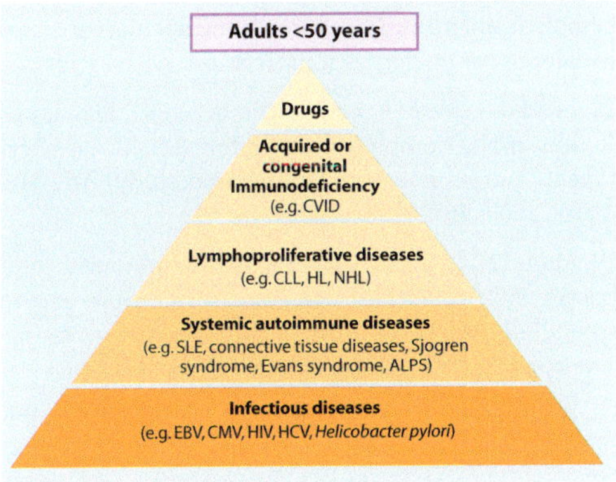


b

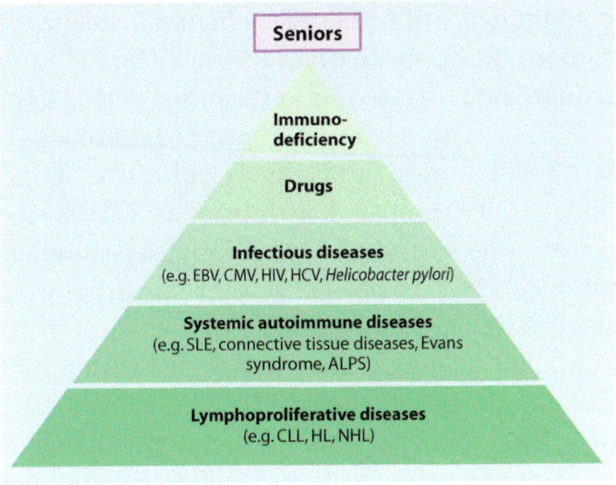


c

***Figure 7.2a-c:*** Proposed illustration of secondary ITP in different age groups. Distribution of secondary ITP causes is dependent on many factors, such as socio-economics and may differ in countries and level of medical services. **ALPS**: autoimmune lymphoproliferative syndrome, **CLL**: chronic lymphocytic leukemia, **CVID**: common variable immunodeficiency, **HL**: Hodgkin lymphoma, **NHL**: non-Hodgkin lymphoma, **SLE**: systemic lupus erythematosus.

In children, secondary ITP or non-IT is rare (2.4 %) [32, 33], and similar to the rate of initial misdiagnosed thrombocytopenia (2.8 %) [23]. Research on secondary ITP in children is limited [8, 31-33, 38]. Recently, an international ITP Registry described a revised diagnosis of secondary ITP or non-IT within 24 months of follow-up in the pediatric population [23]. Secondary ITP and non-IT were reported in only 113 patients out of 3,974 children. Infectious and autoimmune diseases were equally identified as the main causes, with median ages at diagnosis of 3.2 years [IQR: 1.2; 6.7] and 12.4 years [IQR: 7.6; 13.7], respectively. Other causes were malignancies, aplastic anemia, immunodeficiency, and drug use. Patients with malignancies and aplastic anemia had significantly higher initial platelet counts ($37 \times 10^9$/L and $52 \times 10^9$/L, respectively) than did those with infection or autoimmune diseases ($12 \times 10^9$/L and $13 \times 10^9$/L, respectively). Interestingly, the clinical characteristics of children with secondary infection-associated ITP appeared to be very similar to those of children with primary ITP, possibly reflecting a similar disturbance in the immune system. In contrast, the clinical characteristics of all other patients with secondary ITP and non-IT differed from those of children with primary ITP. In accordance with other studies, differences included older age, a predominance of female sex, a higher incidence of comorbidities, positive family history for ITP, and reduced rates of bleeding at the initial diagnosis of ITP [15, 22, 31, 33, 34]. No specific bleeding pattern was found to be distinctly indicative of secondary ITP, compared with primary ITP, in the cohort. The sustained need for platelet-stimulating agents and the need of second-line drugs were significantly higher in patients with an underlying autoimmune disease than in patients with an infectious disease or primary ITP. This corroborates prior findings reported in the literature, highlighting more first-line treatment failures in adult patients with secondary ITP [8, 31, 32, 34].

## 7.6. Conclusions

The pathogenesis of ITP is becoming increasingly understood, and secondary ITP is more likely identified. However, ITP remains to be a syndrome of complex immunological dysfunctions [49]. The overlap between cancer, immunodeficiency, and autoimmune disorders may help define driver immunological pathways, ultimately resulting in possible novel therapeutic strategies (e.g rilzabrutinib, bortezomib).

### References

1. Rodeghiero F, Stasi R, Gernsheimer T, et al. Standardization of terminology, definitions and outcome criteria in immune thrombocytopenic purpura of adults and children: report from an international working group. Blood. 2009;113(11):2386-2393.

2. Liebman HA. Viral-associated immune thrombocytopenic purpura. Hematol Am Soc Hematol Educ Program. 2008:212-218.

3. Papagianni A, Economou M, Tsoutsou E, Athanassiou-Metaxa M. CMV-related immune thrombocytopenic purpura or CMV-induced thrombocytopenia? Br J Haematol. 2010;149:454-5.

4. Cines DB, Liebman H, Stasi R. Pathobiology of secondary immune thrombocytopenia. Semin Hematol. 2009;46(1)(suppl 2):S2-S14.

5. Hamblin TJ. Autoimmune complications of chronic lymphocytic leukemia. Semin Oncol. 2006;33:230-9.

6. Balduini CL, Savoia A, Seri M. Inherited thrombocytopenias frequentlydiagnosed in adults. J Thromb Haemost. 2013;11(6):1006-1019.

7. Fiore M, Pillois X, Lorrain S et al. A diagnostic approach that may help to discriminate inherited thrombocytopenia from chronic immune thrombocytopenia in adult patients. Platelets. 2016;27(6):555-562.

8. Rotz SJ, Ware RE, Kumar A. Diagnosis and management of chronic and refractory immune cytopenias in children, adolescents, and young adults. Pediatr Blood Cancer. 2018;65(10):e27260.

9. Yenicesu I, Yetgin S, Ozyürek E, Aslan D. Virus-associated immune thrombocytopenic purpura in childhood. Pediatr Hematol Oncol. 2002;19(6):433-437.

10. Cines DB, Bussel JB, Liebman HA, Luning Prak ET. The ITP syndrome: pathogenic and clinical diversity. Blood. 2009;113(26):6511-6521.

11. Wu Z, Zhou J, Wei X, Wang X, Li Y, Peng B, Niu T. The role of Epstein-Barr virus (EBV) and cytomegalovirus (CMV) in immune thrombocytopenia. Hematology. 2013 Sep;18(5):295-9.

12. Cirasino L, Robino AM, Cattaneo M, et al. Reviewed diagnosis of primary and secondary immune thrombocytopenic purpura in 79 adult patients hospitalized in 2000-2002. Blood Coagul Fibrinolysis. 2011;22(1):1-6.

13. Johnsen J. Pathogenesis in immune thrombocytopenia: new insights. ASH, the educational programm. Acta Paediatr. 2005;94(2):178-184.

14. Kühne T, Buchanan GR, Zimmerman S, et al. Intercontinental Childhood ITP Study Group. A prospective comparative study of 2540 infants and children with newly diagnosed idiopathic thrombocytopenic purpura (ITP) from the Intercontinental Childhood ITP Study Group. J Pediatr. 2003;143(5):605-8.

15. Consolini R, Costagliola G, Spatafora D. The centenary of immune thrombocytopenia-Part 2: Revising diagnostic and therapeutic approach. Front Pediatr. 2017; 5:179.

16. Liebman H. Other thrombocytopenias. Semin Hematol. 2007;44(suppl 5):S24-S34.

17. Miescher PA, Tucci A, Beris P, et al. Autoimmune hemolytic anemia and/or thrombocytopenia associated with lupus parameters. Semin Hematol. 1992; 29:13-17.

18. Feudjo-Tepie MA, Le Roux G, Beach KJ, Bennett D, Robinson NJ. Comorbidities of idiopathic thrombocytopenic purpura: a population-based study. Adv Hematol. 2009; 963506.

19. Aboud N, Depré F, Salama A. Is autoimmune thrombocytopenia itself the primary disease in the presence of second diseases data from a long-term observation. Transfus Med Hemother. 2017;44(1):23-28.

20. Bussel JB. Therapeutic approaches to secondary immune thrombocytopenic purpura. Semin Hematol. 2009;46(1)(suppl 2):S44-S58.

21. George JN, Aster RH. Drug-induced thrombocytopenia: pathogenesis, evaluation, and management. Hematology. Hematology Am Soc Hematol Educ Program. 2009:153-8.

22. Arnold DM, Nazy I, Clare R, et al. Misdiagnosis of primary immune thrombocytopenia and frequency of bleeding: lessons from the McMaster ITP Registry. Blood Adv. 2017 Nov 28;1(25):2414-2420.

23. Schifferli A, Heiri A, Imbach P, et al. Misdiagnosed thrombocytopenia in children and adolescents: analysis of the Pediatric and Adult Registry on Chronic ITP. Blood Adv. 2021 Mar 23;5(6):1617-1626.

24. Provan D, Arnold DM, Bussel JB, et al. Updated international consensus report on the investigation and management of primary immune thrombocytopenia. Blood Adv. 2019;3(22):3780-3817.

25. Neunert C, Terrell DR, Arnold DM, et al. American Society of Hematology 2019 Guidelines for immune thrombocytopenia. Blood Adv. 2019;3(23):3829-3866.

26. Kühne T, Berchtold W, Michaels LA, et al.; Intercontinental Cooperative ITP Study Group. Newly diagnosed immune thrombocytopenia in children and adults: a comparative prospective observational registry of the Intercontinental Cooperative Immune Thrombocytopenia Study Group. Haematologica. 2011;96(12):1831-7.

27. De Mattia D, Del Vecchio GC, Russo G, et al. Group A-IS. Management of chronic childhood immune thrombocytopenic purpura: AIEOP consensus guidelines. Acta Haematol. 2010;123(2):96-109.

28. Noris P, Klersy C, Gresele P, et al. Platelet size for distinguishing between inherited thrombocytopenias and immune thrombocytopenia: a multicentric, real life study. Br J Haematol. 2013;162(1):112-119.

29. Balduini CL, Savoia A. Genetics of familial forms of thrombocytopenia. Hum Genet. 2012;131(12):1821-32.

30. Buchbinder D, Nugent DJ, Fillipovich AH. Wiskott-Aldrich syndrome: diagnosis, current management, and emerging treatments. Appl Clin Genet. (2014) 7:55–66.

31. Bader-Meunier B, Proulle V, Trichet C, et al. Misdiagnosis of chronic thrombocytopenia in childhood. J Pediatr Hematol Oncol. 2003;25(7):548-52.

32. Lee AC. Isolated thrombocytopenia in childhood: what if it is not immune thrombocytopenia? Singapore Med J. 2018;59(7):390-393.

33. Moulis G, Palmaro A, Montastruc JL, Godeau B, Lapeyre-Mestre M, Sailler L. Epidemiology of incident immune thrombocytopenia: a nationwide population-based study in France. Blood. 2014;124(22):3308-3315.

34. Ayesh MH, Alawneh K, Khassawneh B, Khader Y, Kasasbeh A. Adult primary and secondary immune thrombocytopenic purpura: a comparative analysis of characteristics and clinical course. Clin Appl Thromb Hemost. 2013;19(3):327-330.

35. Drachman JG. Inherited thrombocytopenia: when a low platelet count does not mean ITP. Blood. 2004; 103(2):390-398.

36. Nurden AT, Freson K, Seligsohn U. Inherited platelet disorders. Haemophilia. 2012;18(suppl 4):154-160.

37. Rabbolini DJ, Chun Y, Latimer M, et al. Diagnosis and treatment of MYH9-RD in an Australasian cohort with thrombocytopenia. Platelets. 2018;29(8):793-800.

38. Sipurzynski J, Fahrner B, Kerbl R, et al.Management of chronic immune thrombocytopenia in children and adolescents: lessons from an Austrian national cross-sectional study of 81 patients. Semin Hematol. 201;53 Suppl 1:S43-7.

39. Noris P, Pecci A. Hereditary thrombocytopenias: a growing list of disorders. Hematology Am Soc Hematol Educ Program. 2017;2017(1):385-399.

40. Tangye SG, Al-Herz W, Bousfiha A et al. Human inborn errors of immunity: 2019 update on the classification from the international union of immunological societies expert committee. J Clin Immunol. 2020;40:24-64.

41. Seif AE, Manno CS, Sheen C, et al. Identifying autoimmune lymphoproliferative syndrome in children with Evans syndrome: a multi-institutional study. Blood. 2010;115:2142-2145.

42. Aladjidi N, Leverger G, Leblanc T, et al. New insights into childhood autoimmune hemolytic anemia: a French national observational study of 265 children. Haematologica. 2011; 96:655-663.

43. Teachey DT, Manno CS, Axsom KM, et al. Unmasking Evans syndrome: T-cell phenotype and apoptotic response reveal autoimmune lymphoproliferative syndrome (ALPS). Blood. 2005;105:2443-2448.

44. Savasan S, Warrier I, Buck S, et al. Increased lymphocyte Fas expression and high incidence of common variable immunodeficiency disorder in childhood Evans' syndrome. Clin Immunol. 2007;125:224-229.

45. Heeney MM, Zimmerman SA, Ware RE. Childhood autoimmune cytopenia secondary to unsuspected common variable immunodeficiency. J Pediatr. 2003;143: 662-665.

46. Moulis G, Germain J, Comont T, et al. Group CI. Newly diagnosed immune thrombocytopenia adults: clinical epidemiology, exposure to treatments, and evolution. Results of the CARMEN multicenter prospective cohort. Am J Hematol. 2017;92(6):493-500.

47. Sultan S, Ahmed SI, Murad S, Irfan SM. Primary versus secondary immune thrombocytopenia in adults; a comparative analysis of clinical and laboratory attributes in newly diagnosed patients in Southern Pakistan. Med J Malaysia. 2016;71(5):269-274.

48. Dal MS, Karakus A, Dal T, et al. Assessment of the underlying causes of the immune thrombocytopenia: ten years experience. J Pak Med Assoc. 2017;67(7):1004-1008.

49. Schifferli A, Cavalli F, Godeau B, et al. Understanding Immune Thrombocytopenia: Looking Out of the Box. Front Med (Lausanne). 2021;8:613192.

# 8. Standardization of definitions, terminology and outcome criteria: a common language in ITP

In 2009 an International Working Group (IWG) published a document proposing a consensus-based standardization of definitions, terminology and outcome in immune thrombocytopenia (ITP) that was widely adopted by many clinicians and investigators [1] and substantially adopted for outcome criteria, phases of the disease and major definitions, by the European Medicine Agency (https://www.ema.europa.eu/en/documents/scientific-guideline/guideline-clinical-development-medicinal-products-intended-treatment-chronic-primary-immune_en.pdf). At the time of printing of the third edition of this book, the IWG document still represents a reference tool for the description of ITP and its management. On the other hand, after more than 10 years of use, some issues emerged that make a revision urgent in order to verify if all definitions maintain their validity in the light of the better understanding of the clinical and pathologic aspects of ITP. The scope of this paper is to summarize the current ITP terminology and definitions still based on the 2009 IWG document and to discuss the new aspects needing standardization and the main critical issues that demand revision or integration.

Since the IWG 2009 publication, Immune ThrombocytoPenia (ITP) has been widely used to indicate the disease previously generally known as Immune or Idiopathic Thrombocytopenic Purpura. Indeed, the IWG agreed that the term "Idiopathic" was no longer appropriate and that the "I" should stand for "Immune" since the cause of thrombocytopenia is now identified in a loss of self-tolerance leading to an (auto)immune attack against circulating platelets and megakaryocytes. Similarly, the term "purpura" was also felt misleading, since around half of cases presents without skin bleeding. However, in order to maintain the time-honored acronym ITP, the "P" was assigned a different indication, "Penia" (deficiency) instead of "Purpura". ITP was initially described in 1735 by Werlhof under the name of "Morbus Maculosus Hemorrhagicus", and the studies of its pathophysiology started 70 years ago with the classical, historical experiments of Harrington [2], leading to the discovery of its autoimmune nature. The pathogenetic mechanism consists in the production of auto-antibodies against critical proteins of platelet membrane. There is increasing evidence of the critical role of T-cells and dendritic/macrophagic cells in maintaining the homeostasis of self-tolerance. Opsonized platelets are rapidly and prematurely destroyed by the reticulo-endothelial system [3]. Furthermore, more recent evidence shows that these autoantibodies and cytotoxic T-cells may interfere also with the normal megakaryocytopoiesis. Inadequate levels of circulating unbound thrombopoietin (TPO) further impaired platelet production [4-6]. Despite this long history and its not negligible frequency (with an incidence roughly estimated between 1.6 and 3.9 new cases/$10^5$/year in general population [7-9] and an age-adjusted point prevalence reported between 9.5 [10] to 20.3 in adults [11]), ITP still presents frequent areas of uncertainty regarding epidemiology, natural history, treatment management. The diagnosis remains one of exclusion, the clinical outcomes are poorly defined, the prediction of bleeding risk is not based on clinical or laboratory indicators prospectively validated, the short and long term toxicity of treatments is not prospectively evaluated, the curative potential and the influence of initial treatment on long term outcome are also poorly investigated. Standardization in Patient Reported Outcomes (PRO), Quality of Life (QoL) and fatigue assessment is still in its infancy. Because of the paucity of randomised clinical trials, published guidelines on diagnosis and therapy are still largely based on expert opinion [12-15]. As a consequence, the management may greatly differ among various centers. Furthermore, the comparison of clinical outcomes and of their relationship with the different treatment modalities is obscured by the lack of standardization in definitions and terminology. Unfortunately, this applies also to the few systematic reviews and meta-analyses on the efficacy and safety of splenectomy [16], the treatment of refractory forms [17] or the use of anti CD20 antibodies in chronic cases [18].

Before the publication of the proposal by the International Working Group on ITP [1], authors often used different terminology and criteria to evaluate patient's characteristics and to report outcomes, with an unacceptable heterogeneity for criteria to start the initial therapy, to define the severity of the disease and to evaluate the response to therapy (platelet count, timing of assessment, durability of response) [19].

During the last decade, the need for standardization and harmonization of response criteria has become even more compelling with the development of novel targeted therapies, such as the second generation of thrombopoietin-receptor agonists (TPO-ra) [20] romiplostim [21, 22], eltrombopag [23, 24], avatrombopag [25] and lusutrombopag, the Syc tyrosin kinase fostamatinib [26], the inhibitors of FcRn rozanolixizumab [27] and efgartigimod [28], which may have different mechanisms of action and heterogeneous patterns of response.

Furthermore, the impact of the harmonization on ITP would be of particular relevance in the development and validation of ITP-specific bleeding scales [29, 30] and QoL questionnaires [31-33], which are urgently needed for inclusion in future clinical studies, as also emphasized by the different perspectives that patients and doctors have with regard to the individual burden of ITP [34].

## 8.1. Criteria adopted by the IWG to harmonize terminology and definitions in ITP

The IWG agreed that, in order to be clinically useful, the general criteria and the definitions (☞ Table 8.1) together with the operative principles for the harmonization of ITP terminology should be relevant for the description of the natural history of the disease and should appropriately reflect the effectiveness and benefit/risk ratio of specific interventions with regard to the different phases of the disease. Concerning the relevance for the natural history, the use of surrogate end-points, such as the platelet count, should theoretically be avoided or limited to specific instances, preferring the adoption of clinical end-point, such as a validated bleeding score [29, 30]. Moreover, a personal hemorrhagic risk profile should be considered, taking into account patient's age, sex, life-style, the use of drugs such as antiplatelet therapy or warfarin, the presence of inherited hemorrhagic diathesis, surgery or arterial hypertension. Appropriate definitions, goals, efficacy and safety outcomes should also be defined for "on demand" interventions (like intravenous immunoglobulin infusion) administered to assure a rapid, even if transient, platelet increase sufficient to afford surgery, dentistry, strong physical activity or other risky circumstances.

The definitions and terminology proposed were purposely developed for the primary forms of ITP (as defined below) both in adults and children and so their application to secondary forms may be inappropriate in some instances.

| ITP criteria addressed by the IWG |
|---|
| • Definition and denomination of ITP |
| • Criteria for the different phases of disease |
| • Grading of severity |
| • Platelet count and bleeding symptoms as criteria for response |
| • Aim of treatment (with regard to the different phases) |
| • Criteria for response to therapy |
| • Criteria for response to splenectomy |
| • Refractory ITP (definition, selection for treatment, criteria for response) |
| • Treatment specific criteria for response to old and new agents |
| • Criteria for research purposes and randomized trials |
| • Definitions and terminology in pediatric ITP |

***Table 8.1:*** Main issues addressed by the IWG.

## 8.2. Primary and secondary ITP and diagnostic platelet count threshold

☞ Table 8.2

The distinction between primary and secondary ITP is of great importance since natural history and management are different in the two forms. Treatment is often targeted on the underlying disorder in patients with ongoing medical condition associated to ITP. In drug-induced ITP, it is mainly based on the avoidance of exposure to the inciting drug. The panel recognized that primary ITP could include heterogeneous disorders and that a clear distinction between primary and secondary forms is not always easy. Recently, substantial data indicate that "isolated ITP" may precede by years the

| Primary immune thrombocytopenia (primary ITP) |
|---|
| • Primary immune thrombocytopenia (primary ITP) is an autoimmune disorder characterized by isolated thrombocytopenia (peripheral blood platelet count $<100 \times 10^9$/L) in the absence of other causes or disorders that may be associated with thrombocytopenia. The diagnosis of primary ITP remains one of exclusion; there are currently no robust clinical or laboratory parameters that are able to establish its diagnosis with accuracy. The main clinical problem of primary ITP is an increased risk of bleeding, although bleeding symptoms may not always be present. |
| Secondary immune thrombocytopenia (secondary ITP) |
| • All forms of immune-mediated thrombocytopenia except primary ITP* |
| Phases of the disease |
| • Newly-diagnosed ITP: within three months from diagnosis<br>• Persistent ITP: between 3 to 12 months from diagnosis. Includes patients not reaching spontaneous remission or not maintaining complete response off therapy<br>• Chronic ITP: lasting for more than 12 months |
| Severe ITP |
| • Presence of bleeding symptoms at presentation sufficient to mandate treatment, or occurrence of new bleeding symptoms requiring additional therapeutic intervention with a different platelet-enhancing agent or an increased dose |

***Table 8.2:*** Proposed Definitions of Disease [1] (reproduced with permission).
* The acronym ITP should be followed by the name of the associated disease (for thrombocytopenia after exposure to drugs, the terms "drug-induced" should be used) in parentheses; e.g. Secondary ITP (Lupus-associated), Secondary ITP (HIV-associated), Secondary ITP (Drug-induced). For manuscript titles, abstracts, etc., definitions such as lupus-associated ITP or HIV-associated ITP can also be used.

onset of myelodysplastic syndromes or lymphoproliferative disorders [35, 36]. Furthermore, ITP coexisting with the presence of lupus anticoagulant or antiphospholipid antibodies or with antinuclear antibodies – even in the absence of any related clinical manifestations – might be less responsive to standard treatments and evolve into anti-phospholipid syndrome (APS) with repeated abortions or thrombosis or into an overt collagen disease like systemic lupus erythematosus (SLE). In the absence of a clear demonstration that this is indeed the ultimate development of the majority of these complex forms, the IWG suggested to maintain them within the primary category, before a definite diagnosis of APS or SLE is made. The denomination of thrombocytopenia as "immune" does not require a demonstration of the presence of anti-platelet antibodies recognizing the limitations of the currently available tests. This is in keeping with the recently published international guidelines for ITP [14, 15]. A platelet count $<100 \times 10^9$/L was established as the threshold for diagnosis. Merely selecting the lower limit of the reference interval (usually around 120-150 x $10^9$/L) would have included an unjustified proportion of cases without a clinically relevant disorder and also many cases of pregnancy-related thrombocytopenia, a well-known physiological phenomenon not requiring specific follow up in the absence of additional clinical features.

## 8.3. Definition of the different phases and severity of the disease

In the absence of reliable clinical or laboratory markers able to predict the disease duration, the term "newly-diagnosed ITP" was preferred to "acute ITP" to define the cases diagnosed for the first time. Nevertheless, some of these cases can still be correctly referred to as "newly diagnosed ITP with an acute onset", for example to describe the self-limited forms, mainly present in children with or recovering from viral infections, in which a spontaneous remission could be observed. When an infection is demonstrated, these forms are more appropriately classified as secondary ITP. A new category, called "persistent ITP", was introduced for patients not achieving spontaneous remission or not maintaining their response after stopping treatment between 3 and 12 months from diagnosis. During this phase splenectomy is rarely indicated. The term “chronic ITP” is to be reserved for patients with ITP lasting for more than 12 months. In these patients spontaneous remissions are exceptional and so treatments like immunosuppression or splenectomy, initially deferred for their not negligible toxicity, may become justified.

More recently, with the increasing use of TPO-ra just after an insufficient response to corticosteroids, even in newly diagnosed adult patients and with the current low rate of splenectomy, the distinction among the three phases has been questioned. This Author still holds that the proposed distinction maintains its descriptive usefulness, if not else, for the description of individual cases and for comparison of different studies.

Disease severity (mild, moderate, severe) has been correlated with the degree of thrombocytopenia, which is taken as a surrogate for risk of bleeding. However, the panel agreed that, regardless of the phase of the disease, the term “severe” ITP should only be used in patients who have clinically relevant bleeding. In the absence of an agreed bleeding scale, a bleeding should be considered “clinically relevant” when it mandates treatment at presentation or requires additional therapeutic intervention with a different platelet-enhancing agent or an increased dose for the occurrence of new bleeding symptoms.

To overcome this limitation, the IWG has proposed a consensus-based ITP-specific Bleeding Assessment Tool (ITP-BAT). The ITP-BAT includes a standardized data collection form and a set of precise definitions of the different bleeding manifestations of the disease. Their severity is graded by a consistent severity scale. Bleeding manifestations are grouped into 3 anatomical domains (Skin, visible Mucosae and Organs). The worst-ever grade for each domain occurring during the observation period is recorded to produce a bleeding index (SMOG) [37]. Unfortunately, this system has been rarely adopted in clinical investigations as it is felt sufficiently difficult to implement and more time-consuming in comparison to simpler tools like those based on the WHO scale.

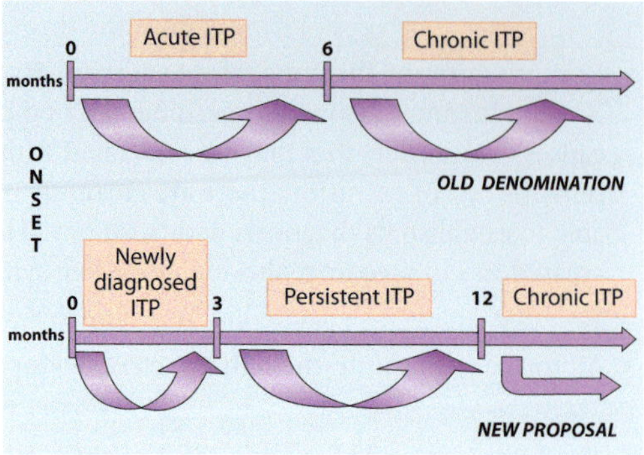


***Figure 8.1:*** Different phases in the natural history of ITP. Old and new definitions are compared.

## 8.4. Therapeutic goals

In newly diagnosed patients or in patients requiring treatment for the first time (initial treatment), management is mainly directed at rapidly obtaining a safe platelet count in order to prevent or stop hemorrhages and at ensuring an acceptable QoL with minimal treatment-related toxicity. Although more than 80 % of patients will reach a safe platelet count, only a minority of them is expected to obtain permanent remission after initial treatment with corticosteroid-based regimen (no more than 20 to 30 %) and most of them will relapse after stopping this treatment in a span of weeks or months. An increase in the rate of long-lasting responses with more robust initial treatments, now made possible with the availability of new therapies (high dose dexamethasone; anti CD-20; TPO-ra), has been attempted. However, in the lack of conclusive results based on prospective randomized trials, this practice should not be used in newly diagnosed patients outside investigational studies. The goal of treatment in persistent or chronic ITP is less well defined and it is often inspired by the desire to defer or avoid the risks of more toxic treatments such as splenectomy or immunosuppression. Thus “on-demand” treatment in anticipation of high risk bleeding situations or surgical procedures is often warranted. Minimal corticosteroid exposure (ideally < 5 mg/day of prednisone) is also often used for chronic ITP. Currently, in affluent countries, TPO-ra, like romiplostim, eltrombopag and avatrombopag, are finding their place for most cases with persistent ITP [20, 43] after their overall good safety has been substantiated in several long-term studies, and long-term durable responses have been observed in 10-15 % of cases after stopping their administration. However, a significant increase of the incidence of venous and arterial thrombosis above that observed in non-exposed ITP patients with similar basal risk factors has been observed [38-40]. Based on current data, we should maintain that a curative approach is not a real goal in persistent phase, yet, and safety should remain a major concern. Splenectomy is best avoided in this phase of ITP and deferred to chronic phase if deemed necessary.

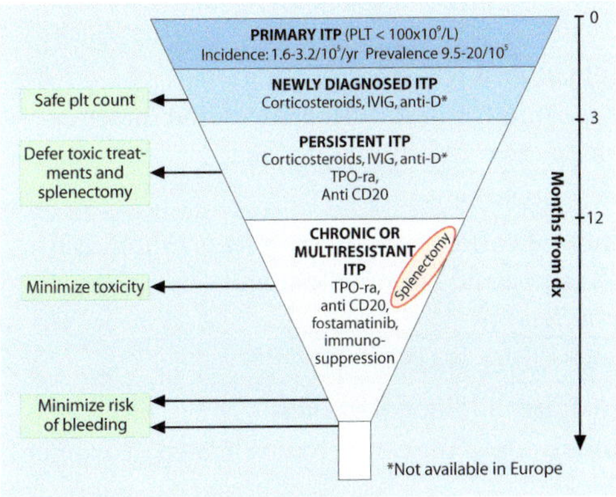


***Figure 8.2:*** Goals of treatment and preferred agents in the different phases of ITP. The proportion of patients in each phase is roughly proportional to the corresponding area of the pyramid.

## 8.5. Definition of response

☞ Table 8.3

"Complete response" (CR) was defined as any confirmed platelet count ≥100 x $10^9$/L. "Response" (R) as any confirmed platelet count ≥30 x $10^9$/L and at least doubling of the baseline count. The definition of response requires concurrent resolution of bleeding symptoms. The threshold of 30 x $10^9$/L corresponds to the level below which active treatment may become indicated according to current international guidelines for ITP. The panel was well aware that the definition of response after a treatment should be preferably based on clinical end points like minimization of bleeding or bleeding risk or amelioration of QoL. However, surrogate end points based on platelet count are objective, clinically relevant, easy to obtain and suitable for comparison. The panel decided to avoid "partial" or "minimal" response categories, often used in scientific papers, because of the wide heterogeneity of these definitions and of the recognition that in some settings less than CR is really a very good achievement. Indeed, even a lower increment of platelet count could be life-saving in refractory patients or patients failing several therapeutic lines. In these cases, an obstinate effort to increase the platelet count above the lowest safe level able to prevent major bleeding may entail the use of disproportionately toxic treatments. CR and R could be on or off the administration of the investigated agent, and this should be specified. In a clinical trial, any ongoing concomitant ITP-specific treatment in addition to the one being investigated, or the time of its discontinuation should be provided. The frequency of platelet count monitoring and the timing of response assessment should be pre-specified and will depend on the expected kinetics of platelet increase after each treatment.

Duration of the response should be calculated from the time of CR or R until loss of CR or R. Two different scenarios are envisioned:

- short-course treatments aimed at curing the disease, or at least at achieving prolonged remissions (e.g., high-dose pulse dexamethasone, rituximab, splenectomy)
- treatments requiring continuous or repeated administration (e.g., TPO-ra, IVIg, anti-D), for which it is anticipated that platelet count could fall temporarily below or increase above the desired threshold for short periods

A Kaplan-Meier analysis based on the product limit estimate is the most useful approach to calculate the overall response duration in a patient cohort in case of short-course treatments (☞ Figure 8.3).

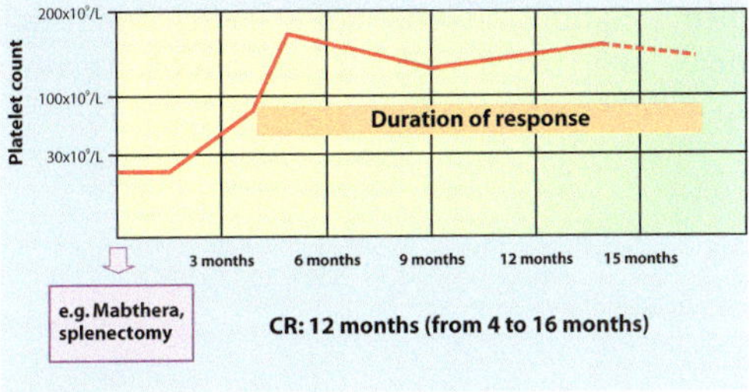


***Figure 8.3:*** Calculation of the duration of response (exemplified for a single patient) to be used for Kaplan-Meier analysis.

| Quality of response §° |
|---|
| • Complete response (CR): platelet count ≥100 x $10^9$/L and absence of bleeding |
| • Response (R): platelet count ≥30 x $10^9$/L and at least 2x increase of baseline platelet count and absence of bleeding |
| • Time to response: time from starting treatment to time of achievement of CR or R# |
| • No response (NR): platelet count <30 x $10^9$/L or less than 2x increase of baseline platelet count or bleeding |
| • Loss of CR or R: platelet count <100 x $10^9$/L or bleeding (from CR) or <30 x $10^9$/L or less than 2x increase of baseline platelet count or bleeding (from R) |
| **Timing of assessment of response to ITP treatments** |
| • Variable, depends on the type of treatment |
| **Duration of response†** |
| • Measured from the achievement of CR or R to loss of CR or R |
| • Measured as the proportion of the cumulative time spent in CR or R during the period under examination as well as the total time observed from which the proportion is derived |
| **Corticosteroid-dependence** |
| • The need for ongoing or repeated doses administration of corticosteroids for at least 2 months to maintain a platelet count at or above 30 × $10^9$/L and/or to avoid bleeding (patients with corticosteroid-dependence are considered non-responders) |
| **Supplemental outcomes (whenever possible)** |
| • Bleeding symptoms measured by a validated scale (requires additional studies) |
| • Health-related quality of life assessment (HRQoL, briefly QoL) measured by a validated instrument (requires additional studies) |

***Table 8.3:*** Proposed criteria for assessing response to ITP treatments* [1] (reproduced with permission).

* For response criteria in refractory ITP ☞ Table 8.4

§ Platelet counts should be confirmed on at least 2 separate occasions (at least 7 days apart when used to define CR, R or 1 day apart when used to define NR or loss of response).

° Baseline platelet count refers to platelet count at the time of starting the investigated treatment; for post-splenectomy response evaluation, basal platelet count refers to the platelet count before the patient was first treated (initial treatment).

# Late responses not attributable to the investigated treatment should not be defined as CR or R.

† The two definitions are not mutually exclusive: the first definition, collectively represented using Kaplan-Meyer analysis, is more suitable for short-course treatments aimed at inducing prolonged remission of the disease, whereas the second one is more suitable to evaluate the overall benefit of continuous or intermittent repeated administration of agents requiring dose adjustments with anticipated temporary losses of CR or R.

Person-years event rates or similar approaches may also be useful, descriptive modalities. For treatments requiring prolonged or repeated administrations, one should calculate the cumulative time spent in CR or R (☞ Figure 8.4).

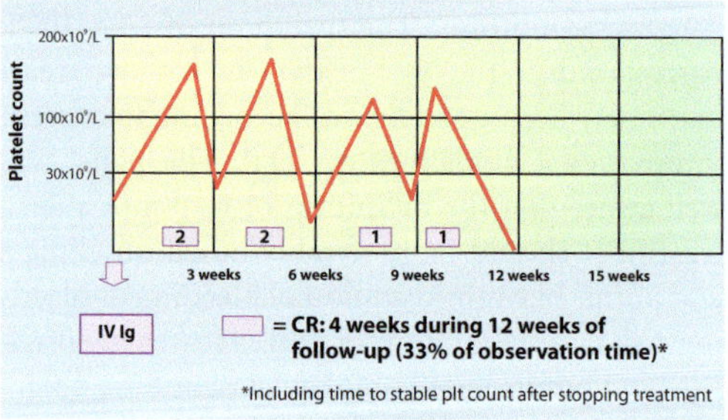


***Figure 8.4:*** Calculation of the cumulative time spent in complete remission (exemplified for a single patient).

This approach is also useful to evaluate the whole impact of a particular treatment plan including different sequential treatments, allowing a more clinically meaningful estimation of response duration. When response duration includes time while on treatment, this should be specified, and CR or R on or off-treatment should be calculated separately. Unfortunately, none of the recently published comparative trials investigating TPO-ra has adopted these more clinically meaningful approaches. We hope that new studies will use the proposed approaches in addition to those that may be imposed by the regulatory agencies.

## 8.6. Refractory ITP: definition, therapeutic goals and response assessment

Based on IWG 2009, but ☞ Chapter 8.8. for some critical comments on the definition of refractory ITP

☞ Table 8.4

To be defined as refractory by 2009 IWG criteria, patients should meet three criteria:

- *First*, they should be confirmed to have primary ITP
- *Second*, they should have failed splenectomy or have relapsed thereafter
- *Third*, they should either exhibit severe ITP or have a risk of bleeding that in the opinion of the attending physician requires therapy.

Refractory patients may have temporary responses to on-demand therapy, like short courses of corticosteroids or IVIg administration. However, during the last years the 2009 IWG definition of refractoriness proved difficult to be used and controversial. The 2009 IWG definition was based on the still true belief that splenectomy remains the only "curative" treatment, with 60 to 70 % of long lasting remissions. On the other hand, we currently recognize that there is increasing reluctance towards splenectomy from both patients and physi-

| Definition (all should be met) |
|---|
| • Failure to achieve at least response (R) or loss of R following splenectomy*<br>• Need of treatment(s) (including, but not limited to, low dose of corticosteroids) to minimize the risk of clinically significant bleeding$^{\S}$. Need of on-demand or adjunctive therapy alone does not qualify the patient as refractory<br>• Primary ITP confirmed by excluding other supervened causes of thrombocytopenia |
| **Definition of on-demand therapy** |
| • Any therapy used to temporarily increase the platelet count sufficiently to safely perform invasive procedures or in case of major bleeding or trauma° |
| **Definition of adjunctive therapy** |
| • Any non-ITP specific therapy that may decrease bleeding e.g., antifibrinolytic agents, hormonal agents, DDAVP, recombinant Factor VIIa, fibrin sealants. Platelet transfusion is also included |
| **Definition of response to therapy in refractory ITP** |
| • Ability to maintain a platelet count sufficient to prevent clinically significant bleeding$^{\S\#}$<br>• Ability to decrease toxic therapy (e.g. corticosteroids) does not qualify for response but should be reported |
| **Definition of response to on-demand therapy** |
| • Control of bleeding in the specific situation<br>• Achievement of a platelet count sufficient to perform procedure or minimize bleeding from trauma |

***Table 8.4:*** Refractory ITP [1] (reproduced with permission).
* May not be applicable in children or in patients with accessory spleen.
§ Bleeding symptoms measured by a validated scale whenever possible (requires further studies).
° Specific platelet thresholds cannot be provided but in most instances a platelet count of 50-70 x $10^9$/L would fulfill this criterion.
\# A strict definition of response in terms of pre-defined platelet count cannot be given and may not be appropriate when considering the risk benefit ratio in refractory ITP because the tradeoff between efficacy of a specific treatment and its short and long term toxicity varies among individuals.

| Eligibility (all should be met) |
|---|
| • Previously treated or untreated patients fitting within one of the different phases of the disease (☞ Table 8.1). Refractory patients defined as in Table 8.4<br>• Entry platelet count: at least <30 x $10^9$/L. At least <50 x $10^9$/L in specific clinical settings or patients on steroids, or in the presence of bleeding symptoms<br>• Patients should be on a stable treatment or off any treatment for a time sufficient to exclude a late effect (☞ Table 8.3) |
| **Supplemental specifications** |
| • Pediatric and adult patients analyzed separately<br>• Response to previous treatment(s), if any, should be reported |
| **End points** |
| • Primary endpoints:<br>- CR or R based on platelet count as in Table 8.2*<br>• Secondary endpoints:<br>- adverse events (safety), need for rescue interventions, corticosteroids/concomitant treatment reduction, rate of splenectomies. Could become primary endpoints according to the design of the clinical trial or patient characteristics.<br>- bleeding scale, HRQoL assessment and, whenever possible, pharmaco-economic analysis should be included |
| **Timing of assessment of primary endpoints and duration of response** |
| • Depends on the type of treatment<br>• Patients enrolled while on a stable treatment with one or more agents must no longer be receiving these treatments for a time sufficient to exclude any protracted effect§<br>• Duration could be calculated as follows depending on study design:<br>- the time from CR or R as defined in Table 8.2 to loss of response°<br>- the cumulative time spent in CR or R or cumulative time spent without meeting a predefined end-point(s) |
| **Adverse events** |
| • Bleeding episodes, rescue interventions, frequency of splenectomy and treatment-related side effects occurring during or after the time of exposure to the experimental agent should always be reported. Duration of side effects monitoring time after the end of experimental treatment should be provided.<br>• For assessment of rebound thrombocytopenia or bleeding, the immediate period following the suspension of the agent up to the attainment of a stable platelet count# or institution of a new treatment should be considered. This treatment should be recorded.<br>• A predefined exceedingly high platelet count induced by treatment could be considered as an adverse event, depending on the agent under investigation. |

***Table 8.5:*** Trial-adapted criteria for eligibility and outcome assessments in ITP [1] (reproduced with permission).
*At variance with Table 8.3 these definitions should be adopted also for refractory cases, considering the experimental nature of clinical trials requiring objective measurements.
§ Specify the duration that a subject should be off other treatments and/or the time elapsed after any rescue medication at the time of response evaluation, ☞ also Table 8.3. For patients enrolled while on a stable concomitant treatment, still requiring it at the time of response evaluation, only secondary endpoints can be assessed
° For some agents requiring continuous administration like TPO-ra an upper limit of acceptable platelet count should be pre-defined and thus cumulative time spent within a therapeutic window is most suitable.
# Defined as a platelet count not requiring treatment or dosage modification for at least 15 days.

cians, with the consequence that the definition could result not applicable to a significant proportion of cases. Accordingly, it seems now agreeable that non-splenectomized patients (adults and children) not responding to medical treatment(s) could be described as having "newly diagnosed, persistent or chronic ITP unresponsive to one or more agents" (with specification of the implicated agents). These patients may have or not severe ITP, a definition referring to clinical symptoms as indicated in Table 8.2.

The aim of a long-term therapy in a refractory ITP should be the achievement of a count sufficient to prevent clinically significant bleeding with the least toxicity. In this population, treatments should be evaluated for their potential to induce a long-lasting response. The net therapeutic benefit of the more "toxic" treatments may be uncertain and critically dependent upon the individual patient characteristics and the specific circumstances. As for any other phase of the disease, adjunctive therapy or platelet transfusion may be required for severe mucosal/organ or life-threatening bleeding.

## 8.7. Clinical trial-adapted criteria for eligibility and outcome assessment

Based on IWG 2009, but ☞ Chapter 8.8. for additional critical comments

☞ Table 8.5

There have been a number of randomized clinical trials performed in adults and children with ITP and their results can be compared only with great difficulty due to differences in the characteristics of the patient populations included (newly-diagnosed vs. persistent or chronic/refractory), study designs and endpoints, as well as to the heterogeneous mechanisms of action and patterns of response to the various investigational treatments. To avoid these limitations in future trials, the panel recommended minimal standardized criteria and definitions to be used in interventional studies (specifically for phase II and III) in order to minimize heterogeneity in study subjects and outcomes. In testing new agents or new approaches, researchers and companies are encouraged to report their results according to the IWG suggestions in addition to the specific requirements of the regulatory agencies.

## 8.8. Application of 2009 IWG proposals in real-word and need for revision

Few studies have examined the current compliance with the IWG proposals. However, recently some selected outcome criteria used in publications between 2010 and 2019 were subject to a systematic literature review to assess their compliance with the outcome criteria originally proposed by the IWG [41]. This comprehensive review included interventional studies with ≥10 patients and observational studies with ≥50 patients describing platelet, bleeding, and/or HRQoL outcome measures in adult and pediatric ITP.

Platelet response outcomes were reported in 141 studies, 57 % of which did not use the strict IWG definitions. This was particularly the case with randomized trials investigating the more recently introduced or still in development treatments favoring a platelet count ≥50 x $10^9$/L instead of ≥30 x $10^9$/L to define response, often without the further requirement of reaching a level at least double the basal one (TPO-ra, fostamatinib, FcRn blocking agents). Furthermore, the term "remission" – not considered in 2009 IWG document – was introduced without a clear definition and rationale, to generally indicate a platelet count ≥100 x $10^9$/L sustained for ≥6 months after tapering off administration of TPO-ra. Bleeding outcomes were reported systematically only in 41 % of studies which used 21 distinct reporting schemes. A plurality of adult studies used the WHO Bleeding Scale, while a number of pediatric ones used the Buchanan and Adix Score. HRQoL outcomes were reported in a very small minority of studies (9 %), which used a total of 8 different HRQoL instruments (2 pediatric instruments and 6 for adults). For further comments on the main issues requiring revision ☞ Table 8.6.

## 8.9. Conclusions

More than 10 years after the publication of the IWG document, some specific outcome definitions are still subject to an unacceptably wide variability. Nevertheless, most conceptual and harmonization recommendations of the IWG have found a favorable acceptance by the investigators in the field of pediatric and adult ITP. Among the most notable examples, the wide acceptance of the new

| Specific issue | IWG 2009 | Comment | Proposal[§] |
|---|---|---|---|
| Response criteria (R and CR) | R ≥ 30.000/μL and doubling basal level<br>CR ≥ 100.000/μL | Prospective trial for new agents have enrolled patients ≤ 30.000/μL and used ≥ 50.000/μL without doubling as response criteria. This platelet threshold has been set as the minimum target for adjusting dose by EMA and FDA | R: maintain ≥ 30.000/μL and doubling basal level for all trials to evaluate clinically meaningful responses, together with ≥ 50.000/μL without doubling for some investigational trials to comply with EMA and FDA<br>CR: ≥ 100.000/μL |
| Duration of R and CR | Separate analysis for R and CR | | Separate analysis advisable for 3 response levels:<br>≥ 30.000/μL and doubling (R)<br>≥ 50.000/μL<br>≥ 100.000/μL (CR) |
| Remission | Generically used to define "spontaneous" years-long responses (particularly after splenectomy) | Recently, with the observation that after TPO-ra a few patients may experience months-long responses, the term remission was introduced but remains poorly defined | Improperly used to indicate months-long response after stopping a previous medical treatment. The term "sustained response off treatment" or similar would be preferable[#] |
| Concomitant treatment(s) in R or CR evaluation | Not specified in detail | A sizable proportion of pts currently enrolled in clinical trials maintain additional associated treatment(s) | Require definition of R or CR in patients receiving more than one treatment to take into account the contribution of the investigational treatment |
| Refractory ITP | Required failure to splenectomy or medical contraindication to surgery in severe ITP | Maintain pathophysiologic validity but no longer applicable with the current low rate of splenectomy | Require detailing lack of response to previous treatments plus specifying if splenectomy was done or not |
| Bleeding assessment | Should be considered the primary end-point but lack of consensus on a universal scale | Persisting major limitation in current ITP evaluation.<br>The SMOG proposed by the IWG found limited acceptance | Widely accepted ITP specific tools considering 3 separate domains (skin, mucosae, organ). Separate tools desirable, one for self-evaluation and one for physicians. User-friendly app welcome |
| HRQoL | Not defined | Criteria for definition and grading required | Widely accepted ITP-specific tools* for self-evaluation. User-friendly app welcome |
| Fatigue | Not defined | Criteria for definition and grading required | Widely accepted ITP-specific tools* for self-evaluation. User-friendly app welcome |

***Table 8.6:*** Main issues requiring modification to meet emerging requirements, or not considered in 2009 IWG document [1]. A personal view.

[§] Based on Author's opinion.

* When comparing ITP patients with normal population or with patients affected by other conditions, non ITP-specific tools should be used.

[#] The term remission or sustained remission implies a "temporary cure" from ITP as an effect of previous treatment so that the more neutral and conservative definitions such as for example "durable or sustained CR/R off treatment," seem more desirable.

name of the disease with the suppression of the old terms "purpura" and "idiopathic". Also the distinction of the ITP course into 3 distinct phases as originally proposed by the IWG is currently adopted in clinical studies and by regulatory agencies and substantially endorsed in the 2019 ASH guidelines [15]. The same applies to principles governing new and old treatments in such phases. On the other hand, some definitions, while conceptually accepted, have shown a limited formal application and need to be revised. Table 8.6 shows the main outcome definition requiring adaptation to the current practice. For other instances like HRQoL and fatigue, new reliable and easily applicable tools to facilitate data collection by the patients or their caregivers seem highly desirable. Indeed, these individual aspects have become of increasing importance at a time when patient's values and perspectives are considered a determinant aspect for a shared management decision.

In addition, it appears of critical importance the integration of the surrogate response criteria based on platelet count with bleeding assessment, considering that reducing bleeding risk and bleeding manifestation with the least toxic agents remains the ultimate goal in ITP treatment. It is quite sad that none of the recent studies was able to clearly demonstrate a reduction in major bleedings, making still actual the major criticism raised by a Cochrane systematic review published shortly after the initial pivotal studies on TPO-ra [42], a criticism that includes also the more recent treatments. These insufficiencies underline the urgent need for a single reliable and easily applicable bleeding assessment tool. In the view of this Author, the SMOG system [37] still represents a good starting point.

## Acknowledgements

The author acknowledges the support of the Hematology Project Foundation (Vicenza) and of Claudia Guzzoni for her invaluable secretarial assistance.

## References

1. Rodeghiero F, Stasi R, Gernsheimer T, Michel M, Provan D, Arnold DM, Bussel JB, Cines DB, Chong BH, Cooper N, Godeau B, Lechner K, Mazzucconi MG, Mc Millan R, Sanz MA, Imbach P, Blanchette V, Kuhne T, Ruggeri M, George JN. Standardization of terminology, definitions and outcome criteria in immune thrombocytopenic purpura of adults and children: report from an international working group. Blood. 2009;113:2386-93.

2. Harrington WJ, Minnich V, Hollingsworth JW, Moore CV. Demonstration of a thrombocytopenic factor in the blood of patients with thrombocytopenic purpura. J Lab Clin Med. 1951;38:1-10.

3. Cooper N, Bussel J. The pathogenesis of immune thrombocytopaenic purpura. Br J Haematol. 2006;133: 364-74.

4. Ballem PJ, Segal GM, Stratton JR, Gernsheimer T, Adamson JW, Slichter SJ. Mechanisms of thrombocytopenia in chronic autoimmune thrombocytopenic purpura. Evidence of both impaired platelet production and increased platelet clearance. J Clin Invest. 1987;80: 33-40.

5. Stasi R, Evangelista ML, Stipa E, Buccisano F, Venditti A, Amadori S. Idiopathic thrombocytopenic purpura: current concepts in pathophysiology and management. Thromb Haemost. 2008;99:4-13.

6. Gernsheimer T, Stratton J, Ballem PJ, Slichter SJ. Mechanisms of response to treatment in autoimmune thrombocytopenic purpura. N Engl J Med. 1989;320: 974-80.

7. Frederiksen H, Schmidt K. The incidence of idiopathic thrombocytopenic purpura in adults increases with age. Blood. 1999;94:909-13.

8. Neylon AJ, Saunders PW, Howard MR, Proctor SJ, Taylor PR, Northern Region Haematology G. Clinically significant newly presenting autoimmune thrombocytopenic purpura in adults: a prospective study of a population-based cohort of 245 patients. Br J Haematol. 2003; 122:966-74.

9. Schoonen WM, Kucera G, Coalson J, Li L, Rutstein M, Mowat F, Fryzek J, Kaye JA. Epidemiology of immune thrombocytopenic purpura in the General Practice Research Database. Br J Haematol. 2009;145:235-44.

10. Segal JB, Powe NR. Prevalence of immune thrombocytopenia: analyses of administrative data. J Thromb Haemost. 2006;4:2377-83.

11. Feudjo-Tepie MA, Robinson NJ, Bennett D. Prevalence of diagnosed chronic immune thrombocytopenic purpura in the US: analysis of a large US claim database: a rebuttal. J Thromb Haemost. 2008;6:711-2

12. Kashiwagi H, Kuwana M, Hato T, Takafuta T, Fujimura K, Kurata Y, Murata M, Tomiyama Y. Reference guide for management of adult immune thrombocytopenia in Japan: 2019 Revision. Int J Hematol. 2020;111: 329-51.

13. Matzdorff A, Meyer O, Ostermann H, Kiefel V, Eberl W, Kuhne T, Pabinger I, Rummel M. Immune Thrombocytopenia - Current Diagnostics and Therapy: Recommendations of a Joint Working Group of DGHO,

OGHO, SGH, GPOH, and DGTI. Oncol Res Treat. 2018; 41 Suppl 5:1-30.

14. Provan D, Arnold DM, Bussel JB, Chong BH, Cooper N, Gernsheimer T, Ghanima W, Godeau B, Gonzalez-Lopez TJ, Grainger J, Hou M, Kruse C, McDonald V, Michel M, Newland AC, Pavord S, Rodeghiero F, Scully M, Tomiyama Y, Wong RS, Zaja F, Kuter DJ. Updated international consensus report on the investigation and management of primary immune thrombocytopenia. Blood Adv. 2019;3:3780-817.

15. Neunert C, Terrell DR, Arnold DM, Buchanan G, Cines DB, Cooper N, Cuker A, Despotovic JM, George JN, Grace RF, Kuhne T, Kuter DJ, Lim W, McCrae KR, Pruitt B, Shimanek H, Vesely SK. American Society of Hematology 2019 guidelines for immune thrombocytopenia. Blood Adv. 2019;3:3829-66.

16. Kojouri K, Vesely SK, Terrell DR, George JN. Splenectomy for adult patients with idiopathic thrombocytopenic purpura: a systematic review to assess long-term platelet count responses, prediction of response, and surgical complications. Blood. 2004;104:2623-34.

17. Vesely SK, Perdue JJ, Rizvi MA, Terrell DR, George JN. Management of adult patients with persistent idiopathic thrombocytopenic purpura following splenectomy: a systematic review. Ann Intern Med. 2004;140: 112-20.

18. Arnold DM, Dentali F, Crowther MA, Meyer RM, Cook RJ, Sigouin C, Fraser GA, Lim W, Kelton JG. Systematic review: efficacy and safety of rituximab for adults with idiopathic thrombocytopenic purpura. Ann Intern Med. 2007;146:25-33.

19. Ruggeri M, Fortuna S, Rodeghiero F. Heterogeneity of terminology and clinical definitions in adult idiopathic thrombocytopenic purpura: a critical appraisal from a systematic review of the literature. Haematologica. 2008;93:98-103.

20. Ghanima W, Cooper N, Rodeghiero F, Godeau B, Bussel JB. Thrombopoietin receptor agonists: ten years later. Haematologica. 2019;104:1112-23.

21. Kuter DJ, Bussel JB, Lyons RM, Pullarkat V, Gernsheimer TB, Senecal FM, Aledort LM, George JN, Kessler CM, Sanz MA, Liebman HA, Slovick FT, de Wolf JT, Bourgeois E, Guthrie TH, Jr., Newland A, Wasser JS, Hamburg SI, Grande C, Lefrere F, Lichtin AE, Tarantino MD, Terebelo HR, Viallard JF, Cuevas FJ, Go RS, Henry DH, Redner RL, Rice L, Schipperus MR, Guo DM, Nichol JL. Efficacy of romiplostim in patients with chronic immune thrombocytopenic purpura: a double-blind randomised controlled trial. Lancet. 2008;371:395-403.

22. Kuter DJ, Bussel JB, Newland A, Wasser JS, Lyons RM, George JN, Macik G, Nie K, Jun S. Long-term efficacy and safety of romiplostim treatment of adult patients with chronic immune thrombocytopenia (ITP): final report from an open-label extension study. Br J Haematol. 2013;161:411-23.

23. Bussel JB, Provan D, Shamsi T, Cheng G, Psaila B, Kovaleva L, Salama A, Jenkins JM, Roychowdhury D, Mayer B, Stone N, Arning M. Effect of eltrombopag on platelet counts and bleeding during treatment of chronic idiopathic thrombocytopenic purpura: a randomised, double-blind, placebo-controlled trial. Lancet. 2009;373 (9664):641-8

24. Wong RSM, Saleh MN, Khelif A, Salama A, Portella MSO, Burgess P, Bussel JB. Safety and efficacy of long-term treatment of chronic/persistent ITP with eltrombopag: final results of the EXTEND study. Blood. 2017; 130(23):2527-2536.

25. Jurczak W, Chojnowski K, Mayer J, Krawczyk K, Jamieson BD, Tian W, Allen LF. Phase 3 randomised study of avatrombopag, a novel thrombopoietin receptor agonist for the treatment of chronic immune thrombocytopenia. Br J Haematol. 2018;183:479-90.

26. Bussel J, Arnold DM, Grossbard E, Mayer J, Trelinski J, Homenda W, Hellmann A, Windyga J, Sivcheva L, Khalafallah AA, Zaja F, Cooper N, Markovtsov V, Zayed H, Duliege AM. Fostamatinib for the treatment of adult persistent and chronic immune thrombocytopenia: Results of two phase 3, randomized, placebo-controlled trials. Am J Hematol. 2018;93:921-30.

27. Robak T, Kazmierczak M, Jarque I, Musteata V, Trelinski J, Cooper N, Kiessling P, Massow U, Woltering F, Snipes R, Ke J, Langdon G, Bussel JB, Jolles S. Phase 2 multiple-dose study of an FcRn inhibitor, rozanolixizumab, in patients with primary immune thrombocytopenia. Blood Adv. 2020;4:4136-46.

28. Newland AC, Sanchez-Gonzalez B, Rejto L, Egyed M, Romanyuk N, Godar M, Verschueren K, Gandini D, Ulrichts P, Beauchamp J, Dreier T, Ward ES, Michel M, Liebman HA, de Haard H, Leupin N, Kuter DJ. Phase 2 study of efgartigimod, a novel FcRn antagonist, in adult patients with primary immune thrombocytopenia. Am J Hematol. 2020;95:178-87.

29. Khellaf M, Michel M, Schaeffer A, Bierling P, Godeau B. Assessment of a therapeutic strategy for adults with severe autoimmune thrombocytopenic purpura based on a bleeding score rather than platelet count. Haematologica. 2005;90:829-32.

30. Page LK, Psaila B, Provan D, Michael Hamilton J, Jenkins JM, Elish AS, Lesser ML, Bussel JB. The immune thrombocytopenic purpura (ITP) bleeding score: assessment of bleeding in patients with ITP. Br J Haematol. 2007;138:245-8.

31. Mathias SD, Bussel JB, George JN, McMillan R, Okano GJ, Nichol JL. A disease-specific measure of health-related quality of life for use in adults with im-

mune thrombocytopenic purpura: its development and validation. Health Qual Life Outcomes. 2007;5: 11.

32. von Mackensen S, Nilsson C, Jankovic M, Mirra N, D'Angelo E, Borkhardt A, Ljung R. Development of a disease-specific quality of life questionnaire for children & adolescents with idiopathic thrombocytopenic purpura (ITP-QoL). Pediatr Blood Cancer. 2006;47:688-91.

33. Klaassen RJ, Blanchette VS, Barnard D, Wakefield CD, Curtis C, Bradley CS, Neufeld EJ, Buchanan GR, Silva MP, Chan AK, Young NL. Validity, reliability, and responsiveness of a new measure of health-related quality of life in children with immune thrombocytopenic purpura: the Kids' ITP Tools. J Pediatr. 2007;150:510-5.

34. Cooper N, Kruse A, Kruse C, Watson S, Morgan M, Provan D, Ghanima W, Arnold DM, Tomiyama Y, Santoro C, Michel M, Laborde S, Lovrencic B, Hou M, Bailey T, Taylor-Stokes G, Haenig J, Bussel JB. Immune thrombocytopenia (ITP) World Impact Survey (iWISh): Patient and physician perceptions of diagnosis, signs and symptoms, and treatment. Am J Hematol. 2021;96:188-98.

35. Rodeghiero F. Immune thrombocytopenia in myeloid and lymphoid clonal disorders: an intriguing association. Haematologica. 2021;106:1231-3.

36. Visco C, Rodeghiero F, Romano A, Valeri F, Merli M, Quaresimini G, Volpetti S, Santi RM, Carli G, Lucchini E, Passamonti F, Rambaldi A, Motta G, Borchiellini A, d'Amore ESG, Ruggeri M. Eltrombopag for immune thrombocytopenia secondary to chronic lymphoproliferative disorders: a phase 2 multicenter study. Blood. 2019;134:1708-11.

37. Rodeghiero F, Michel M, Gernsheimer T, Ruggeri M, Blanchette V, Bussel JB, Cines DB, Cooper N, Godeau B, Greinacher A, Imbach P, Khellaf M, Klaassen RJ, Kuhne T, Liebman H, Mazzucconi MG, Newland A, Pabinger I, Tosetto A, Stasi R. Standardization of bleeding assessment in immune thrombocytopenia: report from the International Working Group. Blood. 2013;121:2596-606.

38. Rodeghiero F. Is ITP a thrombophilic disorder? Am J Hematol. 2016;91:39-45.

39. Bussel JB, Kuter DJ, Pullarkat V, Lyons RM, Guo M, Nichol JL. Safety and efficacy of long-term treatment with romiplostim in thrombocytopenic patients with chronic ITP. Blood. 2009;113:2161-71.

40. Swan D, Newland A, Rodegheiro F, Thachil J. Thrombosis in immune thrombocytopenia - current status and future perspectives. Br J Haematol. 2021;194 (5):822-834.

41. Al-Samkari H, Cronin A, Arnold DM, Rodeghiero F, Grace RF. Extensive Variability in Platelet, Bleeding, and QOL Outcome Measures in Adult and Pediatric ITP: Communication from the ISTH SSC Subcommittee on Platelet Immunology. J Thromb Haemost. 2021;19(9): 2348-2354.

42. Zeng Y, Duan X, Xu J, Ni X. TPO receptor agonist for chronic idiopathic thrombocytopenic purpura. Cochrane Database Syst Rev. 2011:CD008235. 10.1002/14651858.CD008235.pub2.

43. Virk ZM, Kuter DJ, Al-Samkari H. An evaluation of avatrombopag for the treatment of thrombocytopenia. Expert Opin Pharmacother. 2021;22(3):273-280.

# 9. Decision making in the management of children with ITP

It is well known that variation exists, both between and within countries, on the management strategy for children diagnosed with ITP. Data published in 2001 from the Intercontinental Cooperative ITP Study Group (ICIS) indicate that globally, over 70 % of children with newly diagnosed ITP were admitted to hospital following their diagnosis, whereas almost 30 % were discharged home. Similarly, across 38 countries, approximately 1/3 of such children were observed, 1/3 received IVIg, and 1/3 were treated with corticosteroids [1]. More recent publications by the same investigators indicate that only 20 % of children with ITP receive platelet enhancing treatment [22].

How is one to explain such variation?

Differences in local and cultural practices, namely ethnicity, medical and religious beliefs, systems of health care funding, the proximity of patients to medical centers, individual acceptance of therapies and evolving practice patterns over time have all been cited as plausible explanations [2]. In an age of evidence-based guidelines and standardized order sets, should these differences be viewed as problems to be remedied, or practices to be applauded? One may find solace in such practice variation by viewing the management of ITP as a "preference-sensitive decision".

## 9.1. A preference-sensitive decision

Preference-sensitive decisions are ones in which multiple options exist, all of which are medically reasonable to pursue. That is, while there are advantages and disadvantages to each alternative, the benefits of one single option do not clearly outweigh the potential risks of another [3]. Consider, then, a child with newly diagnosed ITP. While natural history dictates spontaneous resolution in 89 % of cases [4, 23], 3 % of patients will present with severe bleeding and intracranial hemorrhage is estimated to occur in 0.17 % [5, 6]. Treatment pathways include observation, an option both well studied and widely practiced, along with IVIg, corticosteroids, and less often anti-D, as the mainstays of traditional, active therapy [7, 8, 22]. Importantly, studies to date have not found a relationship between the various initial therapies (including observation) and the subsequent development of severe bleeding [5, 6]. Provided that patients are stable and not actively bleeding, their management presents the health care provider with a preference-sensitive choice.

Being confronted with a preference-sensitive choice allows one to consider the patient's or family's values in the decision making process. Whereas one family may feel security in a hospital admission, another may feel equal comfort returning to their home following their child's diagnosis. Similarly, how risk averse an individual is may dictate their acceptance of observation versus active treatment. Should active therapy be pursued, some families will have strong beliefs with respect to blood products, whereas others will wish to avoid the adverse effects of corticosteroids. Individual factors also require consideration when thought is given to observation, including discussions regarding health related quality of life (HRQoL), anticipatory guidance with respect to bleeding risk, reliability of follow-up, activity level of the child, and consideration of upcoming procedures [7].

Similar complex decision making is encountered in the setting of chronic ITP with ever expanding options: observation, splenectomy, rituximab and thrombopoetin receptor agonists (TPO-RA) [9]. Each option has its pros and cons. While splenectomy is the most effective approach, the fact that it is "irreversible" causes many patients and families to hesitate choosing this surgical option. Rituximab provides a sustained response in only 20-30 % of patients, but has a fairly good safety profile [10]. TPO-RAs are effective in 60-80 % of patients but are expensive and require an indefinite duration of treatment [11-13]. Consequently, many patients and their families decide to simply "live with it", but are left with sub optimal HRQoL [14, 15]. Updated guidelines published concurrently in 2019 by the American Society of Hematology (ASH) and the international ITP community recommend using TPO-Ras over rituximab and splenectomy but qualify that it is conditional, based on very low certainty in the evidence of effects [24, 25]. The decision making process for chronic ITP involves many factors, including the impact of the illness on the patient and family. When considering splenectomy or rituximab, families must manage the leap from chronic ITP, a disease they know well, to an immune deficient state, about which they are unfamiliar. The uncertainty of response is a difficult reality, since the possibility of proceeding with a treatment or surgery, ultimately with no effect, always exists. Individual differences in how families cope with uncertainty require consideration. TPO-RA therapy requires either weekly subcutaneous injections or significant alterations in diet for the oral preparation [26]. Obtaining approval from drug insurance providers can be challenging, rendering cost a significant barrier for many families.

## 9.2. Shared decision making

How, then, can the health care professional best support a family in making a treatment decision congruent with their personal values? Shared decision making, in which the family and provider work together to reach a decision, is an ideal route to achieve a high quality decision, one that is not only in line with families' values, but is also informed, and associated with minimal regret [16]. Shared decision making encompasses an information exchange between the family and their clinicians, where information is synthesized about medical evidence and patient preferences, and conclusions are drawn about which course of action is most consistent with those preferences [17]. It may be viewed as midway on a spectrum between autonomous (where the patient or parent is fully responsible for making the decision) and paternalistic decision making (where the physician assumes full responsibility); when used effectively, shared decision making can contribute towards genuine patient-centered care [16, 18].

Patient-centered care has been identified as an Institute of Medicine priority for improvement in the United States health care system, defined as "providing care that is respectful of and responsive to individual patient preferences, needs, and values, and ensuring that patient values guide all clinical decisions" [19]. As a global community of health care professionals caring for children with ITP – a true example of a preference-sensitive entity – it behooves us to adopt a shared decision making approach, as a means to achieve patient-centered care.

The provision of such an ideal level of care, however, is complex, and in the pediatric context is at the nascent stage of exploration. The child-parent-physician triad is unique to pediatric decision making, and limits the generalizability of adult-focused literature on decision support [16]. Tools supporting pediatric shared decision making have increased in the literature since 2010, with evidence supporting their role in reducing decisional conflict and increasing knowledge [27, 28]. In their narrative review of pediatric decision making, Lipstein et al. found that overall, parents prefer taking an active role in decision making for their child, and are interested in a collaborative approach, as opposed to either autonomous or paternalistic methods. The role of the child in the decision making process is also a unique consideration, expected to vary based on the patient's age, developmental stage, level of acuity, and with the timeliness with which a choice must be determined [16]. A systematic review of shared decision making in pediatrics found that the majority focus on engaging the caregiver alone, while fewer engaged the patient or the parent-patient dyad in the decision making process [27].

Providing support through the decision making process, both in determining the families' preferences for involvement in decision-making and in effectively providing a shared decision making experience, is warranted. Tools designed to complement physician counseling, such as patient decision aids, are one well researched method of providing decision support [20]. Patient decision aids are developed in an evidence-based manner; provide information about therapeutic options and their associated risks and benefits; and may include values clarification techniques [21]. Through randomized controlled trials, decision aids have been shown to provide effective decision support, resulting in a positive effect on the decision making process [17].

## 9.3. Conclusion

The global variation apparent in the management of children with ITP, a preference-sensitive choice, should be cautiously applauded. Cautiously, as it remains to be determined whether the differences are the result of paternalistic approaches to decision making which vary between centers, or whether variation is due to the practice of patient-centered care via shared decision making. Centers of care would do well to examine their own practice, to consider which approach to decision making is being utilized, and to work toward a process where evidence-based information may be considered alongside individual family values. Through such process improvement, a true family-centered model of care may be realized for children with ITP.

## References

1. Kuhne T, Imbach P, Bolton-Maggs PH, et al. Newly diagnosed idiopathic thrombocytopenic purpura in childhood: an observational study. Lancet 2001;358:2122-2125

2. Imbach P, Kuhne T, Zimmerman S. New developments in idiopathic thrombocytopenic purpura (ITP): cooperative, prospective studies by the Intercontinental Childhood ITP Study Group. J Pediatr Hematol Oncol 2003;25 (Suppl 1):S74-S76

3. Wennberg JE, O'Connor AM, Collins ED, Weinstein JN. Extending the P4P agenda, part 1: how Medicare can improve patient decision making and reduce unnecessary care. Health Aff (Millwood) 2007;26:1564-1574

4. Beck CE, Nathan PC, Parkin PC, et al. Corticosteroids versus intravenous immune globulin for the treatment of acute immune thrombocytopenic purpura in children: a systematic review and meta-analysis of randomized controlled trials. J Pediatr 2005;147:521-527

5. Kuhne T, Buchanan GR, Zimmerman S, et al. A prospective comparative study of 2540 infants and children with newly diagnosed idiopathic thrombocytopenic purpura (ITP) from the Intercontinental Childhood ITP Study Group. J Pediatr 2003;143:605-608

6. Neunert CE, Buchanan GR, Imbach P, Bolton-Maggs PH, et al. Severe hemorrhage in children with newly diagnosed immune thrombocytopenic purpura. Blood 2008;112:4003-4008

7. Neunert C, Lim W, Crowther M, Cohen A, et al. The American Society of Hematology 2011 evidence-based practice guideline for immune thrombocytopenia. Blood 2011;117:4190-4207

8. Provan D, Stasi R, Newland AC, et al. International consensus report on the investigation and management of primary immune thrombocytopenia. Blood 2010;115: 168-186

9. Ghanima W, Godeau B, Cines DB, Bussel JB. How I treat immune thrombocytopenia: the choice between splenectomy or a medical therapy as a second-line treatment. Blood 2012;120:960-969

10. Patel VL, Mahevas M, Lee SY, et al. Outcomes 5 years after response to rituximab therapy in children and adults with immune thrombocytopenia. Blood 2012; 119:5989-5995

11. Bussel JB, Buchanan GR, Nugent DJ, et al. A randomized, double-blind study of romiplostim to determine its safety and efficacy in children with immune thrombocytopenia. Blood 2011;118:28-36

12. Bussel JB, Cheng G, Saleh MN, et al. Eltrombopag for the treatment of chronic idiopathic thrombocytopenic purpura. N Engl J Med 2007;357:2237-2247

13. Kuter DJ, Rummel M, Boccia R, et al. Romiplostim or standard of care in patients with immune thrombocytopenia. N Engl J Med 2010;363:1889-1899

14. George JN, Mathias SD, Go RS, et al. Improved quality of life for romiplostim-treated patients with chronic immune thrombocytopenic purpura: results from two randomized, placebo-controlled trials. Br J Haematol 2009;144:409-415

15. Klaassen RJ, Blanchette VS, Barnard D, et al. Validity, reliability, and responsiveness of a new measure of health-related quality of life in children with immune thrombocytopenic purpura: the Kids' ITP Tools. J Pediatr 2007;150:510-515

16. Lipstein EA, Brinkman WB, Britto MT. What is known about parents' treatment decisions? A narrative review of pediatric decision making. Med Decis Making 2012;32:246-258

17. Stacey D, Bennett CL, Barry MJ, et al. Decision aids for people facing health treatment or screening decisions. Cochrane Database Syst Rev 2011;10:CD001431

18. Epstein RM, Peters E. Beyond information: exploring patients' preferences. JAMA 2009;302:195-197

19. Institute of Medicine, Committee on Quality of Health Care in America. Crossing the Quality Chasm: A New Health System for the 21st Century. Washington, DC: National Academy Press; 2009

20. O'Connor AM, Legare F, Stacey D. Risk communication in practice: the contribution of decision aids. BMJ 2003;327:736-740

21. O'Connor A. Using patient decision aids to promote evidence-based decision making. ACP J Club 2001;135: A11-A12

22. Schifferli A, Holbro A, Chitlur M, Coslovsky M, Imbach P, Donato H, Elalfy M, Graciela E, Grainger J, Holzhauer S, Riccheri C, Rodeghiero F, Ruggeri M, Tamary H, Uglova T, Wu R, Kühne T; Intercontinental Cooperative ITP Study Group (ICIS). A comparative prospective observational study of children and adults

with immune thrombocytopenia: 2-year follow-up. Am J Hematol. 2018;93(6):751-759.

23. Heitink-Pollé KMJ, Uiterwaal CSPM, Porcelijn L, Tamminga RYJ, Smiers FJ, van Woerden NL, Wesseling J, Vidarsson G, Laarhoven AG, de Haas M, Bruin MCA; TIKI Investigators. Intravenous immunoglobulin vs observation in childhood immune thrombocytopenia: a randomized controlled trial. Blood. 2018;132(9):883-891.

24. Neunert C, Terrell DR, Arnold DM, Buchanan G, Cines DB, Cooper N, Cuker A, Despotovic JM, George JN, Grace RF, Kühne T, Kuter DJ, Lim W, McCrae KR, Pruitt B, Shimanek H, Vesely SK. American Society of Hematology 2019 guidelines for immune thrombocytopenia. Blood Adv. 2019;3(23):3829-3866.

25. Provan D, Arnold DM, Bussel JB, Chong BH, Cooper N, Gernsheimer T, Ghanima W, Godeau B, González-López TJ, Grainger J, Hou M, Kruse C, McDonald V, Michel M, Newland AC, Pavord S, Rodeghiero F, Scully M, Tomiyama Y, Wong RS, Zaja F, Kuter DJ. Updated international consensus report on the investigation and management of primary immune thrombocytopenia. Blood Adv. 2019;3(22):3780-3817.

26. Neunert C, Despotovic J, Haley K, Lambert MP, Nottage K, Shimano K, et al. Thrombopoietin Receptor Agonist Use in Children: Data From the Pediatric ITP Consortium of North America ICON2 Study. Pediatr Blood Cancer. 2016;63(8):1407-13.

27. Wyatt KD, List B, Brinkman WB, Prutsky Lopez G, Asi N, Erwin P, Wang Z, Domecq Garces JP, Montori VM, LeBlanc A. Shared Decision Making in Pediatrics: A Systematic Review and Meta-analysis. Acad Pediatr. 2015;15(6):573-83.

28. Boland L, Graham ID, Légaré F, Lewis K, Jull J, Shephard A, Lawson ML, Davis A, Yameogo A, Stacey D. Barriers and facilitators of pediatric shared decision-making: a systematic review. Implement Sci. 2019;14 (1):7.

# 10. ITP in childhood: a problem-oriented review of the management

Immune thrombocytopenia (ITP) is an autoimmune disorder with three forms according to the duration of thrombocytopenia:

- newly diagnosed ITP (3 months)
- persistent ITP (3-12 months), and
- chronic ITP (more than 12 months) [1]

This classification covers both children and adults. ITP occurs in children with a peak age of 1-6 years and the incidence ranges between 2 and 6 of 100,000 children per year. ITP is accompanied by many controversies in diagnosis and management, due to the fact that ITP appears as thrombocytopenia (platelet count <150 x $10^9$/L) with different pathophysiological mechanisms and etiologies. This heterogeneity is one of the reasons of various and sometimes unexpected platelet responses to the various therapeutics. The controversies are further fuelled by a lack of clinical data, particularly with a paucity of investigator-driven controlled randomized clinical trials with an appropriate long-term follow-up time. Furthermore, one of the main goals of treatment, the prevention of patients from serious bleeding, such as intracranial hemorrhage (ICH), is difficult to investigate and will probably never be answered by a prospective trial, as ICH has been shown to be a rare event in patients with ITP and thus, an enormous number of patients would be needed to design an adequately powered trial. Furthermore based on the various pathophysiological mechanisms of ITP it always must be assumed, that the study population is heterogenous demanding large patient numbers.

It has been accepted since decades that the platelet number serves as a treatment endpoint, although its significance is limited. Most of the recent guidelines acknowledge this limitation and recommend a strategy neglecting the platelet count in children with minor bleeding or in patients with chronic ITP. Alternative endpoints other than the platelet count are still poorly defined in clinical every-day situations, and in clinical research. The platelet count is traditionally the main laboratory feature of a patient with ITP and considered to be a gold standard of the assessment of patients with ITP. It is preferred to be an indicator of bleeding risk, and to be a basis for further diagnostic, preventive and therapeutic interventions in clinical situations and in clinical research trials to study the natural history of ITP, to use and study platelet enhancing drugs and to plan new treatment strategies. However, the platelet count is nothing more than a surrogate outcome measure. It does not exactly do what is expected from it: to be an exact indicator of the bleeding risk of an individual patient and to indicate the overall burden of ITP. Although many prospective trials have been designed to assess the dynamics of platelet number increase within a certain time interval upon intervention of study drug against standard treatment or placebo, it has never been shown, that this is of clinical benefit for the patient. Moreover, the assessment of the platelet count is associated with several problems including pre-analytical and analytical difficulties, and the use of different methods of platelet measurements in multi-center trials resulting in difficulties of comparing laboratory results. Bleeding is a symptom with a highly complex hemostaseological background and the result of individual, acquired and inherited factors. Thus, the platelet number reflects an information fragment of the extraordinarily complex system of primary hemostasis. Platelet function may represent a more appropriate measurement. However, it is affected by many endogenous and exogenous factors and remains – although feasible – an analytical problem and is not appropriate as a bedside test, leaving the clinician with the platelet count, which reflects limited information on hemostatic function.

Alternative treatment endpoints other than the platelet count need to be developed and validated (☞ Table 10.1). They may reflect more adequately the individual bleeding risk, the burden of ITP, and the requirements of the patients. Clinical endpoints, such as bleeding, fatigue and health-related quality of life, have been assessed and validated. Pediatric bleeding scores (☞ Table 10.2) have been developed to standardize bleeding symptoms and to assess the bleeding risk [2, 3]. Feasibility of these bleeding scores were demonstrated in an international prospective registry, and may add important information of hemostasis in patients with ITP [4].

Nevertheless, these bleeding scores and their application in the clinical every day situation needs improvement and validation by further research. An international working group under the leadership of F. Rodeghiero [1] developed a tool to adequately investigate and document bleeding. More research should be done in adjusting bleeding scores and the dynamics of bleeding, treatment requirements according to bleeding scores will remain a clinical challenge.

| ITP – Treatment endpoints |
|---|
| • Platelet count |
| • Bleeding signs |
| • Health-related quality of life |
| • Fatigue |
| • Side effects and complications of platelet-enhancing drug treatment |
| • Economic aspects |

***Table 10.1:*** Treatment endpoints in patients with ITP.

| Asymptomatic |
|---|
| A low platelet count was discovered by chance when the child was having a blood test for other reasons |
| Mild symptoms |
| Bruising and petechiae; occasional minor epistaxis, very little or no interference with daily living |
| Moderate |
| More severe skin manifestations with some mucosal lesions and more troublesome epistaxis and menorrhagia |
| Severe |
| Bleeding episodes (epistaxis, melena, and/or menorrhagia) requiring hospital admissions and/or blood transfusions; symptoms seriously interfering with quality of life |

***Table 10.2:*** Clinical classification of ITP according to Bolton-Maggs J, Pediatr Hematol Oncol. 2003;25:S47-S51.

Although health-related quality of life is difficult to assess in patients with ITP, it has been developed for and used in patients with hemophilia and this experience advanced the development of tools for patients with ITP. The Kids' ITP Tools (KIT) [5, 6] is such an instrument, however, there are still many open questions delaying its clinical use. It can be questioned whether health-related quality of life can be measured at all. Nevertheless, different research groups are evaluating current and developing new tools. Side effects and complications of drug treatment should be considered as additional treatment endpoints and are difficult to be assessed in a standardized way. As platelet enhancing drug treatment includes many side effects, which may be serious, e.g. infectious diseases or organ dysfunctions, a systematic assessment of such side effects is an important endpoint, which has to be considered carefully against bleeding risk and quality of life in both clinical practice and clinical trials. Drug treatment cannot be evaluated without assessing economic aspects. Although economic aspects are difficult to assess, it is mandatory to develop tools to adequately assess economics of drugs and management strategies in a standardized manner [7].

Primary ITP is caused by immune dysregulation and represents a diagnosis of exclusion, which makes differential diagnostic considerations particularly important. Once the diagnosis of ITP is made and the clinician is convinced about this diagnosis, the management of children with ITP becomes less stressful and one might choose from the current treatment strategies reflected by guidelines [15, 16, 34] and is discussed later in this chapter. The differential diagnosis of children with newly diagnosed ITP (☞ Table 10.3) who do not respond to first-line therapy or who have chronic primary ITP (thrombocytopenia lasting more than 12 months) represents a challenge. These children should be accompanied by their clinician with continuous careful diagnostic considerations and investigations based on clinical and laboratory characteristics [31]. The diagnosis "primary ITP" should always be challenged and assessed according to the clinical situation of the patient.

## 10.1. Clinical presentation and diagnosis

The male:female ratio is approximately 1:1, however in young children, particularly in infants, males are more often seen than females. ITP is characterized by an abrupt onset of hemorrhagic diathesis in an otherwise healthy child. An infectious disease, often a viral infection of the respira-

| Pre-analytical and analytical reasons of thrombocytopenia | | |
|---|---|---|
| • Pseudothrombocytopenia | | |
| **Acquired peripheral destruction** | | |
| • Primary ITP<br>• Post-transfusion purpura<br>• Drug-induced thrombocytopenia (e.g., drug-induced thrombocytopenia)<br>• Cardiovascular diseases<br>• Antiphospholipid autoantibody syndrome | • Secondary ITP<br>• Disseminated intravascular coagulation<br>• Splenic sequestration<br>• Infectious diseases<br>• Pregnancy | • Neonatal alloimmune thrombocytopenia<br>• Thrombotic thrombocytopenic purpura<br>• Kassabach-Merrit syndrome<br>• Systemic lupus erythematosus |
| **Acquired deficiency of production** | | |
| • Drug-induced thrombocytopenia<br>• Bone marrow infiltration by neoplastic process | • Infectious diseases<br>• Myelodysplastic syndrome<br>• Aplastic anemia | • Alcohol<br>• Hematological neoplasms |
| **Inherited thrombocytopenia** | | |
| • Thrombasthenia Glanzmann<br>• Mediterranean thrombocytopenia<br>• Velocardiofacial syndrome, DiGeorge syndrome<br>• Congenital amegakaryocytemia<br>• Fanconi anemia | • Bernard-Soulier syndrome<br>• Gray platelet syndrome<br>• Wiskott-Aldrich syndrome<br>• Thrombocytopenia with absent or dysplastic radii syndrome<br>• GATA1 mutation | • MYH-9 related (May-Hegglin anomaly, Fechtner, Epstein, Sebastian syndrome)<br>• Paris-Trousseau thrombocytopenia/Jacobsen syndrome<br>• X-linked thrombocytopenia<br>• Autoimmune lymphoproliferative syndrome |

***Table 10.3:*** Differential diagnosis of children with ITP (incomplete list) [32, 33].

tory or gastrointestinal tract, precedes thrombocytopenia days or weeks in approximately two thirds of patients. Whether such events have anything to do with subsequent accelerated platelet destruction resulting in thrombocytopenia is unclear. ITP was reported after immunizations, particularly with life vaccines with an estimated risk of 1 in 24,000 doses [8].

Easy bruising, petechiae and subcutaneous hematomas, but also mucosal bleeding may occur, however major hemorrhage defined by intracranial or other overt internal or mucous membrane bleeding, which results in anemia, or which requires local treatment, seems to be rare, although a majority of children presents with a platelet count of $<20 \times 10^9$/L. The Intercontinental Cooperative ITP Study Group (ICIS) Registry II reported 863 children with newly diagnosed ITP [4]. "Severe bleeding" was defined as bleeding episodes (epistaxis, melena, menorrhagia, and/or intracranial hemorrhage) requiring hospital admission and/or blood transfusions, i.e. symptoms interfering seriously with quality of life. At diagnosis, 25 of 863 children (3 %) experienced a severe hemorrhage, with only one patient having had central nervous system bleeding. The other 24 patients had mucosal bleeding, including epistaxis, mouth, gastrointestinal tract, urinary tract, and uterus bleeding. New severe bleeding events within the first 28 days after the diagnosis of ITP was observed in 3 patients (1.7 %) among 173 patients with moderate bleeding at diagnosis of ITP, and was observed in 3 of 505 patients (0.3 %) with no or mild bleeding and a platelet count of $\leq 20 \times 10^9$/L at diagnosis of ITP.

The initial phase of pediatric ITP is often dramatic and results in fear of life-threatening bleeding in physicians, parents and patients. The presence of an experienced hematologist during this phase of ITP, when diagnosis and management decisions are made, is the basis of an adequate patient-physician relationship. There is growing evidence that severe bleeding in children with ITP is rare and that a minority of patients experiences the most worrisome bleeding type, ICH, often at a time point other than the immediate time following the diagnosis of ITP. Only retrospective data material is available for the description of ICH and relatively little is known about patient characteristics presenting this bleeding type and the outcome of these patients, although ICH represents a main rationale to treat patients with drugs or with splenectomy. Retrospective clinical data indicate that many ICH episodes occur in patients despite they were treated initially and that more than 50% of children reported in the literature did not have a fatal outcome.

Diagnosis of ITP is based on personal and familial history, physical examination and a complete blood count with blood smear. Besides hemorrhagic diathesis the child with ITP occurs healthy with marked thrombocytopenia but otherwise normal blood counts and normal leukocyte differentiation. Additional laboratory tests are indicated,

1) if the clinical history or physical examination reveal any aspects, which deviate from the above mentioned description of ITP, which should direct the clinician to think of other causes of thrombocytopenia (☞ Table 10.3),

2) if other abnormalities of the complete blood count or the blood smear are detected,

3) if thrombocytopenia of treated or untreated patients persists, and

4) in therapy-refractory ITP.

Any atypical findings in history, physical examination or laboratory studies should initiate a differential diagnostic work-up.

Chronic ITP was arbitrarily defined by a duration of thrombocytopenia of more than 6 months, however, a duration of more than 12 months occurs more adequate and was accepted by an International Working Group [1]. This group defined a new group of patients, called persistent ITP, with a duration of thrombocytopenia of 3-12 months, in order to describe patients not reaching spontaneous remission or not maintaining complete response off therapy. It has been shown in childhood ITP, that approximately 25 % of children with thrombocytopenia after 6 months will have a platelet count of >150 x $10^9$/L at 12 months [10] and that remission occurring later than 6 months is always possible [11]. Chronic ITP occurs in children in 20-30 %, depending on its definition, and is rarely associated with severe bleeding. There is a substantial potential of spontaneous or treatment-induced improvement or "remission", however, long-term follow-up data over years are limited.

## 10.2. Prevention from and therapy of bleeding

The management of children with ITP is a subject of ongoing debate and controversies. Once the diagnosis of primary ITP is made, the management of the initial phase of thrombocytopenia is associated with several problems:

1) ITP is a diagnosis of exclusion, however, according to current guidelines, it is not appropriate to include laboratory analyses other than a complete blood count with blood smear. Thus, primary ITP is based on vague presumptions during the time when management decisions are drawn.

2) The individual bleeding risk is unclear and cannot be estimated adequately by clinical signs and by laboratory tests, which makes conversation with the patient and parents difficult and often frustrating. Inexperienced physicians may be forced by patients, parents, but also colleagues to choose an inappropriate management.

3) therapy-refractory ITP. There is now clinical and laboratory information to predict chronic ITP at first presentation of a child with ITP (age ≥11 years, insidious onset of bleeding (more than 2 weeks), no preceding infection and higher platelet counts at presentation, i.e. ≥20 x $10^9$/L).

Various practice guidelines have been published since the 1990's. Since the first guidelines for the management of patients with ITP occurred in the UK [12] and were subsequently revised [13], other national guidelines appeared in United States [14], which were revised in 2019 [15], and in Europe [34] and in Asia, as well as international consensus reports [16]. Problems of these guidelines include

1) Inconsistency in management recommendations, this is particularly true for the management of children with newly diagnosed ITP.

2) It has been demonstrated that guidelines are poorly followed.

3) The heterogeneous background of ITP is poorly reflected in these guidelines yet.

4) Guidelines are based on expert opinion and consensus of selected experts, rather than on clinical evidence.

5) Guidelines cannot solve the problem, that the main treatment endpoint, the avoidance of severe bleeding, particularly ICH, may hardly ever be assessed adequately in a randomized prospective trial, and

6) a certain degree of rigidity, as guidelines need strict methodology and time to be elaborated.

Algorithms have been developed to facilitate the investigations and the management of patients with ITP. While such algorithms may be appropriate in disorders with a common background and a more homogeneous phenotype, they may not reflect the requirements of patients with ITP and tend to over-simplify the management problems encountered in patients with ITP. They should be kept in a general way in order to respect the many aspects and factors affecting the phenotype of ITP [8]. ITP is of heterogeneous background with many possible and often unknown causes, but also with a phenotype affected by different disease modifying endogenous and exogenous factors, making an individual approach more appropriate. This heterogeneity must also be considered, when analyzing and interpreting reports of clinical trials, their methodology, biometrical analyses and results [17].

## 10.3. Non-intervention

Watchful waiting without drug treatment is based on the observation, that severe bleeding in children with ITP is rare although the majority of patients presents with a platelet count of <20 x $10^9$/L. Since the publication of the British and American practice guidelines, several studies, including a population-based study from the Nordic countries [18], audits in the UK [19], a retrospective and prospective surveys in Germany [20, 21], and the ICIS registries [4, 22-24, 36] revealed a very low incidence of severe hemorrhage, particularly ICH, in children with ITP, being less than 0.5 %. There is growing evidence that the risk-benefit ratio is clearly towards benefit, when children with newly diagnosed ITP are observed and be not treated to raise the platelet count. There is no randomized clinical trial which could demonstrate clinical benefit from a rapid platelet raise provoked by platelet-enhancing drugs. However, this management requires

1) an informed consent from patients and parents,

2) an experienced hematologist and

3) an adequate infrastructure.

It should be taken into consideration that the incidence of severe bleeding is not 0 % and that differential diagnostic considerations must always accompany the clinician. This complex situation needs a collaboration of general practitioners with hematologists with referral of the patients to a pediatric hematology/oncology center. A collaboration between general practitioners and hematologists is a basis for a successful management. Further measures to prevent bleeding include avoidance of platelet function inhibiting drugs, such as aspirin and avoidance of head injury, although recommendations to reduce activity in children with ITP are questionable and discussable.

## 10.4. Intervention

As discussed above a trial investigating the main goal of treatment, i.e. preventing a child with ITP from severe bleeding, mainly from ICH, is not feasible, because of the rarity of such severe bleeding events. Therefore, the indication to treat a child with platelet-enhancing drugs remains vague and should be based on individual aspects, including the location and severity of bleeding, patient and parent information, experience of physician, patient-physician relationship and maintenance of follow-up visits by the same care team, including a collaboration of general practitioners and hematologists [38]. The goal of the treatment needs to be always defined and communicated to patients and parents. ITP requires time for conversation of involved persons.

### Treatment goals

Several different treatment goals can be defined and management may be planned and performed accordingly (☞ Table 10.4). Whether non-interventional or interventional strategies are chosen depends on the patient, the available evidence and the experience of the clinician. Again, collaboration with an experienced pediatric hematology/ oncology center is highly advisable. Standard therapy in children with ITP for prevention and treatment of bleeding consists of corticosteroids and polyvalent immunoglobulins and aims to reduce autoantibody production and to interfere with immunological processes (immune modulation), leading to peripheral platelet destruction. Unfortunately, these therapeutic options have many side effects and are described elsewhere. Table 9.5 describes most common treatment regimens with these standard drugs. Corticosteroids and immunoglobulins are also termed "first-line treatments", however, it must be kept into consideration, that these treatments may be effective in patients who are receiving "second-line treatments".

| ITP – Treatment goals in children |
|---|
| • Prevention from severe bleeding<br>• Treatment of bleeding<br>• Emergency treatment<br>• Immune modulation aiming for cure of the autoimmune process of platelet destruction in patients with persistent and chronic ITP<br>• Transient increase of platelets to stabilize hemostasis, e.g. before surgical interventions<br>• Attempts to defer splenectomy<br>• Reduction of concomitant therapies<br>• Reduction of use of rescue therapies<br>• Reduction of corticosteroids as soon as possible |

***Table 10.4:*** Treatment goals in children with ITP.

| | |
|---|---|
| Oral prednisone/ prednisolone | • 4 mg/kg/day for 4 days<br>• 2 mg/kg for 14-21 days |
| Oral or intravenous methylprednisolone | • 30 mg/kg, maximum dose 1g/day for 3 days |
| Intravenous immunoglobulines | • 0.8 g/kg/day for 1-2 days |

***Table 10.5:*** Medical management of children with ITP.

## Life-threatening bleeding

Treatment of life-threatening bleeding is established, although no comparative clinical trials have been performed.

It includes
- platelet transfusions
- intravenous corticosteroids (preferable intravenous methylprednisolone 30 mg/kg, maximum dose 1 g) and
- intravenous immunoglobulins (0.8 g/kg)

Severe bleeding represents the only indication where platelet transfusion may be of clinical benefit. The patient may also benefit from continuous platelet transfusions. These therapies may be repeated on day 2 and 3 according to the clinical situation. Emergency splenectomy has been performed and success was reported in case reports. There is still limited experience with recombinant activated factor VII, although there is a potential of this drug to be effective, reflected by several case series and reports [25]. The new thrombopoietin receptor agonists may be indicated in life-threatening bleeding, however there is no clinical experience yet.

## Immune modulation

Immune modulation aims to target the immune system and to modify dysregulated immune responses resulting in improvement of thrombocytopenia. This treatment goal is particularly important to prevent patients from chronic ITP. It may be achieved with first-line treatments, such as repeated administrations of immunoglobulins or pulse oral dexamethasone . The latter is administered during 6 months with 4 consecutive days per month, independent of the platelet count [26]. Dexamethasone has also been demonstrated to be successful, if it is administered in 4-day pulses every 14 days as first-line treatment [27]. A newer drug interfering with and potentially modulating the immune system is rituximab, a chimeric human and murine monoclonal antibody directed against CD20 antigen expressed on B-lymphocytes of different development stages. Rituximab promotes antibody-dependent cell-mediated cytotoxicity and complement-dependent cytotoxicity and exerts its cytotoxic effects by eliminating most circulating B-cells which recover within 6 to 12 months. It has been approved for treatment of non-Hodgkin's B-cell lymphoma, rheumatoid arthritis, and chronic lymphocytic leukemia, but has also been shown to be effective in a variety of autoimmune disorders. It has been shown to be effective in children with therapy-refractory chronic ITP [28] and is usually given in a regimen approved for the treatment of non-Hodgkin's lymphoma (375 mg/m² as 4 weekly infusions).

### Transient elevation of platelets

A transient elevation of the platelet count is generally required in patients with persistent or chronic ITP and may be achieved by using the standard drugs, such as corticosteroids, polyvalent immunoglobulins and anti-D, or the thrombopoietin receptor agonists romiplostim, eltrombopag and avatrombopag, which are described elsewhere in this book. Experience with these drugs in children with ITP is increasing and romiplostim and eltrombopag are available and approved also for children in many countries. Standard drugs are indicated for short administrations, but not appropriate for long-term use because of side effects and/or high costs.

### Thrombopoietin-receptor agonists

For adults there are now several thrombopoietin-receptor agonists available with 3 (romiplostim, eltrombopag and avatrombopag) for the indication "ITP". Romiplostim and eltrombopag are also approved for children and avatrombopag is currently studied for pediatric ITP. These drugs are successful therapeutic options with strong efficacy and a well-established safety profile, as second-line drugs and are recently introduced in the first-line in adult ITP. Whether they may even have a certain potential to affect the course of ITP is a matter of current research with the hypothesis that the platelet mass may sensitize the immune system and restore tolerance [35].

## 10.5. Splenectomy

Splenectomy has been known for more than a century to be an effective treatment for children and adults with ITP [39]. Although splenectomy is more established in adults than in children with ITP, there is limited experience of indications and timing of splenectomy, pre- and post-operative management, and long-term platelet response in children. Guidelines now recommend deferral of splenectomy for at least 12 months. Table 10.6 shows strategies to defer splenectomy, which is important to consider in children with ITP, because

1) there is a high potential of spontaneous or drug-induced improvement or even cure of ITP,

2) there are risks associated with splenectomy, particularly in young children including increased infectious risk, mainly due to encapsulated bacteria, such as pneumococci, *Haemophilus influenzae* type b, and meningococci, surgical morbidity and mortality, and thromboembolism,

3) splenectomized children need long-term follow-up visits and instructions how to behave, e.g. when there is a fever or clinical deterioration, which may affect quality of life,

4) the pre-, peri- and postoperative management is not standardized [29, 37], and

5) the diagnosis of primary ITP may be inadequate.

| Alternatives to splenectomy |
|---|
| • Watchful waiting (at least 12 months) |
| • Careful individual evaluation of risks and benefit |
| • Immune modulation with dexamethasone |
| • Thrombopoietin-receptor agonists |
| • Rituximab |

***Table 10.6:*** Strategies to defer splenectomy.

Splenectomy is performed in children with chronic symptomatic ITP. Usually the laparoscopic technique is preferred. Immunization with vaccines against encapsulated bacteria should be completed before surgery. Postoperative daily prophylaxis with penicillin or an alternative antibiotic in case of penicillin allergy is recommended. There is limited evidence for the penicillin prophylaxis, many experts recommend performing it particularly in young children and the recommendation for duration of this prophylaxis is from 1 year to several years until adulthood.

## 10.6. Conclusions

ITP is a diagnosis of exclusion and thus requires differential diagnostic work-up at adequate time intervals. The platelet count represents a surrogate marker of bleeding risk, which has been used in most studies investigating drug intervention in patients with ITP, and which is still the main laboratory test based on which management decisions are drawn. Guidelines suggest that the platelet count is a factor used for guiding management of patients with ITP but in children with no or minor bleeding, treatment decisicons may be undertaken independently from the platelet count. Additional and alternative outcome measures should be validated and made available as bed-sidetests, such as bleeding, fatigue, and quality of life. The heterogeneity of ITP and lack of clinical evidence require an individual approach of children with ITP, rather than a standardized algorithm.

## References

1. Rodeghiero F, Stasi R, Gernsheimer T, et al. Standardization of terminology, definitions and outcome criteria in immune thrombocytopenic purpura (ITP) of adults and children. Report from an international working group. Blood. 2009;113:2386-2393.

2. Bolton-Maggs PHB, Moon I. Assessment of UK practice for management of acute childhood idiopathic thrombocytopenic purpura against published guidelines. Lancet. 1997;350:620-623.

3. Buchanan GR, Adix L. Grading of hemorrhage in children with idiopathic thrombocytopenic purpura. J Pediatr. 2002;141:683-688.

4. Neunert CE, Buchanan GR, Imbach P, et al. Severe hemorrhage in children with newly diagnosed immune thrombocytopenic purpura. Blood. 2008;112:4003-4008.

5. Klaassen RJ, Blanchette VS, Barnard D, et al. Validity, reliability, and responsiveness of a new measure of health-related quality of life in children with immune thrombocytopenic purpura: The Kids' ITP Tools. J Pediatr. 2007;150:510-515.

6. Heitink-Pollé KMJ, Haverman L, Annink KV, et al. Health-related quality of life in children with newly diagnosed immune thrombocytopenia. Haematologica. 2014;99(9):1525-1531.

7. Weycker D, Hanau A, Hatfield M, et al. Primary immune thrombocytopenia in US clinical practice: incidence and healthcare burden in first 12 months following diagnosis. J Med Econ. 2020;23(2):184-192.

8. Kühne T, Imbach P. Management of children and adolescents with primary immune thrombocytopenia: controversies and solutions. Vox Sanguinis. 2013;104(1):55-66.

9. Farrington, P, Pugh, S, Colville, A, et al. A new method for active surveillance of adverse events from diphtheria / tetanus / pertussis and measles / mumps/ rubella vaccines. Lancet. 1995;345:567-569.

10. Imbach P, Kühne T, Müller D, et al. Childhood ITP: 12 months follow-up data from the prospective registry I of the Intercontinental Childhood ITP Study Group (ICIS). Pediatr Blood Cancer. 2006;46:351-356.

11. Ducassou S, Gourdonneau A, Fernandes H, et al. Second-line treatment trends and long-term outcomes of 392 children with chronic immune thrombocytopenic purpura: the French experience over the past 25 years. Br J Haematol. 2020;189(5):931-942.

12. Eden OB, Lilleyman JS. Guidelines for management of idiopathic thrombocytopenic purpura The British Paediatric Haematology Group. Arch Dis Child. 1992; 67:1056-1058.

13. British Committee for Standards in Haematology General Haematology Task Force. Guidelines for the investigation and management of idiopathic thrombocytopenic purpura in adults, children and in pregnancy. Br J Haematol. 2003;120:574-596.

14. George JN, Woolf SH, Raskob GE, et al. Idiopathic thrombocytopenic purpura. a practice guideline developed by explicit methods for the American Society of Hematology. Blood. 1996;88:3-40.

15. Neunert C, Terrell D, Arnold D, et al. American Society of Hematology 2019 Guidelines for Immune Thrombocytopenia. Blood Advances. 2019;3(23):3829-3866.

16. Provan D, Arndol DR, Bussel JB, et al. Updated international consensus report on the investigation and management of primary immune thrombocytopenia. Blood Advances. 2019; 3(22):3780-3817.

17. Cines DB, Bussel JB, Liebman HA Luning Prak ET. The ITP syndrome: pathogenic and clinical diversity. Blood. 2009;113:6511-6521.

18. Zeller B, Rajantie J, Hedlund-Treutiger I, et al. Childhood idiopathic thrombocytopenic purpura in the Nordic countries: epidemiology and predictors of chronic disease. Acta Paediatr. 2005;94:178-184.

19. Bolton-Maggs PHB, Moon I. Assessment of UK practice for management of acute childhood idiopathic thrombocytopenic purpura against published guidelines. Lancet. 1997;350:620-623.

20. Sutor AH, Harms A, Kaufmehl K. Acute immune thrombocytopenia (ITP) in childhood: retrospective and prospective survey in Germany. Semin Thromb Hemost. 2001;27:253-267.

21. Dickerhoff R, von Ruecker A. The clinical course of immune thrombocytopenic purpura in children who did not receive intravenous immunoglobulins or sustained prednisone treatment. J Pediatr. 2000;137:629-632.

22. Kühne T, Imbach P, Bolton-Maggs PHB, et al. Newly diagnosed idiopathic thrombocytopenic purpura in childhood: an observational study. Lancet. 2001;358: 2122-2125.

23. Kühne T, Buchanan GR, Zimmerman S, et al. A prospective comparative study of 2540 infants and children with newly diagnosed idiopathic thrombocytopenic

purpura (ITP) from The Intercontinental Childhood ITP Study Group. J Pediatr. 2003;143:605-608.

24. Kühne T, Berchtold W, Michaels LA, et al. Newly diagnosed immune thrombocytopenia in children and adults, a comparative prospective observational registry of the Intercontinental Cooperative Immune Thrombocytopenia Study Group. Haematologica. 2011;96:1831-1837.

25. Salama A, Rieke M, Kiesewetter H, von Depka M. Experiences with recombinant FVIIa in the emergency treatment of patients with autoimmune thrombocytopenia: a review of the literature. Ann Hematol. 2009;88: 11-15.

26. Kühne T, Freedman J, Semple JW, et al. Platelet and immune responses to oral cyclic dexamethasone in childhood chronic immune thrombocytopenic purpura. J Pediatr. 1997;130:17-24.

27. Mazzucconi MG, Fazi P, Bernasconi S, et al. Therapy with high-dose dexamethasone (HD-DXM) in previously untreated patients affected by idiopathic thrombocytopenic purpura: a GIMEMAexperience. Blood. 2007; 109:1401-1407.

28. Parodi E, Rivetti E, Amendola G, et al. Long-term follow-up analysis after rituximab therapy in children with refractory symptomatic ITP: identification of factors predictive of a sustained response. Br J Haematol. 2008; 144, 552-558.

29. Kühne T, Blanchette V, Buchanan GR, et al. Splenectomy in children with idiopathic thrombocytopenic purpura: A prospective study of 134 children from the Intercontinental Childhood ITP Study Group. Pediatr Blood Cancer. 2007;49:829-834.

30. Cines DB, Blanchette VS. Immune thrombocytopenic purpura. N Engl J Med. 2002;346:995-1008.

31. Schifferli A, Heiri A, Imbach P, et al. Misdiagnosed thrombocytopenia in children and adolescents: analysis of the Pediatric and Adult Registry on Chronic ITP. Blood Advances. 2021;5(6):1617-1626.

32. Nurden AT, Nurden P. Inherited thrombocytopenias: history, advances and perspectives. Haematologica. 2020;105(8):2004-2019.

33. Bury L, Falcinelli E, Gresele P. Learning the Ropes of Platelet Count Regulation: Inherited Thrombocytopenias. J Clin Med. 2021;10:533.

34. Matzdorff A, Meyer O, Ostermann H, et al. Immune Thrombocytopenia – Current Diagnostics and Therapy: Recommendations of a Joint Working Group of DGHO, ÖGHO, SGH, GPOH, and DGTI. Oncol Res Treat. 2018; 41(suppl 5):1-30.

35. Schifferli A, Nimmerjahn F, Kühne T. Immunomodulation in primary immune thrombocytopenia: a possible role of the Fc fragment of romiplostim? Front Immunol. 2019;10:1196.

36. Schifferli A, Holbro A, Chitlur M, et al. A comparative prospective observational study of children and adults with immune thrombocytopenia: 2-year follow-up. Am J Hematol. 2018;93(6):751-759.

37. Avila ML, Amiri N, Pullenayegum E, et al. Long-term outcomes after splenectomy in children with immune thrombocytopenia: an update on the registry data from the Intercontinental Cooperative ITP Study Group. Haematologica. 2019;105(11):2682-2685.

38. Kühne T. Advances in chemical pharmacotherapy for the treatment of pediatric immune thrombocytopenia. Exp Op Pharmacother. 2018;19(7):667-676.

39. Ducassou S, Fernandes H, Savel H, et al. Prospective Evaluation of the First Option, Second-Line Therapy in Childhood Chronic Immune Thrombocytopenia: Splenectomy or Immunomodulation. J Pediatr. 2021; 231:223-230.

# 11. ITP in adulthood

Primary immune thrombocytopenia (ITP), previously referred as idiopathic thrombocytopenic purpura, is an immune-mediated acquired disorder characterized by isolated thrombocytopenia, defined as a peripheral blood platelet count <100 x $10^9$/L in the absence of any other cause of thrombocytopenia [1] (☞ Table 11.1). ITP is an orphan disease that can occur at any age with an overall incidence of 1.6 to 3.9/100,000 persons and the male-to-female ratio is close to 1, but with significant differences depending on the age group considered. Indeed, ITP shows an age-specific bimodal distribution for men with two incidence peaks observed in boys (<18 years) and in the elderly. In women, the incidence rate is relatively constant [2, 3]. Signs and symptoms of ITP vary widely and

| Type of disease/ condition | Main causes | Useful tests |
|---|---|---|
| Hematologic disorders | • Lymphoproliferative disorders<br>• Myelodysplastic syndromes, leukemias<br>• Other malignancies and fibrosis<br>• Aplastic anemia<br>• Megaloblastic anemia | Full blood count<br>Reticulocyte count<br>Peripheral blood smear<br>Quantitative immunoglobulin level measurement<br>Bone marrow examination* |
| Infectious disorders | • Human immunodeficiency virus (HIV), hepatitis C virus (HCV) or other infections | HIV, HBV and HCV serologies<br>*Helicobacter pylori* breath-test** |
| Toxic | • Drugs including self-medication<br>• Alcohol abuse<br>• Exposure to environmental toxins | History taking |
| Autoimmune disorders | • Systemic lupus erythematosus | Antinuclear antibodies<br>Direct antiglobulin test |
| Primary immuno-deficiency | | Quantitative immunoglobulin level measurement |
| Inherited thrombo-cytopenia | • MYH9-related disease<br>• ANKRD26-related thrombocytopenia<br>• Bernard-Soulier syndrome<br>• ACTN1-related thrombocytopenia<br>• Thrombocytopenia Absent Radius Syndrome (TAR)<br>• Radioulnar synostosis<br>• Congenital amegakaryocytic thrombocytopenia<br>• Wiskott-Aldrich syndrome<br>• Type 2B von Willebrand disease | Mean platelet volume<br>Peripheral blood smear<br>Familial history<br>NGS (next generation sequencing) |
| Liver disease | • Including alcoholic liver cirrhosis | History taking<br>HCV/HBV testing<br>Sonogram of the abdomen |

***Table 11.1:*** Differential diagnosis of thrombocytopenia.
* Bone marrow examination may be informative in patients with abnormalities in the complete blood count or peripheral blood smear, systemic symptoms, hepatosplenomegaly or lymph node enlargement, or no response to first-line treatment.
** In endemic areas or if digestive symptoms are present

may be asymptomatic in at least one-third of the cases. Among symptomatic patients, many have minimal bruising ± mucocutaneous hemorrhage with purpura. These manifestations mainly occur when the platelet count is below 30 x $10^9$/L. Severe visceral bleeding (hematuria, gastrointestinal hemorrhage or intracranial hemorrhage) may infrequently occur when the platelet count is below 10 x $10^9$/L. Depending on disease duration, ITP is classified as newly diagnosed, persistent (duration of 3-12 months) or chronic (duration of ≥12 months) [1]. Whereas ITP in childhood is usually a self-limited disease within few weeks, ITP has a chronic course in about 70 to 80 % of adults.

The etiology of ITP is unknown. Both increased platelet destruction mainly in the spleen, mediated by autoantibodies, and impaired platelet production, which may be autoantibody- and T-cell mediated, play a role in ITP pathophysiology. No biological test can reliably establish the diagnosis of ITP, which remains a diagnosis of exclusion. A presumptive diagnosis is made when the history, physical examination, complete blood count and examination of the peripheral blood smear do not suggest other etiologies of thrombocytopenia. Although non-specific, a positive response to first-line therapy for ITP, such as intravenous immunoglobulins (IVIg) and/or short course of steroids, is also in favor of the diagnosis. A bone marrow aspirate or biopsy is not systematically required [4, 5]. It must however be performed in case of abnormalities in other blood cells, systemic symptoms, hepatosplenomegaly or lymph node enlargement, or when thrombocytopenia does not respond to first-line treatments. An age >60 years is no longer a criterion to perform a bone marrow examination [4]. In ITP, the bone marrow analysis displays no abnormalities with a normal or increased number of megakaryocytes. Cytogenetic testing may be considered if a myelodysplastic syndrome is suspected. The differential diagnosis includes other causes of isolated thrombocytopenia and mainly drug-induced ITP, ITP secondary to other autoimmune diseases (mainly systemic lupus erythematosus and antiphospholipid syndrome), HIV infection and hepatitis C [1, 4].

The overall prognosis of ITP is good with a mortality rate less than 2 % [6] but mortality can rise to 10 % in a subgroup of selected patients refractory to splenectomy or to conventional treatments [7, 8].

We will focus on the treatment of ITP in adults.

## 11.1. Treatment of adult ITP

### 11.1.1. General rules

guidelines emphasize that the aim of treatment is primarily to prevent bleeding and avoid adverse effects of therapy and not to normalize the platelet count. Usually, only patients with a platelet count <30×$10^9$/L and bleeding symptoms require treatment. Corticosteroids (predniso(lo)ne or dexamethasone) are considered as the first-line treatment. The use of intravenous immunoglobulins (IVIg) may be appropriate in patients who present with severe bleeding symptoms. In the updated version of the guidelines, thrombopoietin-receptor agonists (TPO-RAs) and rituximab are now considered as second-line treatments, in addition to splenectomy. The choice of the second-line treatment must be individualized based on factors related to the patient such as comorbidities, age, lifestyle, preferences, medication adherence, and life expectancy, as well as factors related to treatments, including cost-effectiveness, availability of drugs including potential restriction by health care authorities.

### 11.1.2. First-line therapy (initial treatment for newly diagnosed patients)

#### Corticosteroid therapy

Corticosteroids remain the standard of care for the initial management of ITP in adults in the absence of any contraindication to its use (for example severe diabetes, ongoing infection, psychiatric disorders). The standard practice is to initiate treatment with oral prednisone or prednisolone at a dose of 1 mg/kg/day. The duration of treatment (3-6 weeks) and the mode of tapering (rapid or slow) are not consensual [4, 5]. In our practice, we treat patients for 3 weeks, then we taper the dose over one week. A short-term response to corticosteroids is observed in >60 % of patients, but only 40 % will achieve a durable response [9]. Dexamethasone at 40 mg/day for 4 days is now considered as a valid alternative, as it has the same efficacy and tolerance profile and seems to induce a more rapid rise in platelet count than predniso(lo)ne, and may therefore be preferred in patients with non-life-threatening moderate-to-severe hemorrhage [5, 9].

### Intravenous immunoglobulins

IVIg rapidly increase the platelet count in >70 % of the patients [4]. The effect is however transient and the platelet count returns to its pre-treatment level within 10 to 28 days. The standard dose of IVIg for adults is 1 g/kg given on two consecutive days. A costless strategy is to administer a first infusion of 1 g/kg and to give a subsequent infusion of IVIg at 1 g/kg on day 3 only in case of non-response [10]. A short course of prednisone significantly prolongs the response time to IVIg [11], and should therefore be associated unless contraindicated. Because of the cost and repeated supply tensions of this treatment, the use of IVIg should be reserved for patients with serious bleeding, the severity of which may be assessed using a bleeding score [12], or for those who have contraindication to steroids. In case of risk factors for renal insufficiency (a possible adverse effect of IVIg), such as diabetes, elderly people, pre-existing renal insufficiency, cardiac insufficiency or concomitant use of nephrotoxic drugs, IVIg may be administered at 0.4 g/kg/day for 5 days.

### Intravenous anti-Rh(D) (anti-D)

Anti-D may be used in ITP patients who are rhesus (Rh D) positive, not splenectomized and not severely anemic [13]. However, anti-D is not licensed and not available in many countries, such as in Europa, and may be responsible for hemolytic anemia, disseminated intravascular coagulation and renal failure that may be life-threatening [4]. Therefore, its use is nowadays marginal or even exceptional.

### Life-threatening bleeding

In case of life-threatening bleeding, such as intracerebral hemorrhage bleeding or gynecological or digestive hemorrhage with significant acute anemia, the treatment should include, in addition to general measures, IVIg (1 g/kg/day, on days 1 and 2), steroids (high-dose intravenous methylprednisolone 15 mg/kg/day up to 1 g for 3 days, then prednisone orally), and platelet transfusions (every 8 hours, up to a hemostatic platelet threshold). Whereas platelet transfusions are usually not relevant in ITP because the transfused platelets are removed by platelet auto-antibodies, platelet transfusions may be associated with a transient resolution of bleeding, rapid restoration of adequate platelet counts and minimal adverse effects [14-16]. Vinca alkaloids (vincristine and vinblastine) may be useful in non-responders to this combination therapy [17]. Because of a lower neurologic and digestive toxicity, vinblastine at 5 mg/m² (up to 8 mg) should be in our opinion preferred. The potential neurotoxicity of repeated vinca alkaloid administration is however a limiting factor for their long-term use, especially in the elderly. In addition, full dose TPO-RAs should be discussed for the most severe cases and seems well tolerated in our experience, although an increased risk of thrombo-embolic events is possible [18].

### First-line therapy (summary)

- Oral prednisone remains the first-line treatment for ITP in adults. Prolonged treatment (more than 2 months) is associated with high risk of severe complications and should be strongly avoided.
- High-dose dexamethasone is a valid alternative to oral prednisone/prednisolone.
- IVIg should be reserved for patients with severe bleeding. The recommended dose of 2 g/kg over two days should be reduced to 1 g/kg in a single infusion unless the patient has life-threatening bleeding.
- In life-threatening bleeding, patients should be treated with IVIg, high-dose intravenous methylprednisolone and platelet transfusions. Vinblastine and full-dose TPO-RA may also be useful.

## 11.1.3. Second-line therapy

The goals of second-line treatments are different from those of first-line treatments because the likelihood of durable and complete remission is lower at this stage, and the risks and adverse effects of treatments should be weighed against the risk of no treatment. Therefore, the physician must determine an individual hemostatic platelet count that depends on comorbidities, history of bleeding, concomitant drugs, activity and lifestyle. In the absence of risk factors for bleeding, a platelet count higher than 20-30 x $10^9$/L usually does not require treatment.

### Thrombopoietin-receptor agonists

Rather than modulating the immune system, another therapeutic approach is to stimulate platelet production. Thrombopoietin is the primary factor regulating platelet production and several TPO-RAs have been developed that activate the TPO receptor and increase platelet production. Romiplostim is administered at 1-10 µg/kg/week by subcutaneous injection. Eltrombopag is an oral non-peptide administered at 50-75 mg/day several hours removed from food and polyvalent cations such as calcium. An overall platelet response rate was observed in about 80 % of the patients [19]. About 20 % of the patients under TPO-RA in clinical practice have no significant increase of their platelet count but have an important decrease of their concomitant treatment for ITP or no more bleeding [20].

As long as the treatment is maintained, romiplostim and eltrombopag show sustained response up to 5 to 8 years, with most patients able to decrease or discontinue concurrent corticosteroid therapy [21, 22]. In addition, 20 to 30 % of ITP patients had a sustained response after TPO-RA withdrawal [23, 24].

Romiplostim and eltrombopag appear to be well-tolerated and no severe side effects were observed in the published studies including hundreds of patients [19]. Although most adverse effects were mild, concerns have been raised about an increased risk of venous and arterial thrombotic events [21, 22, 25], although these rates seem to be comparable to those of ITP patients not treated by TPO-RAs, increased bone marrow reticulin deposits [22, 25, 26], but seem to be reversible on treatment withdrawal and with exceptional clinical significance, and a theorical risk of clonal evolution, but long-term results are reassuring. In addition, eltrombopag may induce liver toxicity and cataracts and has interactions with polyvalent cations [21].

Avatrombopag is a small molecule orally-administered at 20 mg/day. It was the third thrombopoietin receptor agonist approved for the treatment of immune thrombocytopenia and the first approved to treat periprocedural thrombocytopenia in patients with chronic liver disease (thereby providing an alternative to blood transfusions for these patients). Unlike eltrombopag, avatrombopag does not require a 4 hr food-restricted window around its use and it has not been associated with hepatotoxicity in ITP patients or portal vein thrombosis in patients with chronic liver disease. In ITP patients it can often be dosed less frequently than once daily. It is overall well-tolerated with a side-effect profile similar to placebo in randomized clinical trials [74].

Fluctuating platelet counts during treatment and rebound thrombocytopenia after cessation of treatment is a matter of concern.

Because of the efficacy and safety of TPO-RAs, these treatments, initially reserved for chronic ITP, may be proposed in persistent ITP [5]. In addition, several studies to evaluate the efficacy of TPO-RAs in newly diagnosed ITP are ongoing, in the hypothesis of a higher rate of sustained remission after withdrawal.

## Rituximab

About 60 %-70 % of patients with ITP show initial response to rituximab [27, 28]. Responses generally occurred after 1-2 weeks to 6-8 weeks after the first infusion. The response rate is similar at 375 mg/m²/week for 4 weeks and at 2 fixed 1,000 mg rituximab infusions on days 1 and 15 [29-31]. However, ITP will eventually relapse in about half of the patients, and sustained response at 5 years is around 30 % [27, 29]. No clear predictive factors of sustained response to rituximab were determined but younger age, female sex and short disease duration were the most frequently and consistently reported. Most patients with a complete response will respond to repeated courses in case of relapse, but the safety of repeated infusions of rituximab needs to be better evaluated [29, 32]. Lower doses of rituximab (100 mg weekly for 4 weeks) may also be effective, although the time to obtain a response seems slower when compared to the standard regimen [33].

To increase the initial and sustained response rates, several combinations with rituximab have been tried. We can mention the combination with dexamethasone, which leads to a longer time to relapse and a higher long-term response rates [34, 35], and with belimumab, which is a monoclonal antibody directed against BAFF. An uncontrolled prospective study suggests that association of rituximab with belimumab may induce a higher initial response rate and a more prolonged response than rituximab alone [36].

Rituximab is contraindicated in patients with evidence of active hepatitis B infection. In patients who receive rituximab, especially before splenectomy, it is recommended to vaccinated against influenza and encapsulated bacteria (*Streptococcus pneumoniae, Haemophilus influenzae,* and *Neisseria meningitidis*) at least 2 weeks before rituximab infusion [4]. It is also strongly recommended during the SARS-CoV2 pandemic to vaccine the patient against COVID19 infection at least 2 weeks before being treated with rituximab. Adverse events associated with rituximab appear usually mild or moderate, with a low incidence of infections and the risk of progressive multifocal leukoencephalopathy initially suspected when rituximab was first used a decade ago has not been confirmed by the most recent registries [29]. The risk of hypogammaglobulinemia is also marginal when rituximab is used alone. However, it can reveal common variable immunodeficiency and we recommend monitoring serum immunoglobulin level before and repeatedly after rituximab infusions [37].

### Splenectomy

Splenectomy has been used for more than 50 years and leads to an overall response in about 80 % of patients and a complete lasting response in 65 % of cases [38-40]. Many patients without a complete response may still expect a partial or transient increase in platelet count. Immediate complications of splenectomy include bleeding, prolonged hospitalization, readmission to the hospital, or requirement for additional intervention with a complication rate of about 10 %; mortality is 1.0 % with laparotomy and 0.2 % with laparoscopy. Splenectomy is associated with lifelong risk of thrombosis (3 to 16 %) and infections (8 to 31 %, with an abrupt onset and a poor outcome) [40-42]. Patients should also be given prophylactic polyvalent pneumococcal, meningococcal and *Haemophilus influenzae* type b vaccines at least 2 weeks prior (preferably) to or 2 weeks after splenectomy and revaccinated according to the country-specific recommendations [4, 43]. In some countries, splenectomized patients are given long-term antibiotic prophylaxis (penicillin V or erythromycin), but the usefulness of this practice is unproven. They should be well-educated about the risk of overwhelming post-splenectomy infection including the need have antibiotics at home (amoxicillin) to be used in case of fever and to contact a physician.

Splenectomy remains a very effective treatment of severe chronic ITP, but because of the initial and long-term risks associated with this treatment and the possibility of spontaneous late remission of ITP of less than 1 year of duration, it should be only proposed for chronic ITP. In addition, because of the efficacy and safety of other second-line treatments (TPO-RAs and rituximab), including a possibility of long-term remission, splenectomy is now proposed after these treatments. Therefore, an increasing number of patients and physicians are now reluctant to consider splenectomy, and splenectomy rate declined over time [44, 45].

### Second-line treatments (summary)

- TPO-RAs are very active in ITP with up to 80 % of response, with a good safety. In addition, 20 to 30 % of ITP patients had a sustained response after TPO-RA withdrawal.
- Rituximab has a sustained response rate at 5 years of almost 30 %. However, no clear predictive factors of sustained response to rituximab were determined to assist the physician in deciding to treat with rituximab on an individual basis.
- Splenectomy remains a good "curative" treatment for adults with chronic ITP with an overall long-term response of 60 %, but should be delayed after 12 months of follow-up. Its initial and long-term risks (mainly thrombosis and infections) and the efficacy and safety of other second-line treatments imply that most teams proposed it as a last resort.

## 11.1.4. Other second-line therapies

A wide variety of medical therapies has been proposed but often with a low level of *evidence-based medicine*. Most studies performed in this setting were retrospective and not controlled and were small case series. Second-line medical therapies are presented here in alphabetical order and thus do not imply a preferred treatment option.

### Azathioprine

Azathioprine is a usually well tolerated immunosuppressive agent that induces a response in about 55-65 % of patients and a 2-year response rate higher than 30 % [46-48]. Onset of action is slow and azathioprine should be continued for up to 3 to 6 months before being considered as ineffective. Relapses are frequent when the drug is discontinued and long-term low-dose maintenance therapy may be required.

## Cyclosporine A

Cyclosporine A (2.5-4 mg/kg/day) has shown efficacy mainly in small uncontrolled series including patients with severe chronic ITP [48, 49]. Its potential toxicity profile may make it unsuitable for patients with renal insufficiency. The frequent adverse effects and especially renal toxicity explain why cyclosporine should be considered only in patients having a truly refractory and severe ITP.

## Cyclophosphamide

Immunosuppression with cyclophosphamide, either orally (1-2 mg/kg daily for at least 16 weeks) or intravenously (0.5-0.7 g/m² for 1-3 doses every 2-4 weeks), has been used for patients refractory to corticosteroids and/or splenectomy [47, 48, 50]. The adverse effects of cyclophosphamide are potentially severe and include bone marrow suppression, bladder cancer, male and female sterility. In view of the severity of the adverse effects, cyclophosphamide should also clearly be reserved for severe refractory ITP.

## Danazol

Danazol, an androgen administered orally at a dose of 200 mg, 2-3 times daily, may be helpful as a corticosteroid-sparing agent, particularly in the elderly [48, 51]. The onset of action is relatively slow (4 to 6 weeks) and danazol should be administered for up to 6 months before to be sure that the treatment is not effective. However, the adverse effects of this treatment (mainly androgenic effects) explain why danazol is rarely used nowadays.

## Dapsone

Dapsone is an antibiotic which may also have an interesting efficacy as steroid-sparing agent in ei-

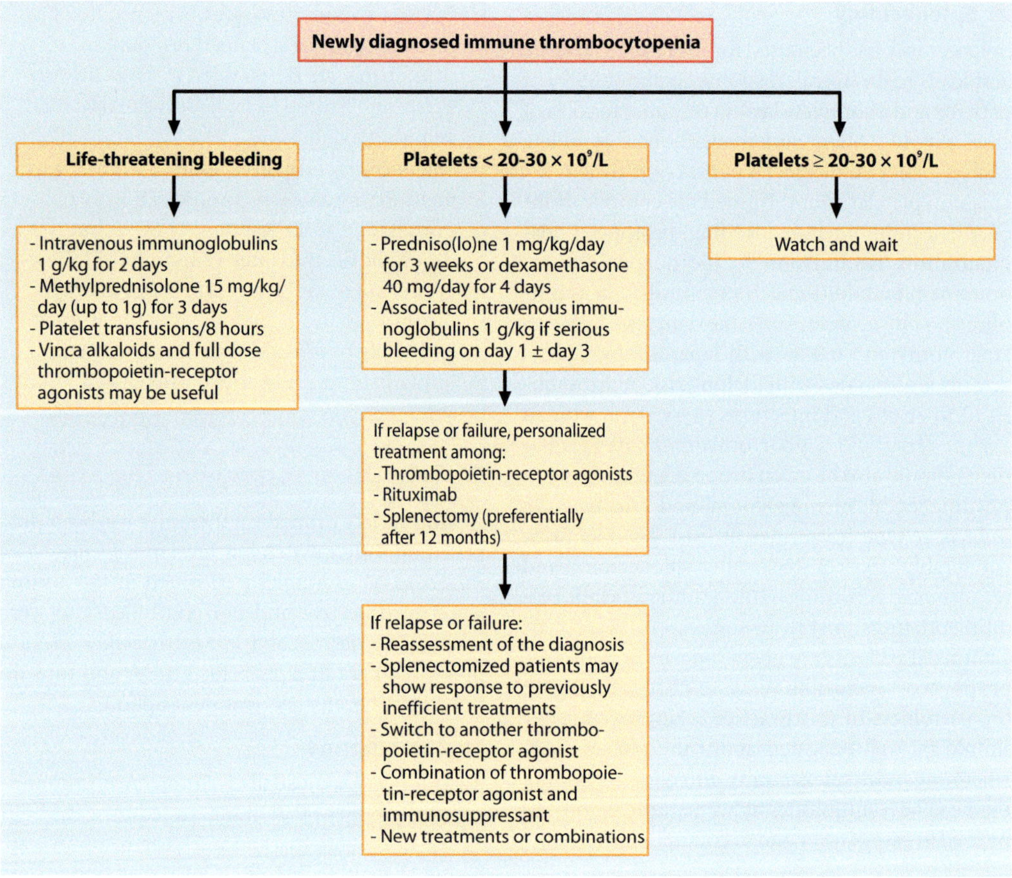


***Figure 11.1:*** Therapeutic strategy for ITP in adult patients.

ther persistent or chronic ITP [47, 48, 52, 53]. It is given orally at a usual dose of 75-100 mg/day. The response rate with dapsone seems similar to that observed with danazol (about 50 % of overall response) but it is likely that many of the patients reported in retrospective studies focusing on dapsone or danazol did not have severe ITP. The rate of response with these two drugs in refractory patients may therefore have been overestimated. Thus, in splenectomized patients, the response rate is lower. Dapsone may be associated with severe toxic side effects including hemolysis (a deficiency in glucose-6-phosphate dehydrogenase deficiency must be ruled out before first administration especially in men of Mediterranean ancestry) and hypersensitivity syndrome with rash and systemic symptoms. This complication is rare but potentially severe and patients should be aware of it.

### Helicobacter pylori

*Helicobacter pylori* infection has been associated with a large spectrum of extra-intestinal diseases including ITP. By using a standard eradication therapy, an overall response was observed in 50 % of ITP cases in Italian and Japanese studies. Focusing the analysis on patients with a baseline platelet count $\leq 30 \times 10^9$/L, the overall response rate was however only 35 % [54]. The response occurred most often within 2 to 4 weeks after the completion of eradication therapy, and exceptional relapses during follow-up have been published [55, 56]. No severe adverse effects of the treatment have been reported. However, the response rate is much lower in countries with a low prevalence of *H. pylori*, and therefore the systematic screening of *H. pylori* in ITP patients should only be performed in appropriate geographical areas or in case of digestive symptoms [4].

### Hydroxychloroquine

In our experience, hydroxychloroquine at 400 mg/day orally can be effective in up to 65 % of patients with lupus or positivity for antinuclear antibodies (titer ≥160 on Hep2 cells) and is well tolerated [57, 58].

### Mycophenolate mofetil

Mycophenolate mofetil (MMF), an antiproliferative immunosuppressant, has been shown to be useful in ITP patients. Administration of MMF at a progressively increasing doses (500 mg twice daily up to optimally 1,000 mg/day bid) produced a platelet increase in 40 to 80 % of patients, and 14 to 45 % of the responders had a sustained response after MMF withdrawal [59, 60]. MMF is associated with a high risk of teratogenicity and therefore an effective contraception is mandatory in women of child-bearing age. When choosing a second-line treatment, some teams consider MMF along with TPO-RAs and rituximab [61]. In addition, the first results of a randomized trial evaluating MMF for newly diagnosed ITP (Flight Trial) have been published as an abstract [62]. These results are very encouraging, with fewer treatment failures in patients treated with MMF for 6 months and corticosteroids than in patients treated with corticosteroids alone (22 vs 44 %, p=0.0064), without an increase in adverse effects. These results, if confirmed, will legitimately raise the question of the early use of an immunosuppressant in ITP to modify its natural history.

### Other second-line medical therapies (summary)

- The second-line treatment must be personalized and it is impossible to propose a rigid algorithm.
- In most guidelines, the choice of the second-line treatment is mainly between TPO-RAs, rituximab and splenectomy, according to comorbidities, concomitant drugs, bleeding history, patient preference and availability of drugs.
- However, the promising results of the Flight Trial evaluating MMF as a first-line treatment could redistribute the roles of immunosuppressants in ITP.
- Dapsone can be considered before splenectomy to delay or avoid splenectomy but with a low level of proof of efficacy.
- Hydroxychloroquine may be indicated in patients with lupus or positivity for antinuclear antibodies
- *H. pylori* screening and eradication may be proposed to patients in *H. pylori*-endemic country.

## 11.1.5. Patients failing multiple therapies

Despite the medical progress represented by TPO-RAs and rituximab, some patients may be refractory to these treatments. Some of them can tolerate severe thrombocytopenia without bleeding and with near normal quality of life. In contrast, others are symptomatic with worse long-term prognosis and increased risk of death [7, 8]. Nowadays, patients are considered as multirefractory if they exhibit no response to at least full dose TPO-RA, rituximab and splenectomy (or patients who are ineligible for or refuse splenectomy) and still require treatment [4]. In these patients, the diagnosis of ITP must be reassessed, and bone marrow examination should be performed. Splenectomized patients may show response to previously inefficient treatments, and if patient failed to respond to a full dose TPO-RA, a switch to another TPO-RA is encouraged, since a response may be seen in 50 % of the patients [63, 64]. A combination of an immunosuppressant with TPO-RA may induce a response in 70 % of the cases [8]. In case of failure, new second-line treatments (see below) may be used, at best in a clinical trial. As last resort, other combination therapy (with several immunosuppressants and/or chemotherapies), alemtuzumab or hematopoietic stem cell transplantation may be attempted, but these treatments have the potential to cause severe, possibly life-threatening immunosuppression and the data supporting their use are limited [4].

### Patients failing multiple therapies (summary)

- In case of multirefractory ITP (failure of at least full dose TPO-RA, rituximab and splenectomy), the diagnostic approach of ITP must be reassessed.
- Patients who relapse after splenectomy may respond to "first-line or second-line" drugs used in initial treatment such as corticosteroids.
- A switch from a TPO-RA to another may induce a response in 50 % of the patients.
- The combination of an immunosuppressant with TPO-RA may induce a response in 70 % of refractory ITP cases.
- More data are needed regarding the new second-line treatments described below to define their place in the therapeutic armamentarium of ITP.

## 11.1.6. New second- or third- or later-line therapies in the management of adults with ITP

### Thrombopoietin-receptor agonists

Avatrombopag is a small molecule, like eltrombopag, which has been firstly FDA-approved for thrombocytopenia in patients with chronic liver diseases, and secondly in chronic ITP. This treatment is still not available in some countries, but the recent approval by the EMA will probably remedy this. Avatrombopag seems to have a similar efficacy than other TPO-RAs, but, unlike eltrombopag, its absorption is not impaired by polyvalent cations and it has not been shown to induce liver toxicity [65]. Thromboembolic events are not uncommon in ITP, and in the phase III study, several thromboembolic events were reported similar to eltrombopag and romiplostim [21, 75] "Real-life" studies are needed to confirm or refute this.

Hetrombopag is also associated with approximately 90 % of overall response, but seems to be associated with infections [66].

Lusutrombopag is another small molecule that has been developed for thrombocytopenia in patients with chronic liver diseases. However, to our knowledge, no data in ITP patients have been published so far.

### Fostamatinib

Fostamatinib is a spleen tyrosine kinase (SYK) inhibitor, which is implicated in the phagocytic function of macrophages and B cell signaling. In phase III studies, long-term overall response is more than 40 % in the patients, who received a median of 3 treatments [67]. The most common adverse effects are hypertension and digestive disorders, but most are mild or moderate. Its efficacy seems better as a second-line treatment than as a third-or-later-line treatment (78 % versus 48 % of responses), raising the question of the place of fostamatinib in the therapeutic armamentarium [68]. It has been firstly FDA-approved and obtained recently also approval by the EMA. Other SYK inhibitors are under development.

### Neonatal fragment crystallizable receptor inhibitors

The neonatal fragment crystallizable receptors (FcRn) are responsible for the recycling of immunoglobulins G and albumin, extending the half-life of these proteins. The inhibition of FcRn results in an accelerate destruction of immunoglobulins G, including pathogenic immunoglobulins G.

Several FcRn inhibitors are under development, such as rozanolixizumab [69] and efgartigimod [70], and seem to induce a response of more than 35 % in persistent and chronic ITP. However, other studies focusing on long-term safety, especially regarding the risks of hypogammaglobulinemia and infections, are needed.

### Bruton Tyrosine Kinase (BTK) inhibitor

Rilzabrutinib is an oral BTK inhibitor that targets underlying mechanisms of platelet destruction without inhibiting platelet aggregation. It represents a new approach for treating patients with ITP and promising results have been recently reported in an open-label phase I/II study including 32 heavily pretreated patients with an overall response rate of 44 % and with a good safety. More data are required to confirm this clinical benefit [71].

### Treatments targeting plasma cells

One of the hypotheses explaining the failure of or relapse after rituximab is the differentiation of B cell into long-lived plasma cells in the spleen [72]. Therefore, several treatments targeting plasma cells in ITP are currently ongoing, including proteasome inhibitors (NCT03013114) or anti-CD38 (NCT04703621). As mentioned above, the combination of rituximab associated with belimumab seems to induce a higher initial response rate than rituximab alone [36].

### Complement inhibition

The preliminary results of a phase I study with sutimlimab, a monoclonal antibody directed against C1s inhibiting the classical complement pathway reported than 40 % of chronic ITP patients achieved an overall response under sutimlimab, with a response sustained for more than 1 year of therapy [73].

## 11.2. Conclusion

Corticosteroids remain the cornerstone of treatment in newly diagnosed ITP and IVIg are still indicated in case of severe bleeding manifestations. Splenectomy has long been the "gold standard" second-line treatment for patients with chronic ITP, but because of its adverse effects and the availability of well tolerated and significantly efficient treatments, splenectomy should probably be reserved for chronic ITP after failure of TPO-RAs and rituximab. The choice of the second-line treatment should consider comorbidities, concomitant drugs, bleeding history, patient preference and availability of drugs. Several new therapeutic pathways are currently being explored, with promising results. It is likely that the therapeutic strategy of ITP will be profoundly modified in the near future.

## References

1. Rodeghiero F, Stasi R, Gernsheimer T, Michel M, Provan D, Arnold DM, et al. Standardization of terminology, definitions and outcome criteria in immune thrombocytopenic purpura of adults and children: report from an international working group. Blood 2009;113:2386-93.

2. Moulis G, Lapeyre-Mestre M, Adoue D, Sailler L. [Epidemiology and pharmacoepidemiology of immune thrombocytopenia]. Rev Med Interne 2017;38:444-9.

3. Moulis G, Palmaro A, Montastruc J-L, Godeau B, Lapeyre-Mestre M, Sailler L. Epidemiology of incident immune thrombocytopenia: a nationwide population-based study in France. Blood 2014;124:3308-15.

4. Provan D, Arnold DM, Bussel JB, Chong BH, Cooper N, Gernsheimer T, et al. Updated international consensus report on the investigation and management of primary immune thrombocytopenia. Blood Adv 2019;3:3780-817.

5. Neunert C, Terrell DR, Arnold DM, Buchanan G, Cines DB, Cooper N, et al. American Society of Hematology 2019 guidelines for immune thrombocytopenia. Blood Adv 2019;3:3829-66.

6. Portielje JE, Westendorp RG, Kluin-Nelemans HC, Brand A. Morbidity and mortality in adults with idiopathic thrombocytopenic purpura. Blood 2001;97:2549-54.

7. McMillan R, Durette C. Long-term outcomes in adults with chronic ITP after splenectomy failure. Blood 2004;104:956-60.

8. Mahévas M, Gerfaud-Valentin M, Moulis G, Terriou L, Audia S, Guenin S, et al. Characteristics, outcome, and response to therapy of multirefractory chronic immune thrombocytopenia. Blood 2016;128:1625-30.

9. Mithoowani S, Gregory-Miller K, Goy J, Miller MC, Wang G, Noroozi N, et al. High-dose dexamethasone compared with prednisone for previously untreated primary immune thrombocytopenia: a systematic review and meta-analysis. Lancet Haematol 2016;3:e489-96.

10. Godeau B, Caulier MT, Decuypere L, Rose C, Schaeffer A, Bierling P. Intravenous immunoglobulin

for adults with autoimmune thrombocytopenic purpura: results of a randomized trial comparing 0.5 and 1 g/kg b.w. Br J Haematol 1999;107:716-9.

11. Godeau B, Chevret S, Varet B, Lefrère F, Zini JM, Bassompierre F, et al. Intravenous immunoglobulin or high-dose methylprednisolone, with or without oral prednisone, for adults with untreated severe autoimmune thrombocytopenic purpura: a randomised, multicentre trial. Lancet 2002;359:23-9.

12. Khellaf M, Michel M, Schaeffer A, Bierling P, Godeau B. Assessment of a therapeutic strategy for adults with severe autoimmune thrombocytopenic purpura based on a bleeding score rather than platelet count. Haematologica 2005;90:829-32.

13. Scaradavou A, Woo B, Woloski BM, Cunningham-Rundles S, Ettinger LJ, Aledort LM, et al. Intravenous anti-D treatment of immune thrombocytopenic purpura: experience in 272 patients. Blood 1997;89:2689-700.

14. Spahr JE, Rodgers GM. Treatment of immune-mediated thrombocytopenia purpura with concurrent intravenous immunoglobulin and platelet transfusion: a retrospective review of 40 patients. Am J Hematol 2008; 83:122-5.

15. Salama A, Kiesewetter H, Kalus U, Movassaghi K, Meyer O. Massive platelet transfusion is a rapidly effective emergency treatment in patients with refractory autoimmune thrombocytopenia. Thromb Haemost 2008; 100:762-5.

16. Goel R, Ness PM, Takemoto CM, Krishnamurti L, King KE, Tobian AAR. Platelet transfusions in platelet consumptive disorders are associated with arterial thrombosis and in-hospital mortality. Blood 2015;125: 1470-6.

17. Stirnemann J, Kaddouri N, Khellaf M, Morin A-S, Prendki V, Michel M, et al. Vincristine efficacy and safety in treating immune thrombocytopenia: a retrospective study of 35 patients. Eur J Haematol 2016;96:269-75.

18. Roumier M, Le Burel S, Audia S, Chauchet A, Gousseff M, Hamidou M, et al. High dose romiplostim as a rescue therapy for adults with severe bleeding and refractory immune thrombocytopenia. Am J Hematol 2021; 96:E43-6.

19. Birocchi S, Podda GM, Manzoni M, Casazza G, Cattaneo M. Thrombopoietin receptor agonists for the treatment of primary immune thrombocytopenia: a meta-analysis and systematic review. Platelets 2021;32:216-26.

20. Khellaf M, Michel M, Quittet P, Viallard J-F, Alexis M, Roudot-Thoraval F, et al. Romiplostim safety and efficacy for immune thrombocytopenia in clinical practice: 2-year results of 72 adults in a romiplostim compassionate-use program. Blood 2011;118:4338-45.

21. Wong RSM, Saleh MN, Khelif A, Salama A, Portella MSO, Burgess P, et al. Safety and efficacy of long-term treatment of chronic/persistent ITP with eltrombopag: final results of the EXTEND study. Blood 2017;130: 2527-36.

22. Rodeghiero F, Stasi R, Giagounidis A, Viallard J-F, Godeau B, Pabinger I, et al. Long-term safety and tolerability of romiplostim in patients with primary immune thrombocytopenia: a pooled analysis of 13 clinical trials. Eur J Haematol 2013;91:423-36.

23. González-López TJ, Pascual C, Álvarez-Román MT, Fernández-Fuertes F, Sánchez-González B, Caparrós I, et al. Successful discontinuation of eltrombopag after complete remission in patients with primary immune thrombocytopenia. Am J Hematol 2015;90:E40-43.

24. Mahévas M, Fain O, Ebbo M, Roudot-Thoraval F, Limal N, Khellaf M, et al. The temporary use of thrombopoietin-receptor agonists may induce a prolonged remission in adult chronic immune thrombocytopenia. Results of a French observational study. Br J Haematol 2014;165:865-9.

25. Cines DB, Gernsheimer T, Wasser J, Godeau B, Provan D, Lyons R, et al. Integrated analysis of long-term safety in patients with chronic immune thrombocytopaenia (ITP) treated with the thrombopoietin (TPO) receptor agonist romiplostim. Int J Hematol 2015;102: 259-70.

26. Brynes RK, Wong RSM, Thein MM, Bakshi KK, Burgess P, Theodore D, et al. A 2-Year, Longitudinal, Prospective Study of the Effects of Eltrombopag on Bone Marrow in Patients with Chronic Immune Thrombocytopenia. Acta Haematol 2017;137:66-72.

27. Ghanima W, Khelif A, Waage A, Michel M, Tjønnfjord GE, Romdhan NB, et al. Rituximab as second-line treatment for adult immune thrombocytopenia (the RITP trial): a multicentre, randomised, double-blind, placebo-controlled trial. Lancet 2015;385:1653-61.

28. Auger S, Duny Y, Rossi JF, Quittet P. Rituximab before splenectomy in adults with primary idiopathic thrombocytopenic purpura: a meta-analysis. Br J Haematol 2012;158:386-98.

29. Deshayes S, Khellaf M, Zarour A, Layese R, Fain O, Terriou L, et al. Long-term safety and efficacy of rituximab in 248 adults with immune thrombocytopenia: Results at 5 years from the French prospective registry ITP-ritux. Am J Hematol 2019;94:1314-24.

30. Mahévas M, Ebbo M, Audia S, Bonnotte B, Schleinitz N, Durand J-M, et al. Efficacy and safety of rituximab given at 1,000 mg on days 1 and 15 compared to the standard regimen to treat adult immune thrombocytopenia. Am J Hematol 2013;88:858-61.

31. Tran H, Brighton T, Grigg A, McRae S, Dixon J, Thurley D, et al. A multi-centre, single-arm, open-label

study evaluating the safety and efficacy of fixed dose rituximab in patients with refractory, relapsed or chronic idiopathic thrombocytopenic purpura (R-ITP1000 study). Br J Haematol 2014;167:243-51.

32. Hasan A, Michel M, Patel V, Stasi R, Cunningham-Rundles S, Leonard JP, et al. Repeated courses of rituximab in chronic ITP: Three different regimens. Am J Hematol 2009;84:661-5.

33. Zaja F, Volpetti S, Chiozzotto M, Puglisi S, Isola M, Buttignol S, et al. Long-term follow-up analysis after rituximab salvage therapy in adult patients with immune thrombocytopenia. Am J Hematol 2012;87:886-9.

34. Zaja F, Baccarani M, Mazza P, Bocchia M, Gugliotta L, Zaccaria A, et al. Dexamethasone plus rituximab yields higher sustained response rates than dexamethasone monotherapy in adults with primary immune thrombocytopenia. Blood 2010;115:2755-62.

35. Gudbrandsdottir S, Birgens HS, Frederiksen H, Jensen BA, Jensen MK, Kjeldsen L, et al. Rituximab and dexamethasone vs dexamethasone monotherapy in newly diagnosed patients with primary immune thrombocytopenia. Blood 2013;121:1976-81.

36. Mahévas M, Azzaoui I, Crickx E, Canoui-Poitrine F, Gobert D, Languille L, et al. Efficacy, safety and immunological profile of combining rituximab with belimumab for adults with persistent or chronic immune thrombocytopenia: results from a prospective phase 2b trial. Haematologica 2020.

37. Levy R, Mahévas M, Galicier L, Boutboul D, Moroch J, Loustau V, et al. Profound symptomatic hypogammaglobulinemia: a rare late complication after rituximab treatment for immune thrombocytopenia. Report of 3 cases and systematic review of the literature. Autoimmun Rev 2014;13:1055-63.

38. Ahmed R, Devasia AJ, Viswabandya A, Lakshmi KM, Abraham A, Karl S, et al. Long-term outcome following splenectomy for chronic and persistent immune thrombocytopenia (ITP) in adults and children: Splenectomy in ITP. Ann Hematol 2016;95:1429-34.

39. Kojouri K, Vesely SK, Terrell DR, George JN. Splenectomy for adult patients with idiopathic thrombocytopenic purpura: a systematic review to assess long-term platelet count responses, prediction of response, and surgical complications. Blood 2004;104:2623-34.

40. Vianelli N, Palandri F, Polverelli N, Stasi R, Joelsson J, Johansson E, et al. Splenectomy as a curative treatment for immune thrombocytopenia: a retrospective analysis of 233 patients with a minimum follow up of 10 years. Haematologica 2013;98:875-80.

41. Thai L-H, Mahévas M, Roudot-Thoraval F, Limal N, Languille L, Dumas G, et al. Long-term complications of splenectomy in adult immune thrombocytopenia. Medicine (Baltimore) 2016;95:e5098.

42. Boyle S, White RH, Brunson A, Wun T. Splenectomy and the incidence of venous thromboembolism and sepsis in patients with immune thrombocytopenia. Blood 2013;121:4782-90.

43. Davies JM, Lewis MPN, Wimperis J, Rafi I, Ladhani S, Bolton-Maggs PHB. Review of guidelines for the prevention and treatment of infection in patients with an absent or dysfunctional spleen: Prepared on behalf of the British Committee for Standards in Haematology by a Working Party of the Haemato-Oncology Task Force: Guideline. Br J Haematol 2011;155:308-17.

44. Michel M, Suzan F, Adoue D, Bordessoule D, Marolleau J-P, Viallard J-F, et al. Management of immune thrombocytopenia in adults: a population-based analysis of the French hospital discharge database from 2009 to 2012. Br J Haematol 2015;170:218-22.

45. Finianos A, Mujadzic H, Peluso H, Mujadzic T, Taher A, Abougergi MS. Temporal trends and outcome of splenectomy in adults with immune thrombocytopenia in the USA. Ann Hematol 2021;100:941-52.

46. Quiquandon I, Fenaux P, Caulier MT, Pagniez D, Huart JJ, Bauters F. Re-evaluation of the role of azathioprine in the treatment of adult chronic idiopathic thrombocytopenic purpura: a report on 53 cases. Br J Haematol 1990;74:223-8.

47. Depré F, Aboud N, Mayer B, Salama A. Efficacy and tolerability of old and new drugs used in the treatment of immune thrombocytopenia: Results from a long-term observation in clinical practice. PLoS ONE 2018;13: e0198184.

48. Vesely SK, Perdue JJ, Rizvi MA, Terrell DR, George JN. Management of adult patients with persistent idiopathic thrombocytopenic purpura following splenectomy: a systematic review. Ann Intern Med 2004;140: 112-20.

49. Emilia G, Luppi M, Morselli M, Forghieri F, Potenza L, Torelli G. A possible role for low-dose cyclosporine in refractory immune thrombocytopenic purpura. Haematologica 2008;93:1113-5.

50. Reiner A, Gernsheimer T, Slichter SJ. Pulse cyclophosphamide therapy for refractory autoimmune thrombocytopenic purpura. Blood 1995;85:351-8.

51. Liu W, Gu X, Fu R, Li Y, Lv M, Sun T, et al. The Effect of Danazol in Primary Immune Thrombocytopenia: An Analysis of a Large Cohort From a Single Center in China. Clin Appl Thromb Hemost 2016;22:727-33.

52. Zaja F, Marin L, Chiozzotto M, Puglisi S, Volpetti S, Fanin R. Dapsone salvage therapy for adult patients with immune thrombocytopenia relapsed or refractory to steroid and rituximab. Am J Hematol 2012;87:321-3.

53. Rodrigo C, Gooneratne L. Dapsone for primary immune thrombocytopenia in adults and children: an evi-

dence-based review. J Thromb Haemost 2013;11:1946-53.

54. Stasi R, Sarpatwari A, Segal JB, Osborn J, Evangelista ML, Cooper N, et al. Effects of eradication of Helicobacter pylori infection in patients with immune thrombocytopenic purpura: a systematic review. Blood 2009; 113:1231-40.

55. Tsumoto C, Tominaga K, Okazaki H, Tanigawa T, Yamagami H, Watanabe K, et al. Long-term efficacy of Helicobacter pylori eradication in patients with idiopathic thrombocytopenic purpura: 7-year follow-up prospective study. Ann Hematol 2009;88:789-93.

56. Kikuchi T, Kobayashi T, Yamashita T, Ohashi K, Sakamaki H, Akiyama H. Eight-year follow-up of patients with immune thrombocytopenic purpura related to H. pylori infection. Platelets 2011;22:61-4.

57. Khellaf M, Chabrol A, Mahevas M, Roudot-Thoraval F, Limal N, Languille L, et al. Hydroxychloroquine is a good second-line treatment for adults with immune thrombocytopenia and positive antinuclear antibodies. Am J Hematol 2014;89:194-8.

58. Mohammadpour F, Kargar M, Hadjibabaie M. The Role of Hydroxychloroquine as a Steroid-sparing Agent in the Treatment of Immune Thrombocytopenia: A Review of the Literature. J Res Pharm Pract 2018;7:4-12.

59. Provan D, Moss AJ, Newland AC, Bussel JB. Efficacy of mycophenolate mofetil as single-agent therapy for refractory immune thrombocytopenic purpura. Am J Hematol 2006;81:19-25.

60. Taylor A, Neave L, Solanki S, Westwood JP, Terrinonive I, McGuckin S, et al. Mycophenolate mofetil therapy for severe immune thrombocytopenia. Br J Haematol 2015;171:625-30.

61. Cooper N. State of the art - how I manage immune thrombocytopenia. Br J Haematol 2017;177:39-54.

62. Bradbury CA, Greenwood R, Pell J, Breheny K, Kandiyali R, Ingram J, et al. A Multicentre Randomised Trial of First Line Treatment Pathways for Newly Diagnosed Immune Thrombocytopenia: Standard Steroid Treatment Versus Combined Steroid and Mycophenolate. the Flight Trial. Blood 2020;136:LBA-2-LBA-2.

63. Khellaf M, Viallard J-F, Hamidou M, Cheze S, Roudot-Thoraval F, Lefrere F, et al. A retrospective pilot evaluation of switching thrombopoietic receptor-agonists in immune thrombocytopenia. Haematologica 2013;98: 881-7.

64. Lakhwani S, Perera M, Fernández-Fuertes F, Ríos de Paz MA, Torres M, Raya JM, et al. Thrombopoietin receptor agonist switch in adult primary immune thrombocytopenia patients: A retrospective collaborative survey involving 4 Spanish centres. Eur J Haematol 2017; 99:372-7.

65. Jurczak W, Chojnowski K, Mayer J, Krawczyk K, Jamieson BD, Tian W, et al. Phase 3 randomised study of avatrombopag, a novel thrombopoietin receptor agonist for the treatment of chronic immune thrombocytopenia. Br J Haematol 2018;183:479-90.

66. Mei H, Liu X, Li Y, Zhou H, Feng Y, Gao G, et al. A multicenter, randomized phase III trial of hetrombopag: a novel thrombopoietin receptor agonist for the treatment of immune thrombocytopenia. J Hematol Oncol 2021;14:37.

67. Bussel JB, Arnold DM, Boxer MA, Cooper N, Mayer J, Zayed H, et al. Long-term fostamatinib treatment of adults with immune thrombocytopenia during the phase 3 clinical trial program. Am J Hematol 2019;94:546-53.

68. Boccia R, Cooper N, Ghanima W, Boxer MA, Hill QA, Sholzberg M, et al. Fostamatinib is an effective second-line therapy in patients with immune thrombocytopenia. Br J Haematol 2020;190:933-8.

69. Robak T, Kazmierczak M, Jarque I, Musteata V, Treliñski J, Cooper N, et al. Phase 2 multiple-dose study of an FcRn inhibitor, rozanolixizumab, in patients with primary immune thrombocytopenia. Blood Adv 2020; 4:4136-46.

70. Newland AC, Sánchez-González B, Rejtõ L, Egyed M, Romanyuk N, Godar M, et al. Phase 2 study of efgartigimod, a novel FcRn antagonist, in adult patients with primary immune thrombocytopenia. Am J Hematol 2020;95:178-87.

71. Kuter DJ, Efraim M, Mayer J, McDonald V, Bird RJ, Regenbogen T, et al. Oral Rilzabrutinib, a Bruton Tyrosine Kinase Inhibitor, Showed Clinically Active and Durable Platelet Responses and Was Well-Tolerated in Patients with Heavily Pretreated Immune Thrombocytopenia. Blood 2020;136:13-4.

72. Mahévas M, Patin P, Huetz F, Descatoire M, Cagnard N, Bole-Feysot C, et al. B cell depletion in immune thrombocytopenia reveals splenic long-lived plasma cells. J Clin Invest 2013;123:432-42.

73. Broome CM, Röth A, Kuter DJ, Scully M, Smith R, Wang J, et al. Long-Term Safety and Efficacy of Sutimlimab in Patients with Chronic Immune Thrombocytopenia. Blood 2020;136:14-5.

74. Cheloff AZ, Al-Samkari H. Avatrombopag for the treatment of immune thrombocytopenia and thrombocytopenia of chronic liver disease. J Blood Med. 2019; 10:313-321.

75. Bussel JB, Provan D, Shamsi T, Cheng G, Psaila B, Kovaleva L, Salama A, Jenkins JM, Roychowdhury D, Mayer B, Stone N, Arning M. Effect of eltrombopag on platelet counts and bleeding during treatment of chronic idiopathic thrombocytopenic purpura: a randomised, double-blind, placebo-controlled trial. Lancet. 2009;373 (9664):641-8.

# 12. Management of ITP in the elderly

The incidence of ITP is characterized by two peaks. Incidence rises in early adulthood, during the twenties, and then again in middle age from the sixties onwards. The incidence reaches 9 in 100,000 person-years in men older than 75 [1].

Generally, around 30-40 % of patients diagnosed with ITP are older than 65 years of age. While there is an overweight of females affected in early adulthood, the second peak is characterized by an approximately equal sex distribution.

The management of ITP in the elderly is more challenging than treating a younger population. Increasing age is associated with higher comorbidity, frailty, risk of falls and polypharmacy, all factors contributing to a higher risk of bleeding [1-4]. Conditions requiring anticoagulation agents or platelet inhibitors, such as atrial fibrillation, venous thrombosis, coronary artery and cerebrovascular diseases increase with age [5]. All these aspects represent challenges which require particular attention in managing ITP patients over 60 years of age [5, 6].

The pathophysiology of primary ITP in the elderly does not differ from that of the general population. However, the underlying causes of secondary ITP may differ. Diseases like chronic lymphocytic leukemia and indolent lymphomas, known to cause secondary ITP, increase with age. Higher use of various medications makes this population more susceptible to drug-induced ITP. The list of drugs associated with ITP is long, and this possibility should be explored whenever suspected, such as recent initiation of a new drug prior to the diagnosis of ITP [6]. Discontinuation of suspected drugs or testing for drug-dependent antibodies when available should be considered.

## 12.1. Diagnosis of ITP in the elderly

Diagnosing ITP in the elderly may be challenging. The presence of comorbidities causing cytopenia associated with or mimicking ITP increase with age. A wider panel of tests should be considered, if anemia, leukopenia/leukocytosis, or abnormal cellular morphology are found. Conditions such as megaloblastic anemia, iron deficiency anemia, myelodysplastic syndrome and acute leukemias should be excluded. Managing myelodysplastic syndrome and leukemia as ITP may be directly harmful. The importance of ruling out these diseases warrants a more liberal approach to bone marrow biopsy and aspirate for morphology, flow cytometry, and cytogenetic and molecular genetic testing. A confusing factor is that autoimmune disorders, including ITP, can be associated with MDS or chronic myelomonocytic leukemia-associated immune thrombocytopenia [6]. Regardless of patients age, it is currently recommended to perform a bone marrow examination in the presence of abnormalities in the blood count or cell morphology that raises the suspicion of other disorders, or if the patient does not respond adequately to ITP treatment.

## 12.2. Treating ITP in the elderly

Patients presenting with acute bleeding require prompt treatment even before establishing the exact diagnosis. First-line therapies that may be indicated include measures to secure local hemostasis, platelet and blood transfusion (if needed), as well as tranexamic acid. The effect of platelet transfusion is transient and often lasts only for a few hours. Prolonged elevation of platelet count after transfusion supports the presence of other conditions like MDS, rather than ITP. IVIg and steroids should be administered concurrently.

Steroids and often IVIg should also be initiated without delay in patients with no active bleeding but having very low platelet counts, e.g. $<10 \times 10^9$/L and/or at high risk of bleeding. Thrombopoietin receptor agonists and vinca alkaloids (vinblastine or vincristine) are other medications that should be considered when a rapid elevation of the platelet count is needed.

For patients presenting with minor mucocutaneous bleeding or no bleeding, or who have a low to moderate risk of bleeding, the goals of therapy are to maintain a hemostatic platelet count to reduce future risk of major bleeding and to improve health-related quality of life. The target platelet count should be individualized based on bleeding risk.

Although studies have shown higher risk of bleeding in patients over 60 years of age, there is no consensus on platelet threshold to start and maintain treatment. Keeping the platelet count at >30 x $10^9$/L seems to be a safe level for both. A higher count should be considered in the presence of comorbidities, previous bleeding, particularly if recurrent ITP, or comedications are present [6]. In the case of concurrent anticoagulation therapy, there is general consensus on aiming for a higher platelet count >50 x $10^9$/L is typically considered a safe level. If it is not possible to increase the platelet count to >30 x $10^9$/L and in the presence of a strong indication for treatment, a single anticoagulant agent or platelet inhibitor can be used at that level [7]. Occasionally even a lower threshold is accepted for a short period, if the indication for anticoagulation is very strong and anticoagulation or platelet inhibitors cannot be postponed awaiting a higher count as in case of newly diagnosed venous thrombosis, myocardial infarction or stroke; however, every effort should be made to elevate the platelet count to a safer level as soon as possible.

### 12.2.1. Intravenous immunoglobulins (IVIg)

IVIg is a rapid-onset, effective drug raising platelet counts within 12-24 hours in around 80 % of treated patients [8]. However, studies suggest it may be less effective in the elderly population, although reliable data are lacking. IVIg is indicated in patients with active bleeding or in those with very high risk of bleeding where a rapid elevation of the platelet count is mandated pending the effects of other therapies.

The main safety concerns of IVIg in the elderly population include the risk of thrombosis, fluid overload and renal failure [6]. The latter was mainly observed in sucrose containing IVIg, and dose reduction should be considered in patients with renal insufficiency. The risk of thrombosis should not delay or prevent the use of IVIg if needed, instead prompting prophylactic measures like hydration and thromboprophylaxis to prevent thrombosis.

### 12.2.2. Corticosteroids

The elderly population is more prone to the side effects of steroids including glucose intolerance, psychological disturbances and accelerated osteoporosis. High dose prednisolone and dexamethasone may cause delirium. Dexamethasone should be administered with caution in patients >60-70 years of age and preferably at doses not higher than 20 mg daily for a maximum of 4 days. Administration of corticosteroids to patients with diabetes requires special attention and often adjustment of antidiabetic agents.

> Generally, prednisolone use should be limited to a maximum of 6-8 weeks and dexamethasone to a maximum of 2 to 3 cycles [7, 9]. Switching to a second-line therapy is recommended, if the patient becomes steroid-dependent (requiring more than 5 mg of prednisolone daily) to maintain an adequate platelet count.

Quicker tapering is recommended, if there is no response to therapy. Some patients need a low dose of prednisolone, e.g. 2.5 mg to 5 mg, to maintain a satisfactory long-term platelet count. If low-dose prednisolone is continued for a prolonged period of time, it is important to monitor side effects regularly, and to provide patients with calcium and vitamin-D supplementation, as well as bisphosphonates to prevent osteoporosis.

### 12.2.3. Managing treatment failure and corticosteroid dependency

The choice of a second-line therapy should be individualized and based on patient education and shared decision-making [7, 9]. It is recommended to use therapies with robust evidence first, i.e. therapies that have been evaluated in randomized controlled trials. Therapy options are increasing and currently include the three thrombopoietic agents, rituximab and fostamatinib [7]. If these therapies fail or are unavailable, other medications, mainly other immunomodulators like dapsone, danazol, mycophenolate mofetil can be used.

The absence of biomarkers and/or accurate clinical markers to guide the decision-making process limits parameters to be used to those related to the therapy itself, including availability of therapy, response and safety, mode and onset of action.

### 12.2.4. Thrombopoietin receptor agonists

Romiplostim, eltrombopag, and avatrombopag are the three thrombopoietic agents licensed for the treatment of ITP [10]. They act by stimulating thrombopoiesis. Romiplostim and eltrombopag have been used for nearly 15 years and have undergone meticulous evaluation in randomized controlled trials [11]. The drugs are considered by most guidelines first choice in patients failing to respond to or becoming steroid-dependent. They have a high level of evidence for efficacy, safety, and effect on health-related quality of life [7, 9, 12]. In addition to elevating platelet counts, the medications are effective in reducing bleeding, use of rescue and concomitant medications and improving health-related quality of life [11].

Furthermore, sustained response rates are high, reaching 60-70 % [13]. The actual response rates may be even higher. Many patients did not meet the response criteria in the clinical trials, yet they had an increase in platelet count and reduction in bleeding that was clinically significant, raising the clinical response rates to approximately 85 % [6]. Several post-hoc analyses and observational trials indicate that thrombopoietic agents might be slightly more effective in the elderly population compared to younger ITP patients [14-16].

Romiplostim is a peptide administered as weekly injections, whereas eltrombopag and avatrombopag are small molecules given as daily tablets. Because of interaction with dairy products and polyvalent cations (calcium, magnesium, iron) and antacids, such products should not be taken four hours before and two hours after eltrombopag. Particular attention should be paid to the use of calcium supplementation, which is frequent in the elderly, and may reduce the effect of eltrombopag, if taken within this time interval. These interactions do not exist with avatrombopag, hence no such precautions are needed. Administration of romiplostim might be challenging in the elderly population, who may require help to administer the injections, although most of the patients manage to administer the injections themselves [13].

The dose should be titrated to maintain a platelet count between 50-150 x $10^9$/L. Sometimes the tablets can be given every other or every third day, if platelet counts exceed the upper bound of the range. On the other hand, lower platelets counts are sometimes accepted, if the lower boundary cannot be achieved with highest recommended dose. If no response is achieved, switching to the other agent is often helpful. Thrombopoietic agents can be discontinued after some time without losing response in approximately 10-30 % of treated patients [10, 13].

The drugs are safe and well-tolerated in the elderly population with a couple of exceptions. One concern is the increased risk of thromboembolism, venous thromboembolism in particular. This side effect has not been shown to be associated with platelet count, the dose of the thrombopoietic agent, or the duration of treatment. According to the literature, older patients, patients with history of previous thrombosis, or patients with risk factors for venous or arterial thromboembolism are generally at higher risk of developing thromboembolism [6, 13, 14, 16]. In these patients, other less thrombogenic agents, such as rituximab or fostamatinib, may be better suited. Another possible side effect pertinent to this population is cataract, which has been reported with use of eltrombopag. Patients should be counseled and monitored properly to prevent and/or manage these side effects.

### 12.2.5. Rituximab

Rituximab, an anti-CD 20 monoclonal antibody, is one of the most widely used second-line therapies for ITP, despite of not being licensed for this indication. It is administered in two or four intravenous infusions and can provide relatively long-lasting treatment-free responses in 60 % of treated patients. However, half of responders lose the effect within two years [17]. Younger age, female gender and patients with short duration of ITP seem to have higher response rates in some studies, but the prognostic value of these factors is still uncertain [8]. Given its properties, rituximab may be a good choice in those who fail thrombopoietin-receptor agonists or even before these agents, if patients prefer treatment-free responses, or are at a high risk of thromboembolism. Apart from infusion-related reactions, rituximab is generally safe. However, a slight increase in the risk of infection after infusion has been reported by some studies [16]. Vaccination against pneumococcal pneumonia is recommended in older ITP patients. Patients with a history of HBV infection should not receive rituximab due to the risk of viral reactivation. Since rituximab reduces the effects of vaccines, vaccination is not recommended four weeks prior to or six months after rituximab administration. This is particularly pertinent to COVID-19 and pneumococcal, HIB and meningococcal vaccines.

### 12.2.6. Fostamatinib

Fostamatinib is a SYK tyrosine kinase inhibitor that has shown response rates of approximately 20 % in randomized controlled trials (RCTs) [18]. However, there are observations that higher rates can be achieved when administered to patients with ITP who have received no more than two previous ITP drugs [19]. Fostamatinib is administered orally, and response is maintained as long as treatment continues. The main side effects of fostamatinib are diarrhea and hypertension. Since the latter is common in the elderly, particular care should be taken with regards to monitoring blood pressure in this population. Fostamatinib has not been found to increase the risk of thromboembolism. Thus, it may be a good alternative in patients at high risk of thromboembolism [20].

### 12.2.7. Splenectomy

Splenectomy is a highly effective remission inducing therapy in 60-70 %. However, there are two main concerns that need to be taken into consideration in the elderly population:

- *First*, splenectomy may be less effective in the elderly, as demonstrated in several studies [21]
- *Secondly*, older patients have a greater risk of surgical complications [21]

The rates of splenectomy have decreased substantially in the last two decades with safe and effective medical therapies becoming available. It is currently recommended to delay splenectomy for at least one year after the diagnosis of ITP, and preferably to be used as a last resort after medical alternatives have been exhausted [7, 9]. It should be kept in mind that remission rates for splenectomy in such a refractory population should not be expected to be as high as they have previously been reported when splenectomy was applied as a second-line therapy. On the other hand, it may have become safer to splenectomize elderly patients given the wide use of laparoscopic splenectomy and the advances in the pre- and post-operative care.

Measures to prevent the risk of overwhelming post-splenectomy infections are important, such as annual immunization against influenza, anti-pneumococcal immunization, and immediate antibiotics in case of fever.

### 12.2.8. Other medications

Several other immunosuppressives/immune modulatory agents exist including mycophenolate mofetil, cyclosporine, danazol, dapsone, and azathioprine. These agents have varying response rates ranging between 30-60 % in single arm studies but require several weeks (dapsone) to months (mycophenolate mofetil, danazol, azathioprine) of treatment before effects can be observed. The safety profiles are also variable.

Danazol may be more effective in the elderly population, particularly in women. Of note, it is contraindicated in patients with prostate cancer. Side effects include liver toxicity and increased risk of thromboembolism.

Dapsone induces skin reactions, and patients should be screened for glucose-6-phosphate dehydrogenase deficiency before starting treatment. Additionally, they should be monitored for hemolysis, methemoglobinemia and liver damage during treatment [6, 16].

Mycophenolate mofetil is an immunosuppressant that is effective in ITP. Its main side effects include headache, gastrointestinal symptoms, fungal skin infections, and increased risk of cancer.

Due to availability of many other medications with well-documented response and safety in ITP, the use of these agents should be reserved for ITP patients failing to respond to or do not tolerate medications having high-quality evidence. They may be used either as single agents, or in combination with other drugs like thrombopoietin-receptor agonists.

### 12.2.9. Investigational therapies

Several new medications are under development, including BTK inhibitors, FcRn receptor inhibitors, and complement inhibitors. Including older patients in clinical trials should be encouraged to assess the safety and efficacy aspects of new therapies in the elderly. However, a major impediment to including elderly patients are comorbidities that often render these patients ineligible.

## References

1. Moulis G, Palmaro A, Montastruc JL, Godeau B, Lapeyre-Mestre M, Sailler L. Epidemiology of incident immune thrombocytopenia: a nationwide population-based study in France. Blood. 2014;124(22):3308-15.

2. Cohen YC, Djulbegovic B, Shamai-Lubovitz O, Mozes B. The bleeding risk and natural history of idiopathic thrombocytopenic purpura in patients with persistent low platelet counts. Arch Intern Med. 2000;160(11):1630-8.

3. Piel-Julian ML, Mahevas M, Germain J, Languille L, Comont T, Lapeyre-Mestre M, et al. Risk factors for bleeding, including platelet count threshold, in newly diagnosed immune thrombocytopenia adults. J Thromb Haemost. 2018;16(9):1830-42.

4. Adelborg K, Kristensen NR, Norgaard M, Bahmanyar S, Ghanima W, Kilpatrick K, et al. Cardiovascular and bleeding outcomes in a population-based cohort of patients with chronic immune thrombocytopenia. J Thromb Haemost. 2019;17(6):912-924.

5. Palandri F, Santoro C, Carpenedo M, Cantoni S, Barcellini W, Carli G, et al. Management of elderly patients with immune thrombocytopenia: Real-world evidence from 451 patients older than 60 years. Thromb Res. 2020;185:88-95.

6. Mahevas M, Michel M, Godeau B. How we manage immune thrombocytopenia in the elderly. Br J Haematol. 2016;173(6):844-56.

7. Provan D, Arnold DM, Bussel JB, Chong BH, Cooper N, Gernsheimer T, et al. Updated international consensus report on the investigation and management of primary immune thrombocytopenia. Blood Adv. 2019;3(22):3780-817.

8. Cooper N, Ghanima W. Immune Thrombocytopenia. N Engl J Med. 2019;381(10):945-955.

9. Neunert C, Terrell DR, Arnold DM, Buchanan G, Cines DB, Cooper N, et al. American Society of Hematology 2019 guidelines for immune thrombocytopenia. Blood Adv. 2019;3(23):3829-66.

10. Ghanima W, Cooper N, Rodeghiero F, Godeau B, Bussel JB. Thrombopoietin receptor agonists: Ten Years Later. Haematologica. 2019;104(6):1112-1123.

11. Birocchi S, Podda GM, Manzoni M, Casazza G, Cattaneo M. Thrombopoietin receptor agonists for the treatment of primary immune thrombocytopenia: a meta-analysis and systematic review. Platelets. 2021;32(2):216-226

12. Matzdorff A, Meyer O, Ostermann H, Kiefel V, Eberl W, Kuhne T, et al. Immune Thrombocytopenia - Current Diagnostics and Therapy: Recommendations of a Joint Working Group of DGHO, OGHO, SGH, GPOH, and DGTI. Oncol Res Treat. 2018;41 Suppl 5:1-30.

13. Palandri F, Rossi E, Bartoletti D, Ferretti A, Ruggeri M, Lucchini E, et al. Real-world use of thrombopoietin receptor agonists in elderly patients with primary immune thrombocytopenia. Blood. 2021;138(7):571-583.

14. Michel M, Wasser J, Godeau B, Aledort L, Cooper N, Tomiyama Y, et al. Efficacy and safety of the thrombopoietin receptor agonist romiplostim in patients aged >/= 65 years with immune thrombocytopenia. Ann Hematol. 2015;94(12):1973-80.

15. Steurer M, Quittet P, Papadaki HA, Selleslag D, Viallard JF, Kaiafa G, et al. A large observational study of patients with primary immune thrombocytopenia receiving romiplostim in European clinical practice. Eur J Haematol. 2017;98(2):112-120.

16. Lucchini E, Fanin R, Cooper N, Zaja F. Management of immune thrombocytopenia in elderly patients. Eur J Intern Med. 2018;58:70-6.

17. Ghanima W, Khelif A, Waage A, Michel M, Tjonnfjord GE, Romdhan NB, et al. Rituximab as second-line treatment for adult immune thrombocytopenia (the RITP trial): a multicentre, randomised, double-blind, placebo-controlled trial. Lancet. 2015;385(9978):1653-61.

18. Bussel J, Arnold DM, Grossbard E, Mayer J, Trelinski J, Homenda W, et al. Fostamatinib for the treatment of adult persistent and chronic immune thrombocytopenia: Results of two phase 3, randomized, placebo-controlled trials. Am J Hematol. 2018;93(7):921-30.

19. Boccia R, Cooper N, Ghanima W, Boxer MA, Hill QA, Sholzberg M, et al. Fostamatinib is an effective second-line therapy in patients with immune thrombocytopenia. Br J Haematol. 2020;190(6):933-8.

20. Cooper N, Altomare I, Thomas MR, Nicolson PLR, Watson SP, Markovtsov V, et al. Assessment of thrombotic risk during long-term treatment of immune thrombocytopenia with fostamatinib. Ther Adv Hematol. 2021;12:20406207211010875.

21. Kojouri K, Vesely SK, Terrell DR, George JN. Splenectomy for adult patients with idiopathic thrombocytopenic purpura: a systematic review to assess long-term platelet count responses, prediction of response, and surgical complications. Blood. 2004;104(9):2623-34.

# 13. Chronic refractory ITP

Chronic immune thrombocytopenia (ITP), as defined by the international working group at the Vincenza Consensus Conference, is ITP (primary or secondary), lasting >12 months (following an intermediate phase of "persistent ITP" lasting 3-12 months from diagnosis).

> Refractory ITP is currently defined by a failure to achieve a durable clinical response despite splenectomy (truly refractory disease cannot be diagnosed before splenectomy is performed although this definition is being changed), and is characterized by an ongoing requirement for disease-specific treatment (i.e., including adjuncts and frequent on-demand therapy) to minimize the risk of clinically significant bleeding [1].

It is estimated that refractory ITP may account for up to 25% of all chronic ITP patients [2]. In this chapter, refractory ITP will be addressed in detail. Topics to be covered include cases of thrombocytopenia that are NOT ITP, infectious and many other causes of secondary ITP, inherited thrombocytopenias, marrow failure states, immunodeficiency, and refractory ITP. An approach to management will be discussed. Outcomes and sequelae are strongly linked to what the starting population is.

## 13.1. Practical Considerations of Refractory ITP

Refractory is defined as "resisting ordinary methods of treatment". "Resisting" is not exactly defined. In ITP, it would likely mean that a safe adequate count cannot be maintained. This would be a combination of a lack of clinical efficacy and/or an inability to tolerate an efficacious dose without unacceptable toxicity. To be refractory, the number of front line and second line treatments that would need to be tried before defining someone as refractory are relatively many. As a minimum, they would include prednisone and dexamethasone, IVIg, a TPO agent and anti-CD20 antibodies. Using these treatments and determining non-responsiveness is not as straightforward as it might superficially seem.

First, what degree of response means "not refractory"? How do you decide? What if the platelets don't change much but there is clearly less bleeding? What if the count increases by 10,000/μL; is that enough? Does the count have to achieve a "response" i.e. increase by 20,000/μL or doubling to a count >30,000/μL? In certain very difficult patients, as an example, going from 5,000 to 20,000/μL would make sophisticated doctors and patients happy. Bleeding is perhaps more important but harder to assess. If there, for example, is a patient with epistaxis and it is a major problem but treated successfully with tranexamic acid without changing the platelet count: how does this rate? This case illustrates the problems with using bleeding as an assessment. A similar setting with heavy menstrual bleeding could be another example. A further complication is: what if the platelets go up "some" but the patient is very fatigued and the fatigue fails to improve?

Second, how the treatments are used including all of: at what dose, for how long, and with what requirements. Examples include several below. It is not uncommon to have a patient take azathioprine for 6 weeks, not respond and be taken off as "refractory". This is too short a time although this reflects a real flaw in azathioprine: it takes so long to have an effect.

A common problem is when eltrombopag is taken. It appears that a crucial feature of its mechanism of effect is chelation (of intracellular iron). If eltrombopag is taken with food containing divalent cations (dairy, broccoli, red meat, etc.) then it is ineffective. A patient may be thought to be "refractory" to it but it may just be how it is administered. In contrast, avatrombopag is recommended to be taken with food so that it has more consistent absorption. If this is not adhered to the effect of the avatrombopag may vary and make establishing a dose difficult.

Furthermore, if one TPO agent is tried and there is no response, some of the data from so-called "switch" studies would suggest that lack of response to one agent does not exclude response to another TPO agent. Many anecdotal cases and several studies established this for romiplostim and eltrombopag. Recent smaller studies have included avatrombopag in this finding. This almost means that at least 2 TPO agents at full dose for several weeks each have to be used to say a patient is refractory to "TPO agents".

Rituximab and dexamethasone can be used separately; however, they could possibly be better when used together. The "theory" would be that rituximab depletes the B cells and dexamethasone would be effective against plasma cells. This should be brilliant but it has been hard to demonstrate a clear advantage of the combination. The fact that hypogammaglobulinemia occurs in 20% of ITP patients when dexamethasone and rituximab are combined but in essentially no ITP patients with just rituximab seems to confirm this hypothesis of an effect of dexamethasone on plasma cells. The crossover study by Zaia in *Blood* 2010 clearly showed that dexamethasone alone was not as effective as the dexamethasone-rituximab combination and Ghanima et al have emerging data on dexamethasone-rituximab compared to rituximab alone suggesting superiority of the combination. Other less well-documented examples exist.

The above relates to the definition of refractoriness. An even bigger problem is the difficulty of accurately diagnosing ITP. The classical definition is an isolated thrombocytopenia without another explanation.This is said to be a diagnosis of exclusion. What else can be added? First response to ITP specific treatment especially but not only IVIg is very helpful. Again the degree of response should ideally be unequivocal and, in a perfect world, be a transient response repeated at least once. The Canadian group led by Arnold and Kelton has advanced the role of more severe thrombocytopenia as more consistent with ITP. This would be in the form of platelet count < 20,000/μL and more bleeding.

The same group explored misdiagnosis among a network of experienced hematologists and identified 17% or approximately 50 of just over 300 patients who had been considered to be ITP to not be primary ITP. While some of the "misdiagnosed" cases were those with secondary ITP, a major category involved myelodysplastic syndrome (MDS). Of note, there were apparently no cases of inherited thrombocytopenia identified. Studies of prevalence suggest that for every 10 cases of ITP, 1 case of inherited thrombocytopenia exists. This means that these cases are vastly underdiagnosed.

When do you suspect an **inherited thrombocytopenia?**

Inherited thrombocytopenias (IT) should be suspected in patients who:
- **show little or no response to standard ITP therapy,**
- have family histories of thrombocytopenia,
- have relatively stable platelet counts over time,
- have no known "normal" platelet counts antecedent to the development of "ITP,
- have any syndromic features of an IT.

Another diagnostic feature that may be the most useful simple screen across the spectrum of ITs is having large platelets [Carlo Balduini, personal communication]. This of course requires review of the smear by an experienced morphologist. It always used to be the hallmark of ITP diagnosis to emphasize seeing large platelets on the smear. However, too many too large platelets should not be thought to be ITP but instead suggests IT. Also "family history" of thrombocytopenia may be complicated: in families with ITP, there may often be cousins who are affected. However, first degree relatives, e.g. siblings or parent-child, is extremely rare in primary ITP. Rarely there can be secondary ITP in first degree relatives. Obviously, THE question is: how do you know the cousins are ITP and not IT? They respond to IVIg. Obviously, as discussed above, treatment response is not always black and white.

The focus on IT is for several reasons. First, they may be the easiest patients to misdiagnose. Second, they are relatively common forms of isolated thrombocytopenia (10% of ITP); like large platelets isolated thrombocytopenia is another hallmark of ITP. In addition, secondary ITP may be a presentation of certain inherited forms of thrombocytopenia, e.g. Wiskott-Aldrich syndrome, DiGeorge/VeloCardioFacial (VCF) syndrome and others. Finally, there are now well-described more than 30 types of IT, each with separate molecular pathogenesis and a range of clinical presentations. A recent study from experienced centers using standard morphologic approach and whole exome sequencing was able to identify a specific diagnosis in <50% of cases.

In summary, this means that ITs are among the most prevalent causes of "refractory" ITP.

Which **inherited thrombocytopenias** are most common?

Perhaps the most prevalent are the MYH9-related disorders (previously called May-Hegglin, Sebastian, Ebstein, Fechtner, and Alport syndromes). On the one hand they often have moderate but not severe thrombocytopenia, no obvious other manifestations, and large platelets, features which could all be consistent with ITP. However, the platelets are too large (unique for eliminating patients with ITP by finding too many too large platelets); needless to say, this requires careful review of the smear by an experienced morphologist. Many other things could be identified on the smear but, in certain patients with MYH9-related disorders, there would also be Döhle bodies visible on the peripheral smear, i.e. light blue inclusions located in the cytoplasm of neutrophils. Certain patients will have other features of MYH9-related disorders: early onset cataracts, high tone hearing loss, and/or renal disease that can lead to kidney failure.

Another relatively common inherited thrombocytopenia is Wiskott-Aldrich syndrome (WAS); it can be confused with ITP, especially the XLT-form (isolated thrombocytopenia). The sine qua non is the small platelet size but we have had experience seeing normal platelet size in a newborn; this may reflect the need for maturation of splenic phagocytosis, in order for the platelet size to become small. In addition, one diagnostic clue is milk allergy, which contributes to GI bleeding along with thrombocytopenia in the newborn. The first two XLT patients that I saw (in the 1980's) had mothers' brothers who had undergone splenectomy for "ITP"; both died of sepsis which, along with the X-linked inheritance, was suggestive in retrospect of WAS.

There are several other forms that are particularly likely to be confused with ITP and thus contribute to refractory ITP.

- The first is cyclical thrombocytopenia. The usual periodicity is in the neighborhood of 21-28 days and thus a patient can be thrombocytopenic, appear to have responded to therapy, and then appear to have relapsed. The optimal approach remains to be clarified when treatment is needed and does overlap with treatments of ITP.
- The second type is von Willebrand disease 2B which can have variable thrombocytopenia often aggravated by stress including hormonal stimulation of release of von Willebrand multimers from endothelial cells. This can be further complicated by the essentially identical clinical picture seen with platelet type von Willebrand disease. Treatment is different with provision of normal von Willebrand factor versus normal platelets.
- The third type is Bernard Soulier syndrome (BSS) both heterozygote and homozygote. The confusion with ITP is partly artifactual: the analyzer platelet count is often lower than the real count because the platelets are so large. Combined with the bleeding secondary to platelet dysfunction, it appears to be difficult ITP. Cases of splenectomy and cyclophosphamide treatment of BSS have been reported. As indicated, VCF may be clinically subtle and associated with autoimmune thrombocytopenia. There may be no history of neonatal hypercalcemia, chest X-ray (if performed) may be read as normal (since a right-sided arch alone is considered a variant of normal), and thus a VCF patient may resemble a patient with primary ITP. While they may not be refractory to treatment, they may be at increased risk of sepsis. In addition, there is an extremely rare form of DiGeorge in which there is a large deletion which incorporates glycoprotein IIIa; this causes a non-immune thrombocytopenia.

Within the spectrum of inherited thrombocytopenias are bone marrow failure states. While careful examination would normally identify these cases, they can present with a predominant or sole cytopenia of low platelets. Clues can come from a number of features: family history, anemia especially with macrocytosis, neutropenia and/or lymphopenia, and/or specific features, such a absent radii or hypoplasia of the thenar eminence. In addition, there is an entity of acquired megakaryocytic thrombocytopenia. The latter would appear very similar to ITP but treatment would need to be heavily immunosuppressive i.e. cyclosporin. These and some of the many other inherited thrombocytopenias are reviewed in greater detail elsewhere [3-4].

The other "common" cause of misdiagnosis occurring in patients older than 60 years of age, unlike patients with inherited thrombocytopenias who are younger, is myelodysplastic syndrome (MDS). This entity may be particularly confusing in that there may initially be a pronounced autoimmune component which diminishes over time, creating the appearance of increasingly refractory ITP. Also, MDS may be difficult to diagnose, especially in its early stages, and serial bone marrow aspirations and biopsies may be required until overt dysplasia or aberrant cytogenetics allows a specific diagnosis.

## 13.2. Infection-related thrombocytopenia

Mechanisms for post-infectious ITP are not clearly delineated, but may include molecular mimicry [5], immune dysregulation [6], induction of platelet phagocytosis [7], direct infection of megakaryocytes [8], or induction of inhibitory cytokine secretion by infected leukocytes and marrow stromal cells [9]. Implicated agents include not only cytomegalovirus (CMV), but also varicella, rubella, mumps, Epstein-Barr virus, HHV-6, HHV-8, parvovirus B19 [10]), and even HIV (see below). The wide variety of viruses implicated in initiating childhood ITP suggests that in general they disrupt the immunoregulatory network rather than all being associated with molecular mimicry, but the latter has been well-demonstrated in certain cases, e.g. varicella.

*Helicobacter pylori* infection has been associated with chronic ITP in multiple studies, and is reviewed in detail elsewhere [23]. It is most clinically relevant in areas of high background infection. Prevalence of *H. pylori* infection varies widely by geographical area, ranging from 22% in North America [24] to 50% in Italy [25] and 70% in Japan [26]. Reported clinical characteristics of ITP patients infected with *H. pylori* have included older age [27], dyspepsia [28] perhaps especially while on steroids, and bone marrow hyperplastic megakaryocytosis [29]. *In vitro* studies have shown that antibodies to *H. pylori* can cross-react with human platelet glycoprotein IIIa [30]. The *H. pylori* surface protein CagA has been implicated in this mechanism of molecular mimicry; the prevalence of the *H. pylori* CagA gene was significantly higher in patients with ITP than in a control group. Potentiation of FcR-mediated platelet phagocytosis by *H. pylori* LPS has also been proposed as a mechanism for *H. pylori*-induced ITP with downregulation of FcγRIIB, the inhibitory FcγR [31].

Multiple international phase II and phase III trials of triple therapy (amoxicillin, clarithromycin, and a proton pump inhibitor, e.g. lansoprazole) have demonstrated clear increases in platelet counts in patients receiving triple therapy (response rates range from 33% to 100% of patients); results in North American studies have not been nearly as successful [24, 32]. The presence or absence of CagA, which is more prevalent in Japan, has been correlated with platelet response to treatment [33-34]. Platelet response has even been seen in several patients who failed eradication therapy, raising the question of whether triple therapy may have a separate immunomodulatory effect [35]. The use of triple therapy for the treatment of ITP has been validated by international prospective studies, but its role in regions where background prevalence of *H. pylori* is low remains less clear. Given the relatively low toxicity of triple therapy (primarily gastrointestinal adverse effects, e.g. diarrhea), its short duration (7-14 days), and likelihood of increasing the platelet count, all patients with ITP in high prevalence areas, should be screened and treated if *H. pylori* positive. If therapy is initiated, predictors of platelet response to eradication therapy include short duration of ITP, platelet count >30 x $10^9$/L, and CagA positivity. In long-term outcome studies, the response has been durable with a very low rate of relapse at five years [36].

There are other categories in consideration of apparent refractory ITP. A prime cause here of truly refractory ITP is CMV. The scenario is most troublesome in a patient with pre-existing ITP. CMV has been reported to both cause and perpetuate ITP, sometimes resulting in a "refractory" clinical presentation. CMV viremia in the setting of ITP can present with associated findings, such as neutropenia [11]), peripheral atypical lymphocytosis [12-14]), presentation with CMV-like illness (headache, fever, throat pain, malaise) [13-14], or hepatomegaly/transaminitis [15-16] but may be clinically "silent" as well. Paradoxical decline in platelet count following administration of corticosteroids is a hallmark of active CMV-related ITP

[17-22]. Improvement in platelet count has been seen following treatment with anti-CMV agents, such as ganciclovir and/or CMV-specific immune globulin [14, 17-18, 21] and has been correlated with decreasing CMV PCR. Treatment of CMV-related refractory ITP is aimed toward rapidly reducing CMV viral load, with agents such as ganciclovir and anti-CMV immune globulin; second-line agents such as foscarnet or cidofovir can be used, if myelosuppression is seen with ganciclovir. Immunosuppression is tapered briskly, with the use of IVIg and/or thrombopoietic agents as necessary to maintain adequate platelet counts while awaiting the effect of anti-CMV agents. Once CMV is undetectable by PCR, the efficacy of routine agents for the treatment of ITP (such as IVIg, anti-D, and splenectomy) is typically restored.

Other viral infections such as EBV, are typically more clinically evident.

Hematological complications of HIV were often very difficult to manage, thrombocytopenia in particular in late stage disease. At this relatively late stage of HIV disease; however, thrombocytopenia was rarely "isolated" and there might typically be lymphadenopathy, as well anemia and/or leukopenia. In HIV-associated thrombocytopenia (HIV-TP), as previously reviewed [37], thrombocytopenia has been well-described in 10% of HIV-infected patients (30% of AIDS patients), and is characterized by accelerated platelet destruction and ineffective platelet production by infected megakaryocytes. Pathophysiologically, for HIV-TP, Hepatitis C-TP (see below), and certain cases of drug-related thrombocytopenia, a novel anti-platelet antibody has been described, which may be the result of molecular mimicry. The antibody is directed against the region of GPIIIa involving amino acids 49-66 and apparently mediates thrombocytopenia by intravascular lysis rather than by FcγR-mediated clearance. This may explain some of the lack of response to conventional ITP therapy (such as IVIg) in these settings [38]. In general, thrombocytopenia responds to HIV-directed and also to ITP-directed therapy (immunosuppressants, TPO-like agents, anti-D, splenectomy, etc.), but currently the widespread use of highly active antiretroviral therapy (HAART) has made this entity (HIV-TP) relatively uncommon. A significant fraction of HIV-TP may be related to co-infection with hepatitis C and/or advanced liver disease [39]. While antiviral agents are the unequivocal first line of therapy, treatment must be tailored to each individual due to the comorbidities and increased risk of infection in this population. Anti-D has been used with adequate duration of response (50% respond for >3 weeks), significantly greater than the response to IVIg [40]. The reported superiority of IV anti-D to IVIg both for platelet increase as well as duration of response in a retrospective analysis was confirmed in a small cross-over study [41].

Hepatitis C infection is a well-known cause of secondary ITP, likely via HCV core envelope I mimicry of platelet glycoprotein GPIIIa. It has been found in as many as 30% of chronic ITP patients in an area of high prevalence, and is more common in older patients [42]. Since at least 1-2% of the population of the USA is hepatitis C infected, it is not surprising that the co-incidence of ITP and hepatitis C infection is relatively common. In these patients, bleeding may be seen at higher platelet counts, which has been attributed to cryoglobulinemia-mediated vasculitis as well as to DIC; in addition, if the liver is cirrhotic, other coagulation abnormalities may be present. Thrombocytopenia itself may be caused by the stimulation of autoimmunity by hepatitis C infection, as well as by hypersplenism and reduced levels of thrombopoietin, the latter in cases of advanced cirrhosis. Hypersplenism, if present, will make the thrombocytopenia refractory to standard treatments.

Suppression of HCV viral load has not been well-correlated with improvement in platelet count, in contrast to what has been seen in HIV infection. HCV-specific therapy with interferon exacerbates thrombocytopenia, which may precipitate severe hemorrhage. Thrombopoietin-receptor agonists, in particular eltrombopag, may provide a beneficial effect for the thrombocytopenic patients in particular, allowing them to tolerate pegylated-interferon-based antiviral strategies that have achieved overall cure of hepatitis C in greater than 50% of infected patients. However, this type of hard-to-tolerate treatment has been largely replaced by newer antivirals and is rarely used.

Finally, it is important to consider COVID and COVID vaccination. Two cases of refractory ITP in conjunction with COVID infection resulted in intracranial hemorrhage. These were both newly-diagnosed cases. Similarly a well-publicized case of intracranial hemorrhage after a COVID vaccination occurred with the patient presenting to the emergency room 2 days after vaccination. He remained refractory to multiple treatments over 2 weeks before dying from the hemorrhage. To the best of our knowledge, the great majority of cases following COVID infection and vaccination have not usually been very refractory although in certain cases we have resorted to use of vincristine combined with TPO agents to increase the count acutely before continuing with TPO agents as needed. Rituximab was often used in these difficult cases but if they develop immediately after vaccination, the drawback of rituximab is that it might eliminate the antiviral antibody response to vaccination while postponing the ability to be vaccinated for another 6-12 months.

## 13.3. Drug-induced thrombocytopenia

Drug-induced thrombocytopenia is a particularly murky area especially in older patients who may be on multiple medications. There are certainly well-recognized causes of drug-induced thrombocytopenia that include heparin, quinidine, valproic acid, glycoprotein IIb/IIIa inhibitors, such as abciximab and eptifibatide. Other causes include exogenous estrogens, antibiotics, such as linezolid, trimethoprim/sulfamethoxazole, vancomycin, and nitrofurantoin; and anti-viral agents, such as ganciclovir. However, a much larger number of medications including acetaminophen, amoxicillin and many others have been reported to cause thrombocytopenia in at least one case each. The same is true for certain foods and food additives, e.g. certain "natural" substances, such as Chinese herbal remedies. Quinine is commonly thought of because of its resemblance to quinidine, but also because it is in tonic water and is a commonly used remedy for restless legs syndrome. Testing for drug-specific platelet antibodies is possible but is not widely available and rarely used in part because there are possible reasons for false negative testing, such as metabolites of the drug causing the immune thrombocytopenia rather than the drug itself. Concurrent medications can often (and should if possible) be discontinued, if there is any suspicion of effect on platelets, with replacement with an alternative medication if necessary. One ongoing rule of thumb is to discontinue or change all medications that have been started within the past year. Fortunately, this is easier than it had been in the past because of the current availability of alternative medications for almost all indications. Special cases include heparin (in which alternative anticoagulation is often mandatory), valproate (in which dose reduction may be sufficient) and estrogen (in which a relative increase in the progesterone to estrogen ratio of the administered agent may be sufficient or a shift from estrogen to progesterone depending upon the reason for the hormonal treatment). Since estrogens may often not be thought of as "medications" they may been omitted in consideration of drug induced TP. However, a small series emphasized how they can make ITP "refractory" either when used as oral contraceptives or for post-menopausal management.

## 13.4. Secondary ITP

There are many causes of secondary ITP including

- common variable immune deficiency (CVID);
- collagen vascular disease, such as SLE;
- lymphoproliferative syndromes including benign (ALPS), as well as malignant disorders (CLL, Hodgkin and non-Hodgkin lymphoma);
- paroxysmal nocturnal hemoglobinuria (PNH);
- thrombotic thrombocytopenic purpura (TTP) – hemolytic uremic syndrome (HUS); and
- antiphospholipid syndrome (APLS).

There should be a low threshold to specifically exclude these entities, if there are any indications that they might be present. All can be considered "game changers" in that they may well increase the likelihood of "refractory ITP" and require specific management directed at the underlying condition in addition to whatever may be needed to manage the thrombocytopenia.

There are a number of considerations to the above. CVID is like ITP in being a "final common pathway" disease identified by a laboratory abnormality i.e. hypogammaglobulinemia instead of thrombocytopenia. CVID can be roughly divided into 2 groups:

a) ones who primarily have hypogammaglobulinemia and thus do very well with IV or subcutaneous immunoglobulins; and

b) more complex immunodeficiencies, which also have granulomatous disease, interstitial pulmonary disease, and/or autoimmunity.

The latter may have identifiable underlying genetic defects which, if identified, may be directly treated. These cases, especially the "complex" ones, may be relatively refractory to ITP management, although in one study treatment with rituximab was extremely effective albeit requiring probably lifelong IgG replacement (which may well have been required anyway). An interesting feature of CVID-ITP is that it may not only respond to steroids but actually go into remission for years but then relapse. This scenario should lead to measurement of immunoglobulins.

In cases with SLE and APLS, ITP can be relatively refractory, especially in the former. This may be because of a so-called "hostile" marrow environment reducing platelet production, likely based on inflammation. Therefore, immunosuppression is probably more likely to be helpful here than in other secondary causes of ITP.

How hard to look for lymphoma is uncertain but in more refractory cases of ITP, radiologic investigation is likely warranted. I have seen one case of refractory ITP in a patient with Hodgkin disease who died from an intracranial hemorrhage. It is also important to realize that an underlying immune defect may link ITP and lymphoma in a patient. Finally, CLL may not be overt and review of the smear may reveal a too large population of small mature-appearing lymphocytes. Flow cytometry would confirm that these are B-cells. In cases of CLL, in addition to ITP per se, there may also be thrombocytopenia based on the CLL cells "crowding out" normal hematopoietic elements and, if for example fludarabine is used, AIHA and ITP may develop as a side effect.

One study of ITP patients to explore ALPS with genetic testing, identified 2 unsuspected cases among more than 100 cases of "ITP". If ALPS is identified, even without concomitant AIHA and lymphadenopathy, possibly this would suggest the use of mycophenolate mofetil and especially sirolimus.

### Summary of Secondary ITP

These examples raise the critical but unanswered question of which "routine" laboratory tests should be sent in which patients. It is our position that especially refractory patients deserve a full round of testing to uncover any "unusual" etiologies, because many of these etiologies will determine specific therapeutic approaches, which otherwise would have been neither obvious nor chosen for the management of "idiopathic" refractory ITP. One could suggest that in women of childbearing age screening for autoimmunity including thyroid testing is especially warranted, whereas in older patients, lymphoproliferative etiologies may be more important. Finally, CVID can present at any age. How many of these cases of secondary ITP appear refractory is not clear but their identification allows for "targeted" therapy in some cases.

### Summary of (Mis)Diagnosis of Refractory ITP

Especially in refractory ITP, it is important to cast a wide net in considering the potential etiologies of the thrombocytopenia. The most obvious cause of refractoriness is that it is not ITP at all. This has recently become more complicated in that many different etiologies of thrombocytopenia will respond to TPO agents and this response, unlike response to IVIg, is NOT diagnostic of ITP. It is likely that the most common causes of misdiagnosis are MDS (older patients) and inherited thrombocytopenias (young adults). A particularly tricky cause is cyclical thrombocytopenia, because it can readily appear to be ITP with response to treatment and then loss of response.

## 13.5. Therapeutic approach

Once re-evaluation of the patient, including bone marrow aspiration, biopsy, flow cytometry and cytogenetics is completed, management needs to be implemented in those cases requiring treatment. As stated in the beginning, while we would no longer include failing splenectomy in the definition of refractoriness, arbitrarily we would include lack of sustained response to steroids, IVIg, TPO agents and rituximab as a minimum for the definition. With this definition, there is no consensus approach for treatment of refractory ITP, as individualized treatment is required based on each patient's history and preferences. An overall approach as outlined in Figure 8.1 could be considered. As noted above, "refractory" has been defined as lack of response to splenectomy [1]. In clinical practice, patients without any response to fewer treatments may be more difficult to treat (more refractory to therapy), than those with intermediate but transient response to a greater number of treatments. Finally, the goal of therapy should be to maintain a platelet count at which at most minor bleeding symptoms (petechiae, bruises, oral mucosal bleeding) occur; treatment-related toxicities are acceptable; and the risk of life-threatening hemorrhage (GI, intracranial bleeding) is minimal, while incorporating patient choice and quality of life factors especially depression and fatigue.

### 13.5.1. General approach to refractory ITP

#### 13.5.1.1. Observation

Despite a low platelet count, observation without therapy could be employed in certain cases. Unlike views espoused by some practitioners, we do not believe that very low platelet counts (e.g., <20 x $10^9$/L) should be treated with observation only. This is because of the risk of severe hemorrhage and because health related quality of life is typically lower than optimal in these patients. The willingness to treat these patients is also based on the high efficacy and low apparent toxicity of the newer therapies, such as the thrombopoietic receptor agonists and rituximab. This recommendation is different than the setting of newly diagnosed childhood ITP where spontaneous platelet improvement is expected in the majority of patients in the not too far distant future. Even adults with ITP may improve over time so there may still be improvement 1 year from diagnosis.

The use of agents to minimize bleeding even if they do not impact the platelet count may be important here. The most commonly used ones are hormonal treatments to limit vaginal bleeding and antifibrinolytic agents for mucosal bleeding. For the former, as discussed, progestational treatment is better than estrogenic treatment. For the latter, it appears that the risk of thrombosis is less than had been anticipated.

#### 13.5.1.2. Standard therapy

Even in refractory patients, low dose corticosteroids (5 mg daily or every other day), or periodic infusions of IVIg may be useful to achieve platelet count increases sufficient to minimize minor bleeding. The use of long-term steroids for maintenance treatment of ITP is limited by toxic side effects such as osteopenia, early-onset diabetes mellitus, gastric distress, hypertension, weight gain, and increased risk of infection, all of which can occur even on low dose continuous therapy.

The spleen is the primary site of peripheral platelet destruction in most patients with chronic ITP. $^{111}$In-labelled autologous platelet studies have suggested that over 90% of patients with primarily splenic platelet destruction achieved remission; suboptimal platelet responses were seen in 60 or more per cent of patients with hepatic or diffuse platelet destruction [43]. Overall, splenectomy is curative in 60-70% of patients with chronic ITP at 5 years from surgery, and the majority of relapses occur in the first 2-5 years [44]. Relapse post-splenectomy may be due to the presence of an accessory spleen, if there has been an initial response lasting years [45]. With the emergence of alternative therapies as described below, the rate of splenectomy in ITP is decreasing, allowing more time for spontaneous or treatment-based improvement in chronic patients [46].

A major concern for splenectomy is that in the patients who need it the most, those unresponsive to other treatments, will likely benefit the least, i.e. have the lowest response rate to splenectomy. However, if splenic sequestration studies are available, then their predictive ability may advance the utility of splenectomy. A recent study from the national French Hematology group suggested that certain patients unresponsive for example to TPO agents pre-splenectomy might respond to them post-splenectomy.

#### 13.5.1.3. Therapy for refractory disease

**First-line therapy**

These agents include high-dose dexamethasone, danazol, azathioprine, mycophenolate mofetil, rituximab, and thrombopoietin (TPO) receptor agonists (romiplostim, eltrombopag and avatrombopag; ☞ Table 13.1). Of these, rituximab and the TPO receptor agonists appear to have the most favorable risk/benefit profile, and are discussed further below.

Rituximab is a monoclonal anti-CD20 chimeric antibody that induces transient depletion of B cells (but spares plasma cells). T cells are affected indi-

| Agent | Dose/Regimen | Toxicity | Efficacy | Notes |
|---|---|---|---|---|
| | | First-line therapy | | |
| Dexametha-sone pulse | 4 mg daily x 4 days<br>28 mg/m²/day | Immunosuppression<br>GI<br>Hypertension<br>Hyperglycemia [47] | Temporary | Useful when rapid rise in platelets is needed.<br>Little data for "curative" effect when used at diagnosis in patients with refractory disease |
| Danazol | 800 mg daily | Hepatotoxicity | Variable durable response [48-49] | Down-regulates monocyte Fc receptors[50]<br>Monthly LFT monitoring<br>Suppression of menses |
| Azathioprine | 150 mg daily | Leukopenia<br>Hepatotoxicity | Variable durable response [51] | Delayed response<br>Best used in combination with danazol |
| Mycophenolate mofetil | 250 mg BID to 2,000 mg BID | Immunosuppression<br>Headache<br>GI upset | Variable durable response [52-56] | Well-tolerated with minimal side effects |
| Rituximab (Anti-CD20 mAb) | 375 mg/m² weekly x 4 weeks | Infusion reaction in 77% of first infusions [57-58]<br>Progressive multifocal leukoencephalopathy (PML) [59] | Variable durable response [60] | Decreased response to splenectomy following rituximab therapy [57].<br>Consider vaccination (i.e. prior to splenectomy) at least 2 weeks prior to administration |
| Romiplostim | 1-15 μg /kg subcut weekly<br>Mean dose 5.9 μg/kg/week | Thromboses<br>Muscle aches<br>GI discomfort<br>Bone marrow reticulin formation | 80% overall response [61, 63] | Responses lower in splenectomized patients |
| Eltrombopag | 25-75 mg daily | Thromboses<br>Muscle aches<br>GI discomfort<br>Hepatotoxicity (transient)<br>Vision changes<br>Bone marrow reticulin formation | 81% response at highest dose<br>73% durable response | Responses lower in splenectomized patients |
| Avatrombopag | 20 mg weekly to 40 mg daily | Thromboses<br>Headache<br>Contusion<br>Upper respiratory tract infections | up to 80-90% | Responses lower in splenectomized patients |
| | | Second- and third-line agents | | |
| Cyclosporine A | 5 mg/kg/day (Goal 100-200 ng/mL) | Immunosuppression<br>Nephrotoxicity<br>Neurotoxicity<br>GI distress<br>Gingival hyperplasia<br>Hirsutism<br>Lymphoma (long-term use) | 50% response in subsets of refractory patients [75-77] | Calcineurin inhibitor |

| Agent | Dose/Regimen | Toxicity | Efficacy | Notes |
|---|---|---|---|---|
| Cyclophos-phamide | 1,000-1,500 mg/m²/dose IV intermittent pulse (Oral dosing titrated to avoid leukopenia) | Neutropenia<br>Sterility<br>Secondary malignancy<br>Bladder fibrosis (oral dosing) | 85% response<br>Variable durable response [78] | SIADH and hemorrhagic cystitis are uncommon at low doses |
| Etanercept (Enbrel®) | 25 mg subcut twice weekly (3-month courses) | Extensive side effect profile:<br>• Infection (sinus/URI)<br>• Injection site reaction<br>• Heart failure<br>• Neurotoxicity<br>• Autoimmune disease<br>• Malignancy | Limited number of responses [79-80] | Soluble TNF-alpha receptor<br>Used in combination with IVIg |
| Alemtuzumab (CAMPATH-1H, humanized anti-CD52 mAb) | Slow dose escalation (3 mg to 30 mg) 3 x weekly<br>Subcut preferred over IV [80] | Extensive side effect profile:<br>• Infusion reactions<br>• Dyspnea<br>• Hypo/hypertension<br>• GI toxicity<br>• CNS toxicity<br>• Infection<br>• Blood/bone marrow toxicity | Mixed/delayed responses in small numbers of patients [82] | Experience in CLL [83-84], post-bone marrow transplant [85], and in cytopenias, such as AIHA, cold agglutinin disease, pure red cell aplasia, and ITP [86] |
| IDEC-131<br>Hu5c8<br>(Anti-CD40 Ligand mAb) | 5-20 mg/kg/dose IV | Thromboembolism | 24% complete or partial response [87] | Modulates B cell/T cell interaction [88]<br>Agents no longer available due to thromboembolic side effects |
| SYK inhibitors (R406 and related compounds) | 75-175 mg PO Q12 h | GI toxicity: vomiting, diarrhea, transaminitis | 75% response, 50% durable response [89] | SYK is required for signal transduction by IgG Fc receptors<br>Use is limited by GI toxicity |

***Table 13.1:*** First-line, second-line and third-line agents for refractory ITP disease

rectly as well. Recent studies have demonstrated that the combination of rituximab and dexamethasone is likely more effective than either agent alone. Curative effects are primarily seen in young women of child-bearing age. Refractory patients would normally have received rituximab already. If there has been a transient response (months), especially if it was a complete response (count > 100,000/ml), then rituximab may be repeated. If response continues, this may be an avenue to management. However, the likelihood of hypogammaglobulinemia probably increases with time and therefore IgG replacement may also be needed.

A mechanism for lack of response to rituximab in an antibody-mediated ITP would be failure to affect plasma cells. In addition to dexamethasone, trials of anti-plasma cell agents have included bortezomib and more recently daratumumab, the latter with promising results.

Following the cloning of **thrombopoietin** in 1994, recombinant human thrombopoietin (rhTPO) and pegylated recombinant human megakaryocyte growth and development factor (PEG-rHuMGDF), entered clinical trial in 1995. High, even very high platelet counts achieved in certain patients confirmed the efficacy of these agents. However, in a subset of multiply-dosed patients, antibodies to exogenous, with cross-reactivity to endogenous thrombopoietin, these first generation thrombopoietic agents were found to cause severe thrombocytopenia, requiring immunomodulatory therapy to suppress the antibody and restore adequate platelet counts.

Development of these agents was discontinued, but newer agents lacking strong homology to endogenous TPO are now in use without development of antibody-mediated tachyphylaxis involving endogenous thrombopoietin. Romiplostim (AMG-531), eltrombopag (SB-497115), and avatrombopag are thrombopoietin (TPO) receptor agonists that have been shown to be effective in the treatment of ITP. These agents target decreased platelet production as an alternative mechanism of thrombocytopenia not addressed by other therapies.

In the pivotal trial of romiplostim in splenectomized patients, overall response (platelet count of 50,000/μL or more in 24 weeks) was seen in almost 80% of patients [61] however durable responses were seen in only 38%. Eltrombopag is one of several small (400-900 Da) molecules found through screening libraries to bind the human TPO receptor with great specificity. Of note these agents bind the transmembrane region of the TPO receptor, possibly rendering their biologic effect additive to endogenous TPO, which binds the more distal hematopoietic receptor domain (HRD) region. In phase II/III randomized placebo-controlled studies of eltrombopag 50mg and 75mg in adults with ITP, a majority of even splenectomized patients responded [70, 71]. A phase III trial randomizing 197 patients 2:1 to eltrombopag or placebo for 6 months has been completed and results, appear to be similar to those seen in the pivotal studies of romiplostim [61, 62]. Further description of mechanism, efficacy, and safety are described in a recent review [Ghanima,W et al. Haematologica 2019].

The primary toxicity of concern is thrombosis. While this has been seen in less than 6% of patients in any of the controlled trials, it is nonetheless an area requiring careful monitoring. Studies of platelet function have revealed that the current agents do not appear to activate platelets. However, while ITP is clearly hemorrhagic, it is also pro-thrombotic and virtually any agent that has normalized platelet counts in ITP has been associated with thromboembolic events in certain patients who were otherwise pre-disposed for this to occur. These agents do however increase the number of circulating young platelets so that even though they do not activate these platelets, there may be a greater potential for thrombosis. At least a theoretical area of concern with thrombopoietic agents is induction of malignancy, which has been seen with the use of romiplostim to alleviate thrombocytopenia and the need for platelet transfusion in patients with MDS. Concomitant use of 5-azacytidine appears to have alleviated this effect. Eltrombopag has also been associated with a low incidence of abnormal liver tests. In most of the infrequent such cases in the 6 month-study, the abnormalities resolved despite continued treatment.

Avatrombopag has been reported in two studies [106, 107] with very good results. Long-term data is still missing.

## Second-line and third-line therapy

Agents reserved for persistently refractory disease despite first-line therapy, as outline above, are summarized in Table 11.1. Combination therapy and stem cell transplantation are discussed separately below.

## Combination therapy

Multiple first- and second-line agents can be used together or in succession to induce remission in severely refractory patients. Significant acute but short-lived platelet increases have been obtained using the combination of IVIg (1 g/kg), methylprednisolone (30 mg/kg), anti-D (50-75 μg/kg), and vincristine (0.03 mg/kg, max. 1.5 mg). In certain cases, this combination was followed by maintenance therapy with azathioprine (2 mg/kg) and danazol (10-15 mg/kg) [90]. The combination of danazol (200 to 400 mg daily), colchicine (0.6 mg daily) and prednisone (10 to 15 mg daily) has also been used to improve platelet counts [91]. A number of other combination treatments have been used including

- MMF, azathioprine, and cyclosporin

- rituximab-dexamethasone-cyclophosphamide
- MMF and romiplostim
- IVIg-MMF-TPO agent
- CHOP and R-CHOP

and a number of others. Recently several studies form China have explored combination treatments by comparing treatment A to treatments A + B. These studies (danazol + ATRA, rituximab + TPO agent, eltrombopag + dexamethasone) all suggested a benefit of the combination compared to a single agent.

At present there are rationales for usage:

- different mechanisms to add together
- similar mechanisms to have a bigger effect in a given area, e.g. FcR inhibition or immuno-suppresssion
- combination of short-acting medications to increase the platelet count, and
- combinations based on availability.

The area of combination therapy remains to be further explored. Ideally, this approach would be combined with a better approach to understanding pathophysiology, so that it could be specifically targeted.

### Stem cell transplantation

Huhn et al. reported on a series of 14 patients with chronic ITP who received high-dose cyclophosphamide 200 mg/kg divided in 30-90 minute-infusions of 50 mg/kg each over four days [94]; 6 patients obtained durable complete responses (platelets >100,000/µL), and two had partial responses (platelets >50,000/µL). Complications (e.g., sepsis) were common and several patients expired from different causes.

At present the availability of novel agents with several in development has pushed stem cell transplantation further to the back burner to where it is rarely even considered let alone employed.

## 13.6. Outcomes and sequelae

Portielje J.E. et al. showed that chronic ITP that remains refractory to therapy 2 years after diagnosis carries a 4-fold increase in mortality (secondary to bleeding and infection), compared with the general population, and a 4-fold increase in morbidity compared with other ITP patients [97]. In a prospective long-term follow-up study of 105 patients with refractory ITP, almost 30% of patients remained unresponsive to all therapy (platelets <30,000/µL) [98]. Morbidity was highest in this subset of patients, with 10 deaths secondary to intracranial hemorrhage, and one death due to generalized post-operative bleeding. There were six deaths attributable to treatment complications in the entire cohort. Three were due to sepsis associated with immunosuppression and asplenia, one due to postoperative pancreatitis and sepsis, and two deaths from transfusion-related hepatitis C with liver failure. Mean time from splenectomy to death was 63 months. Fifteen patients died of causes apparently unrelated to ITP. This study illustrates in part what can happen when too much in the way of steroids are given for too long. The narrative that treatment causes as much with complications as it saves is only true with overuse of steroids. Current treatments have far better long-term safety profiles.

Within refractory patients could be included those with major bleeding or special circumstances. Several such special cases are described below.

- Intracranial hemorrhage needs to be prevented rather than treated but that is not always possible. In the event of an apparent ICH, one key element is platelet transfusion. Since it is not anticipated that a single platelet transfusion will be effective in a patient with difficult ITP, the best approach is likely to be a bolus followed by continuous infusion. Simultaneously, treatment to increase the patient's own platelet count should be initiated. A minimum would by 1 gram of IV methylprednisolone and 1 gm/kg of IVIg. If this is given with platelet transfusion, it may have the added benefit of protecting the transfused platelets. Additional treatment could include 1.5 mg IV push vincristine, 75 micrograms/kg of IV anti-D, and 10 micrograms/kg of subcutaneous romiplostim. Additional options, such as recombinant factor VIIa could be used, if needed as could anti-fibrinolytics. Further ITP treatment could be pursued, if the above does not bring up the platelet count rapidly and/or the count starts to relapse.

- Two potential emergency treatments are plasmapheresis and splenectomy. Both are likely to be effective but each has a major drawback. Plasmapheresis requires anticoagulation which is potentially dangerous in the setting of an ongoing ICH. Splenectomy requires a major operation, even if done laparoscopically, which could destabilize a patient. Evidence of benefit for each of these are lacking. That may be in part because they are only used as the last resort and thus are selected for use in the worst patients. Alternatively, they may not have enough benefit to be worthwhile. An option could be to use "medical" plasmapheresis by injecting or infusing an FcRn inhibitor to dramatically lower IgG levels, likely including IgG anti-platelet antibodies. This would be of less risk but takes longer, e.g. several days, to lower IgG levels.

- Prevention involves treatment such that the platelet count does not remain dangerously low. It is thought that platelets may provide a tonic nourishment of endothelial cells. This could explain in part why hemorrhage may occur in the setting of unremitting severe thrombocytopenia. The role of antibody specificity in the pathogenesis of ICH is uncertain; GPIIIa is expressed on endothelial cells and anti-GPIIIa antibodies are common in ITP.

## 13.7. Summary

For patients with apparent refractory chronic ITP, as reviewed above, the first and most important consideration is to determine as best as possible whether the patient has ITP or another diagnosis. Furthermore, working with "refractory" patients requires a new, widely accepted definition of refractoriness. Even those with refractory ITP likely represent a heterogeneous subset of ITP patients. The presence of contributing factors should be ruled out and/or eliminated prior to escalating therapy in these patients. With the development of targeted therapy such as rituximab and alemtuzumab, and newer agents such as the thrombopoietin receptor agonists and syk inhibitors, more options are available both to minimize the use and thus the toxicity of long-term corticosteroids, and to reserve the use of cytotoxic immunosuppressive therapy for patients refractory to these agents, first line agents, and possibly splenectomy. Further studies, particularly combination treatments, are needed to more clearly define the role of these medications in the refractory population.

## References

1. Rodeghiero F, et al., Standardization of terminology, definitions and outcome criteria in immune thrombocytopenic purpura of adults and children: report from an international working group. Blood. 2009;113:2386-2393.

2. Berchtold P, McMillan R. Therapy of chronic idiopathic thrombocytopenic purpura in adults. Blood. 1989;74:2309-2317.

3. Drachman JG. Inherited thrombocytopenia: when a low platelet count does not mean ITP. Blood. 2004; 103:390-398.

4. Balduini CL, et al. Inherited thrombocytopenias: a proposed diagnostic algorithm from the Italian Gruppo di Studio delle Piastrine. Haematologica. 2003;88:582-592.

5. Wright JF, et al., Characterization of platelet-reactive antibodies in children with varicella-associated acute immune thrombocytopenic purpura (ITP). Br J Haematol. 1996;95:145-152.

6. Cooper N, Bussel J. The pathogenesis of immune thrombocytopaenic purpura. Br J Haematol. 2006;133: 364-374.

7. Sawanobori M, et al., Severe thrombocytopenia after cytomegalovirus infection in an immunocompetent host – correlation between CMV infection and platelet count in immunocompetent host. Nihon Rinsho Meneki Gakkai Kaishi. 1997;20:134-138.

8. Amitai Y, Granit G. Thrombocytopenic purpura during the incubation period of rubella. Helv Paediatr Acta. 1986;41:55-57.

9. Miyahara M, Shimamoto Y, Yamada H, Shibata K, Matsuzaki M, Ono K. Cytomegalovirus-associated myelodysplasia and thrombocytopenia in an immunocompetent adult. Ann Hematol. 1997;74:99-101.

10. Srivastava A, et al. Parvovirus B19-induced perturbation of human megakaryocytopoiesis in vitro. Blood. 1990;76:1997-2004.

11. Ikehara S, Mizutani H, Kurata Y. Autoimmune thrombocytopenic purpura. Crit Rev Oncol Hematol. 1995;19:33-45.

12. Garcia-Suarez J, et al. Persistent lymphocytosis of natural killer cells in autoimmune thrombocytopenic purpura (ATP) patients after splenectomy. Br J Haematol, 1995;89:653-655.

13. Ichiche M, Fontaine C, Lacor P. Severe thrombocytopenia secondary to cytomegalovirus infection in an immunocompetent adult. Eur J Intern Med. 2003;14:56-59.

14. DiMaggio D, Anderson A, Bussel JB. Cytomegalovirus can make immune thrombocytopenic purpura refractory. Br J Haematol. 2009;146:104-112.

15. Wright JG. Severe thrombocytopenia secondary to asymptomatic cytomegalovirus infection in an immunocompetent host. J Clin Pathol. 1992;45:1037-1038.

16. van Spronsen DJ, Breed WP. Cytomegalovirus-induced thrombocytopenia and haemolysis in an immunocompetent adult. Br J Haematol. 1996;92:218-220.

17. Arruda VR, et al. Cytomegalovirus infection as cause of severe thrombocytopenia in a nonimmunosuppressed patient. Acta Haematol. 1997;98:228-230.

18. Alliot C, Barrios M. Cytomegalovirus-induced thrombocytopenia in an immunocompetent adult effectively treated with intravenous immunoglobulin: a case report and review. Hematology. 2005;10:277-279.

19. Sahud MA, Bachelor MM. Cytomegalovirus-induced thrombocytopenia. An unusual case report. Arch Intern Med. 1978;138:1573-1575.

20. Gural A, et al., Massive intracranial bleeding requiring emergency splenectomy in a patient with CMV-associated thrombocytopenia. Haemostasis. 1998;28: 250-255.

21. Harris AI, Meyer RJ, Brody EA. Letter: Cytomegalovirus-induced thrombocytopenia and hemolysis in an adult. Ann Intern Med. 1975;83:670-671.

22. Fiala M, Kattlove H. Letter: Cytomegalovirus mononucleosis with severe thrombocytopenia. Ann Intern Med. 1973;79:450-451.

23. Stasi R, et al. Effects of eradication of Helicobacter pylori infection in patients with immune thrombocytopenic purpura: a systematic review. Blood. 2009;113: 1231-1240.

24. Michel M, et al. Does Helicobater pylori initiate or perpetuate immune thrombocytopenic purpura? Blood. 2004;103:890-896.

25. Russo A, et al. Determinants of Helicobacter pylori seroprevalence among Italian blood donors. Eur J Gastroenterol Hepatol. 1999;11:867 873.

26. Graham DY, et al. Helicobacter pylori infection in Japan: current status and future options. Eur J Gastroenterol Hepatol. 1994;6 Suppl 1:S1-4.

27. Franchini M, et al. Effect of Helicobacter pylori eradication on platelet count in idiopathic thrombocytopenic purpura: a systematic review and meta-analysis. J Antimicrob Chemother. 2007;60:237-246.

28. Michel M, et al. Autoimmune thrombocytopenic Purpura and Helicobacter pylori infection. Arch Intern Med. 2002;162:1033-1036.

29. Fujimura K, et al. Is eradication therapy useful as the first line of treatment in Helicobacter pylori-positive idiopathic thrombocytopenic purpura? Analysis of 207 eradicated chronic ITP cases in Japan. Int J Hematol. 2005;81:162-168.

30. Bai Y, et al. Cross-reaction of antibody against Helicobacter pylori urease B with platelet glycoprotein IIIa and its significance in the pathogenesis of immune thrombocytopenic purpura. Int J Hematol. 2009;89:142-149.

31. Asahi A. et al. Helicobacter pylori eradication shifts monocyte Fcgamma receptor balance toward inhibitory FcgammaRIIB in immune thrombocytopenic purpura patients. J Clin Invest. 2008;118:2939-2949.

32. Leibman H, Personal Communication.

33. Suzuki M, et al. Interaction of CagA with Crk plays an important role in Helicobacter pylori-induced loss of gastric epithelial cell adhesion. J Exp Med. 2005;202: 1235-1247.

34. van Doorn LJ, et al. Distinct variants of Helicobacter pylori cagA are associated with vacA subtypes. J Clin Microbiol. 1999;37:2306-2311.

35. Tamaoki J, Kadota J, Takizawa H. Clinical implications of the immunomodulatory effects of macrolides. Am J Med. 2004;117 Suppl 9A:5S-11S.

36. Emilia G, et al. Helicobacter pylori infection and chronic immune thrombocytopenic purpura: long-term results of bacterium eradication and association with bacterium virulence profiles. Blood. 2007;110:3833-3841.

37. Scaradavou A. HIV-related thrombocytopenia. Blood Rev. 2002;16:73-76.

38. Zhang W, et al. Role of molecular mimicry of hepatitis C virus protein with platelet GPIIIa in hepatitis C-related immunologic thrombocytopenia. Blood. 2009 113:4086-4093.

39. Marks KM, et al. Risk Factors for Thrombocytopenia in HIV-Infected Persons in the Era of Potent Antiretroviral Therapy. J Acquir Immune Defic Syndr. 2009;52: 595-9.

40. Scaradavou A, et al. Intravenous anti-D treatment of immune thrombocytopenic purpura: experience in 272 patients. Blood. 1997;89:2689-2700.

41. Scaradavou A. et al. Superior effect of intravenous anti-D compared with IV gammaglobulin in the treatment of HIV-thrombocytopenia: results of a small, randomized prospective comparison. Am J Hematol. 2007; 82:335-341.

42. Rajan SK, Espina BM, Liebman HA. Hepatitis C virus-related thrombocytopenia: clinical and laboratory characteristics compared with chronic immune thrombocytopenic purpura. Br J Haematol. 2005;129: 818-824.

43. Najean Y, Rain JD, Billotey C. The site of destruction of autologous 111In-labelled platelets and the efficiency of splenectomy in children and adults with idiopathic thrombocytopenic purpura: a study of 578 patients with 268 splenectomies. Br J Haematol. 1997; 97:547-550.

44. Kojouri K, et al. Splenectomy for adult patients with idiopathic thrombocytopenic purpura: a systematic review to assess long-term platelet count responses, prediction of response, and surgical complications. Blood. 2004;104:2623-2634.

45. Schwartz J, et al. Long term follow-up after splenectomy performed for immune thrombocytopenic purpura (ITP). Am J Hematol. 2003;72:94-98.

46. George JN. Management of patients with refractory immune thrombocytopenic purpura. J Thromb Haemost. 2006;4:1664-1672.

47. Andersen JC. Response of resistant idiopathic thrombocytopenic purpura to pulsed high-dose dexamethasone therapy. N Engl J Med. 1994;330:1560-1564.

48. Ahn YS. Efficacy of danazol in hematologic disorders. Acta Haematol. 1990;84:122-129.

49. Edelmann DZ, et al. Danazol in non-splenectomized patients with refractory idiopathic thrombocytopenic purpura. Postgrad Med J. 1990;66:827-830.

50. Schreiber AD, et al. Effect of danazol in immune thrombocytopenic purpura. N Engl J Med. 1987;316: 503-508.

51. Quiquandon I, et al. Re-evaluation of the role of azathioprine in the treatment of adult chronic idiopathic thrombocytopenic purpura: a report on 53 cases. Br J Haematol. 1990;74:223-228.

52. Provan D, et al. Efficacy of mycophenolate mofetil as single-agent therapy for refractory immune thrombocytopenic purpura. Am J Hematol. 2006;81:19-25.

53. Howard J, et al. Mycophenolate mofetil for the treatment of refractory auto-immune haemolytic anaemia and auto-immune thrombocytopenia purpura. Br J Haematol. 2002;117:712-715.

54. Hou M, et al. Mycophenolate mofetil (MMF) for the treatment of steroid-resistant idiopathic thrombocytopenic purpura. Eur J Haematol. 2003;70:353-357.

55. Kotb R, et al. Efficacy of mycophenolate mofetil in adult refractory auto-immune cytopenias: a single center preliminary study. Eur J Haematol. 2005;75:60-64.

56. Zhang WG, et al. Mycophenolate mofetil as a treatment for refractory idiopathic thrombocytopenic purpura. Acta Pharmacol Sin. 2005;26:598-602.

57. Cooper N, et al. Should rituximab be used before or after splenectomy in patients with immune thrombocytopenic purpura? Curr Opin Hematol. 2007;14:642-646.

58. Arnold DM, et al. Systematic review: efficacy and safety of rituximab for adults with idiopathic thrombocytopenic purpura. Ann Intern Med. 2007;146:25-33.

59. Carson KR, et al. Progressive multifocal leukoencephalopathy after rituximab therapy in HIV-negative patients: a report of 57 cases from the Research on Adverse Drug Events and Reports project. Blood. 2009;113: 4834-4840.

60. Cooper N, et al. The efficacy and safety of B-cell depletion with anti-CD20 monoclonal antibody in adults with chronic immune thrombocytopenic purpura. Br J Haematol. 2004;125:232-239.

61. Kuter DJ, et al. Efficacy of romiplostim in patients with chronic immune thrombocytopenic purpura: a double-blind randomised controlled trial. Lancet. 2008; 371:395-403.

62. Cheng G, Saleh MN, Marcher C, et al. Eltrombopag for management of chronic immune thrombocytopenia (RAISE): a 6-month, randomised, phase 3 study. Lancet. 2011;377:393-402.

63. Bussel JB, et al. Safety and efficacy of long-term treatment with romiplostim in thrombocytopenic patients with chronic ITP. Blood. 2009;113:2161-2171.

64. Stasi R, et al. Response to B-cell depleting therapy with rituximab reverts the abnormalities of T-cell subsets in patients with idiopathic thrombocytopenic purpura. Blood. 2007;110:2924-2930.

65. Stasi R. et al. Analysis of regulatory T-cell changes in patients with idiopathic thrombocytopenic purpura receiving B cell-depleting therapy with rituximab. Blood. 2008;112:1147-1150.

66. Yu J, et al. Defective circulating CD25 regulatory T cells in patients with chronic immune thrombocytopenic purpura. Blood. 2008;112:1325-1328.

67. Sakakura M, et al. Reduced Cd4+Cd25+ T cells in patients with idiopathic thrombocytopenic purpura. Thromb Res. 2007;120:187-193.

68. Ling Y, et al. Circulating dendritic cells subsets and CD4+Foxp3+ regulatory T cells in adult patients with chronic ITP before and after treatment with high-dose dexamethasome. Eur J Haematol. 2007;79:310-316.

69. Wang B, Nichol JL, Sullivan JT. Pharmacodynamics and pharmacokinetics of AMG 531, a novel thrombopoietin receptor ligand. Clin Pharmacol Ther. 2004;76: 628-638.

70. Bussel JB, et al. Effect of eltrombopag on platelet counts and bleeding during treatment of chronic idiopathic thrombocytopenic purpura: a randomised, double-blind, placebo-controlled trial. Lancet. 2009;373: 641-648.

71. Bussel JB, et al. Eltrombopag for the treatment of chronic idiopathic thrombocytopenic purpura. N Engl J Med. 2007;357:2237-2247.

72. Kuter DJ, et al. Bone marrow fibrosis: pathophysiology and clinical significance of increased bone marrow stromal fibres. Br J Haematol. 2007;139:351-362.

73. Kuter DJ, et al. Evaluation of bone marrow reticulin formation in chronic immune thrombocytopenia (ITP) patients treated with romiplostim. Blood. 2009;114: 3748-56.

74. Douglas VK, et al. Thrombopoietin administered during induction chemotherapy to patients with acute myeloid leukemia induces transient morphologic changes that may resemble chronic myeloproliferative disorders. Am J Clin Pathol. 2002;117:844-850.

75. Kappers-Klunne MC, van't Veer MB. Cyclosporin A for the treatment of patients with chronic idiopathic thrombocytopenic purpura refractory to corticosteroids or splenectomy. Br J Haematol. 2001;114:121-125.

76. Perrotta S, et al. Treatment with short-term, high-dose cyclosporin A in children with refractory chronic idiopathic thrombocytopenic purpura. Br J Haematol. 2003;121:143-147.

77. Zver S, Zupan IP, Cernelc P. Cyclosporin A as an immunosuppressive treatment modality for patients with refractory autoimmune thrombocytopenic purpura after splenectomy failure. Int J Hematol. 2006; 83:238-242.

78. Reiner A, Gernsheimer T, Slichter SJ. Pulse cyclophosphamide therapy for refractory autoimmune thrombocytopenic purpura. Blood. 1995;85:351-358.

79. McMinn JR Jr, et al. Complete recovery from refractory immune thrombocytopenic purpura in three patients treated with etanercept. Am J Hematol. 2003;73: 135-140.

80. Litton G. Refractory idiopathic thrombocytopenic purpura treated with the soluble tumor necrosis factor receptor etanercept. Am J Hematol. 2008;83:344.

81. Frampton JE, Wagstaff AJ. Alemtuzumab. Drugs. 2003;63:1229-1243; discussion 1245-1246.

82. Lim SH, et al. CAMPATH-1 monoclonal antibody therapy in severe refractory autoimmune thrombocytopenic purpura. Br J Haematol. 1993;84:542-544.

83. Ammatuna E, et al. Successful treatment of steroid resistant autoimmune thrombocytopenia associated with chronic lymphocytic leukemia with alemtuzumab. Eur J Haematol. 2004;73:225-226.

84. Otton SH, et al. Autoimmune thrombocytopenia after treatment with Campath 1H in a patient with chronic lymphocytic leukaemia. Br J Haematol. 1999; 106:261-262.

85. Chao MM, et al. Successful treatment of refractory immune hemolysis following unrelated cord blood transplant with Campath-1H. Pediatr Blood Cancer. 2008;50:917-919.

86. Willis F, et al. The effect of treatment with Campath-1H in patients with autoimmune cytopenias. Br J Haematol. 2001;114:891-898.

87. Patel VL, Schwartz J, Bussel JB. The effect of anti-CD40 ligand in immune thrombocytopenic purpura. Br J Haematol. 2008;141:545-548.

88. Xu Y, Song G. The role of CD40-CD154 interaction in cell immunoregulation. J Biomed Sci. 2004;11:426-438.

89. Podolanczuk A, et al. Of mice and men: an open-label pilot study for treatment of immune thrombocytopenic purpura by an inhibitor of Syk. Blood. 2009;113:3154-3160.

90. Boruchov DM, et al. Multiagent induction and maintenance therapy for patients with refractory immune thrombocytopenic purpura (ITP). Blood. 2007; 110: 3526-3531.

91. McMillan R. Long-term outcomes after treatment for refractory immune thrombocytopenic purpura. N Engl J Med. 2001;344:1402-1403.

92. Figueroa M, et al. Combination chemotherapy in refractory immune thrombocytopenic purpura. N Engl J Med. 1993;328:1226-1229.

93. Kaufman M, et al. A combination of rituximab, cyclophosphamide and dexamethasone effectively treats immune cytopenias of chronic lymphocytic leukemia. Leuk Lymphoma. 2009;50:892-899.

94. Huhn RD, et al. High-dose cyclophosphamide with autologous lymphocyte-depleted peripheral blood stem cell (PBSC) support for treatment of refractory chronic autoimmune thrombocytopenia. Blood. 2003;101:71-77.

95. Raetz E, Beatty PG, Adams RH. Treatment of severe Evans syndrome with an allogeneic cord blood transplant. Bone Marrow Transplant. 1997;20:427-429.

96. Urushihara N, et al. Secondary sclerosing cholangitis and portal hypertension after O157 enterocolitis: Extremely rare complications of hemolytic uremic syndrome. J Pediatr Surg. 2001;36:1838-1840.

97. Portielje JE, et al. Morbidity and mortality in adults with idiopathic thrombocytopenic purpura. Blood. 2001;97:2549-2554.

98. McMillan R, et al. Suppression of in vitro megakaryocyte production by antiplatelet autoantibodies from adult patients with chronic ITP. Blood. 2004;103: 1364-1369.

99. Butros LJ, Bussel JB. Intracranial hemorrhage in immune thrombocytopenic purpura: a retrospective analysis. J Pediatr Hematol Oncol. 2003;25:660-664.

100. Psaila B, Petrovic A, Page LK, et al. Intracranial hemorrhage (ICH) in children with immune thrombocytopenia (ITP): study of 40 cases. Blood. 2009;114: 4777-4783.

101. Gernsheimer T, McCrae KR. Immune thrombocytopenic purpura in pregnancy. Curr Opin Hematol. 2007;14:574-580.

102. Michel M, Novoa MV, Bussel JB. Intravenous anti-D as a treatment for immune thrombocytopenic purpura (ITP) during pregnancy. Br J Haematol. 2003;123: 142-146.

103. Gross Z, Rodriguez JJ, Stalnaker BL. Vincristine for refractory autoimmune thrombocytopenic purpura in pregnancy. A case report. J Reprod Med. 1995;40:739-742.

104. Varghese L, Viswabandya A, Mathew AJ. Dapsone, danazol, and intrapartum splenectomy in refractory ITP complicating pregnancy. Indian J Med Sci. 2008;62:452-455.

105. Webert KE, et al. A retrospective 11-year analysis of obstetric patients with idiopathic thrombocytopenic purpura. Blood. 2003;102:4306-4311.

106. Bussel J, et al. A randomized trial of avatrombopag, an investigational thrombopoietin-receptor agonist, in persistent and chronic immune thrombocytopenia. Blood. 2014;123(25):3887-3894.

107. Jurczak W, et al. Phase 3 randomised study of avatrombopag, a novel thrombopoietin receptor agonist for the treatment of chronic immune thrombocytopenia. Br J Haematol. 2018;183(3):479-490.

# 14. Immune thrombocytopenia in pregnancy

Thrombocytopenia is a very common finding in pregnancy, occurring in approximately 10% of women [1, 2]. Although most women maintain a normal platelet count throughout gestation, the normal range of platelet counts decreases during pregnancy. Most low platelet counts observed in the pregnant patient are due to normal physiologic changes of pregnancy [3], while some disorders associated with thrombocytopenia occur with a higher frequency during pregnancy and some causes are exclusive to pregnancy [4]. All of these must be considered and ruled out in turn when considering the diagnosis and management of the thrombocytopenic parturient and her fetus.

## 14.1. The differential diagnosis of thrombocytopenia during pregnancy

### Gestational thrombocytopenia

"Incidental" or gestational thrombocytopenia is the most common cause of pregnancy-associated thrombocytopenia and accounts for 65 to 80% of cases [1, 4]. Increased blood volume, an increase in platelet activation and increased clearance contribute to a "physiologic" decrease in the platelet count [3]. The consequence of these changes is generally only a mild decrease in the platelet count, typically approximately 10% [5]. In pregnant women at term, mean platelet count was 213,000/µL compared to 248,000/µL in age matched control women [1, 6]. Gestational thrombocytopenia tends to occur late, usually during the third trimester [7]. Platelet counts <70,000-80,000/µL or occurring during the first or early in the second trimester suggest an etiology other than gestational thrombocytopenia and require further evaluation [8].

### Disorders associated with thrombocytopenia in pregnancy

Many disorders are exacerbated by pregnancy or may be quiescent until the immunologic stimulation that occurs with pregnancy provokes their recurrence.

Autoimmune disorders such as systemic lupus erythematosus may first appear or worsen during pregnancy and hypothyroidism may first manifest during gestation. The antiphospholipid antibody syndrome, which is accompanied by thrombocytopenia in approximately 10-30% of cases [9], need be considered because of its association with fetal loss and the indication for anticoagulation [10].

Women with thrombocytopenia first noted in the second or third trimester should be evaluated for preeclampsia, HELLP syndrome (Hemolysis, Elevated Liver function tests, Low Platelets), acute fatty liver, disseminated intravascular coagulation and thrombotic thrombocytopenic purpura (TTP) or hemolytic uremic syndrome (HUS). These and nutritional and primary bone marrow disorders are generally accompanied by additional clinical and laboratory abnormalities and can be distinguished from ITP on that basis.

Thrombocytopenia may be the primary manifestation of viral infections such as human immunodeficiency virus, viral hepatitis, EBV and CMV. Thrombocytopenia is a common adverse reaction to many drugs and supplements. Women treated with low molecular weight or unfractionated heparin are at risk of heparin induced thrombocytopenia (HIT) and should undergo testing, particularly in the presence of new or worsening thrombosis.

- Gestational (incidental) thrombocytopenia
- Preeclampsia
- HELLP syndrome
- Acute fatty liver of pregnancy
- Thrombotic thrombocytopenic purpura
- Hemolytic uremic syndrome
- Systemic lupus erythematosus
- Antiphospholipid antibody syndrome
- Disseminated intravascular coagulation
- Viral infection
- Nutritional deficiency
- Drug induced
- Primary bone marrow disorder

***Table 14.1:*** Causes of thrombocytopenia in pregnancy.

### Evaluation of the pregnant patient with thrombocytopenia

The history and physical exam may provide clues to the diagnosis, either by disclosure of preexisting thrombocytopenia or bleeding symptoms, or findings of hypertension, edema, or signs of autoimmune disease. Frequent childhood infections may suggest immune deficiency which can be associated with ITP [11]. A careful history of all drug, supplement and toxin exposure should be undertaken. Nutritional status should be ascertained. A family history of thrombocytopenia may suggest a congenital rather than acquired thrombocytopenia. Patients with ITP diagnosed during pregnancy are usually relatively asymptomatic or have only mild symptoms and physical signs related to their thrombocytopenia [12, 13]. Rarely is severe bleeding seen in ITP associated with pregnancy and may at least in part be explained by physiologic changes of the hemostatic system that occur in pregnancy such as increased levels of fibrinogen, factor VIII and von Willebrand factor and decreased fibrinolysis and protein S activity [14].

### Laboratory investigations for the diagnosis of thrombocytopenia in pregnancy

A complete blood count with review of the peripheral blood smear is mandatory in evaluating the thrombocytopenic patient. Although by definition thrombocytopenia is an isolated hematologic abnormality in ITP, anemia of pregnancy or associated with chronic bleeding may also be present. Platelets in the peripheral blood may occasionally be large, but very large and/or hypogranular platelets may suggest a congenital disorder. The presence of schistocytes in the peripheral blood suggests microangiopathic hemolysis. A direct antiglobulin test (DAT) will help to rule out complicating autoimmune hemolysis. Coagulation screening (prothrombin time[PT], activated partial Thromboplastin time [APTT], fibrinogen), liver function tests (Bilirubin, albumin, total protein, transferases and alkaline phosphatase), antiphospholipid antibodies and lupus anticoagulant, thyroid function testing and SLE serology may all be helpful in differentiating ITP from other disorders with associated low platelet counts. Thyroid disorders are associated with significant pregnancy related complications and fetal risk but respond well to therapy. Viral screening (HIV, HCV, HBV), as in the evaluation of non-pregnant women with ITP [15], is recommended. Testing for quantitative immunoglobulins to rule out an immune deficiency syndrome should be considered.

Bone marrow examination is not required to make the diagnosis of ITP in pregnancy. At present, the measurement of maternal anti-platelet immunoglobulin is too insensitive and nonspecific to be of value in the routine diagnosis of ITP in pregnancy and does not predict neonatal thrombocytopenia [16].

| Recommended |
|---|
| • Peripheral blood smear |
| • Reticulocyte count |
| • Direct antiglobulin test |
| • Coagulation screening |
| • Liver function tests |
| • Antiphospholipid antibody and lupus anticoagulant |
| • Systemic lupus erythematosus serology |
| • Thyroid function tests |
| • Viral screening (HIV, HBV, HCV, CMV) |
| **Consider testing** |
| • Quantitative immunoglobulins |
| **Not routinely recommended** |
| • Antiplatelet antibody testing |
| • Bone marrow examination |

***Table 14.2:*** Recommended testing in the differential diagnosis of thrombocytopenia in pregnancy.

## 14.2. ITP in pregnancy

### Presentation of ITP during pregnancy

ITP occurs in approximately 2 per 1,000pregnant women [17]. While ITP may develop at any time during pregnancy, it is often initially recognized in the first trimester and is the most common cause of isolated thrombocytopenia in this time period. In some cases, the initial presentation of ITP may occur during pregnancy, while preexisting cases of ITP may either worsen or remain quiescent [18, 19]. A review of the clinical courses of 92 women with ITP during 119 pregnancies over an 11 year period found that women with previously diagnosed ITP were less likely to require therapy for ITP than those with newly diagnosed ITP12 but the clinical course varies widely.

## Management of ITP during pregnancy

Treatment of ITP in the first and second trimesters is generally undertaken because the patient is symptomatic with bleeding, platelet counts are in the 20-30,000/μL range, or as prophylaxis for planned procedures. Webert and colleagues found in a retrospective analysis of 119 pregnancies in ITP patients that only 89 % had platelet counts <150,000/μL [11]. Although most patients had only mild to moderate thrombocytopenia and the pregnancies were uneventful, 31 % required intervention to increase the platelet count. During the third trimester platelet counts can fall despite remaining relatively stable through most of the pregnancy and monitoring should be more frequent [15]. Therapy late in pregnancy is generally based on the risk of maternal hemorrhage at delivery.

First line therapy for ITP in pregnancy is similar to the management of acute ITP, utilizing corticosteroids [20], intravenous immunoglobulins (IVIg) [21] or a combination of the two when a patient does not respond to a single agent alone [15]. There are no comparative trials of the two agents but responses seem to be similar to that in non-pregnant patients.

Prednisone or prednisolone is generally started at a low dose (10-20 mg by mouth daily) and adjusted to maintain the platelet count in a safe range. Although prednisone is generally safe in pregnancy it can increase weight gain and exacerbate hypertension and hyperglycemia which can have an adverse effect of the outcome of the pregnancy [22]. In addition the emotional effect in the postpartum period should be carefully monitored and dosage should be tapered to avoid a rapid drop in the platelet count after delivery. Very high doses of corticosteroids may have an effect on the fetus. Antenatal corticosteroids have not been found to have an effect on the platelet count on the neonatal platelet count [23] and should not be administered to the near term mother with this objective.

IVIg can be used for a rapid increase in platelet count or to maintain safe platelet counts when patients are not responsive to steroids or they are poorly tolerated. Because of concerns of acute hemolysis and anemia if the antibody crosses the placenta, anti-RhD immuneglobulin is generally not used as a first line agent but has been used in refractory cases throughout pregnancy with successful outcomes [24]. If anti-RhD (50-75 μg/kg) is administered the neonate should be carefully monitored for a positive DAT, anemia and jaundice.

Patients who are only partially responsive or refractory to first line therapy may respond to azathioprine which has been safely administered during pregnancy [25, 26]. High dose methylprednisolone may also be used in combination with IVIg or azathioprine for the patient refractory to oral corticosteroids or IVIg alone.

Many agents that are frequently used in non-pregnant ITP patients such as vinca alkaloids and cyclophosphamide cannot be used because of known or concern for teratogenicity. Cyclosporine A has not been associated with significant toxicity to mother or fetus during pregnancy when used for inflammatory bowel disease [27], but there is no published experience on its use in ITP in the pregnant female.

Although there are case reports of treatment of lymphoproliferative disorders with rituximab early in pregnancy [18, 29], experience is limited and its use for pregnancy associated ITP cannot be recommended because of its potential for crossing the placenta. Danazol in combination with high dose IVIg and corticosteroids has been used for short-term treatment in the third trimester in refractory thrombocytopenia [30], but longer term use is likely to be teratogenic. There are no data on the use of thrombopoietin receptor agonists in pregnancy and their effects on the fetus are unknown.

For patients who remain refractory to therapy or who incur significant toxicity, splenectomy may induce a remission. Splenectomy can be safely performed during the second trimester [31, 32], when the risk of anesthesia to the fetus is minimal and uterine size will not complicate the procedure.

## Management of delivery

The mode of delivery in a pregnant patient with ITP is based on obstetric indications and ITP in the mother is not an indication for Caesarian section [33]. Most neonatal hemorrhage occurs at 24-48 hours [34, 35] and is not related to trauma at the time of delivery. Methods to determine the fetal platelet count such as periumbilical blood sampling [36] or fetal scalp vein blood draws present a potential hemorrhagic risk to the fetus and may inaccurately predict a low platelet count [16]. For this reason fetal platelet count measurement is not recommended.

Maternal anesthesia must be based on safety of the mother. The risk of spinal hematoma at lower platelet counts is unknown, but the general practice is to withhold spinal anesthesia for women with platelet counts below 75,000/μL [37-39]. Thromboelastograms have been suggested as evaluating the entire hemostatic state of the mother [40], however their usefulness is unclear. The bleeding time has also been suggested as a mode of establishing the safety of the platelet count [4], but most centers no longer offer this test and the experience in using it to predict bleeding at delivery is limited. A short course of corticosteroids for 1 to 2 weeks or IVIg may help to prepare the mother if an increase in the count is required for epidural anesthesia. Platelet transfusion is not appropriate as post-transfusion increments are frequently inadequate and likely to be short-lived. Platelet transfusion should be only used to treat bleeding.

### Monitoring and management of the neonate

Neonatal ITP accounts for only 3% of all cases of thrombocytopenia at delivery [42]. There is no accurate predictor of fetal platelet count; correlation between maternal and fetal platelet counts is poor [1, 43, 44] and appears to relate to the presence of alloantibody (in neonatal alloimmune thrombocytopenia) but not autoantibody. The best predictor of thrombocytopenia in the neonate may be whether there was a previously affected sibling [45]. Severe thrombocytopenia in the neonate delivered to a mother with ITP is uncommon and platelet counts <50,000/μL occur in 8.9-14.7% [34, 35, 46]. A retrospective study of 127 pregnancies in 88 women with ITP in Japan showed a trend toward lower platelet counts in offspring when the mothers' platelet counts were less than 100,000/μL but was not statistically significant [47]. Mortality in neonates of mothers with ITP is rare (<1 %) and estimates of the incidence of intracranial hemorrhage range from 0-1.5%. A cord blood platelet count should be obtained at the time of delivery to determine if immediate therapy is indicated. Injections such as intramuscular vitamin K should be avoided unless the neonate is known to have a safe platelet count. The nadir platelet count frequently occurs 2-5 days after birth and may last weeks to months [48]. Unsafe platelets counts in neonates of ITP mothers may be treated with IVIg 1g/kg and can be repeated every few weeks as necessary to maintain a safe platelet count until spontaneous recovery.

## 14.3. Conclusion

ITP is a fairly common complication in otherwise normal pregnancies, but must be distinguished from more commonly occurring incidental gestational thrombocytopenia or other disorders requiring directed therapy. ITP in pregnancy is managed similarly to ITP in the non-pregnant adult patient but choice of therapy must take into account risks to the developing fetus. A history of ITP or ITP in a previous pregnancy is not a contraindication to pregnancy and the vast majority of patients are delivered of non- or only mildly thrombocytopenic infants.

### References

1. Sainio S, Kekomaki R, Riikonen S, Teramo K. Maternal thrombocytopenia at term: a population-based study. Acta Obstet Gynecol Scand 2000;79:744-749

2. Burrows RF, Kelton JG. Incidentally detected thrombocytopenia in healthy mothers and their infants. N Engl J Med 1988:319:142-145

3. Matthews JH, Benjamin S, Gill DS, Smith NA. Pregnancy-associated thrombocytopenia: definition, incidence and natural history. Acta Haematol 1990;84:24-29

4. Burrows RF, Kelton JG. Thrombocytopenia at delivery: a prospective survey of 6715 deliveries. Am J Obstet Gynecol 1990;162:731–734

5. Verdy E, Bessous V, Dreyfus M et al. Longitudinal analysis of platelet count and volume in normal pregnancy. Thromb Haemost 1997;77:806-807

6. Boehlen F, Hohlfeld P, Extermann P, et al. Platelet count at term pregnancy: A reappraisal of the threshold. Obstet Gynecol 2000;95:29-33

7. Gernsheimer T, McCrae KR. Immune thrombocytopenic purpura in pregnancy. Curr Opin Hematol 2007;14:574-580

8. British Committee for Standards in Haematology General Haematology Task Force. Guidelines for the investigation and management of idiopathic thrombocytopenic purpura in adults, children and in pregnancy. Br J Haematol 2003;120:574-596

9. Godeau B, Piette JC, Fromont P, et al. Specific antiplatelet glycoprotein autoantibodies are associated with the thrombocytopenia of primary antiphospholipid syndrome. Br J Haematol 1997:98:873-879

10. Oshiro BT, Silver RM, Scott JR, et al. Antiphospholipid antibodies and fetal death. Obstet Gynecol 1996; 87:489-493

11. Cines DB, Liebman HA. The immune thrombocytopenia syndrome: a disorder of diverse pathogenesis and clinical presentation. Hematol Oncol Clin North Am 2009;23:1155-1161

12. Webert KE, Mittal R, Sigouin C, et al. A retrospective 11-year analysis of obstetric patients with idiopathic thrombocytopenic purpura. Blood 2003;102:4306-4311

13. Fujimura K, Harada Y, Fujimoto T, et al. Nationwide study of idiopathic thrombocytopenic purpura in pregnant women and the clinical influence on neonates. Int J Hematol 2002;75:426-33.

14. Calderwood C. Thromboembolism and thrombophilia in pregnancy. Curr Obstet Gynaecol 2006;16:321-326

15. Provan D, Stasi R, Newland AC, et al. International consensus report on the investigation and management of primary immune thrombocytopenia. Blood 2010;115: 168-186

16. Boehlen F, Hohlfeld P, Extermann P, de Moerloose P. Maternal antiplatelet antibodies in predicting risk of neonatal thrombocytopenia. Obstet Gynecol 1999;93-169-173

17. Gill KK, Kelton JG. Management of idiopathic thrombocytopenic purpura in pregnancy. Semin Hematol 2000;37:275-289

18. Won YW, Moon W, Yun YS, et al. Clinical aspects of pregnancy and delivery in patients with chronic idiopathic thrombocytopenic purpura (ITP). Korean J Intern Med 2005; 20:129–134

19. Fujimura K, Harada Y, Fujimoto T, et al. Nationwide study of idiopathic thrombocytopenic purpura in pregnant women and the clinical influence on neonates. Int J Hematol 2002;75:426-433

20. Karpatkin S. Autoimmune thrombocytopenic purpura. Sem Hematol 1985;22:260-288

21. Besa EC, MacNab MW, Solan AJ, et al. High-dose intravenous IgG in the management of pregnancy in women with idiopathic thrombocytopenic purpura. Am J Hematol 1985;18:373-379

22. The HAPO Study Cooperative Research Group. Hyperglycemia and adverse pregnancy outcomes. N Engl J Med 2008;358:1991-2002

23. Christiaens GCML, Nieuwenhuis HK, von dem Borne AEGKr, et al. Idiopathic thrombocytopenic N Engl J Med purpura in pregnancy: A randomized trial on the effect of antenatal low dose corticosteroids on neonatal platelet count. Br J Obstet Gynaecol 1990;97:893-898

24. Michel M, Novoa MV, Bussel JB. Intravenous anti-D as a treatment for immune thrombocytopenic purpura (ITP) during pregnancy. Br J Haematol 2003;123:142-146

25. Alstead EM, Ritchie JK, Lennard-Jones JE, et al. Safety of azathioprine in pregnancy in inflammatory bowel disease. Gastroenterology 1990;99:443-446

26. Price HV, Salaman JR, Laurence KM, Langmaid H. Immunosuppressive drugs and the foetus. Transplantation 1976;21:294-298

27. Reddy D, Murphy SJ, Kane SV, et al. Relapses of inflammatory bowel disease during pregnancy: in-hospital management and birth outcomes. Am J Gastroenterol 2008;103:1203-1209

28. Kimby E, Sverrisdottir A, Elinder G. Safety of rituximab therapy during the first trimester of pregnancy: a case history. Eur J Haematol 2004;72:292-295

29. Herold M, Schnohr S, Bittrich H. Efficacy and safety of a combined rituximab chemotherapy during pregnancy. J Clin Oncol 2001;19:3439

30. Orisaka M, Shukunami K, Orisaka S, et al. Combination therapy for a pregnant woman with severe refractory ITP. Eur J Obstet Gynecol Reprod Biol 2005;121:119-120

31. Anglin BV, Rutherford C, Ramus R, et al. Immune thrombocytopenic purpura during pregnancy: laparoscopic treatment. JSLS 2001;5:63-67

32. Griffiths J, Sia W, Shapiro AM, et al. Laparoscopic splenectomy for the treatment of refractory immune thrombocytopenia in pregnancy. J Obstet Gynaecol Can 2005;27:771-774

33. Laros RK, Kagan R. Route of delivery for patients with immune thrombocytopenic purpura. Am J Obstet Gynecol 1984;148:901

34. Kaplan C, Daffos F, Forestier F, et al. Fetal platelet counts in thrombocytopenic pregnancy. Lancet 1990; 336:979-982

35. Bussel JB, Druzin ML, Cines DB, Samuels P. Thrombocytopenia in pregnancy. Lancet 1991;337:251

36. Scioscia AL, Grannum PA, Copel JA, Hobbins JC. The use of percutaneous umbilical blood sampling in immune thrombocytopenic purpura. Am J Obstet Gynecol 1988;159:1066-1068

37. Beilin Y, Zahn J, Comerford M. Safe epidural analgesia in thirty parturients with platelet counts between 69,000 and 98,000 mm3. Anesth Analg 1997;85:385-388

38. Choi S, Brull R. Neuraxial Techniques in Obstetric and Non-Obstetric Patients with Common Bleeding Diatheses. Anesth Analg 2009;109:648-660

39. Van Veen JJ, Nokes TJ, Makris M. The risk of spinal haematoma following neuraxial anaesthesia or lumbar

puncture in thrombocytopenic individuals. Br J Haematol 2010;148:15-25

40. Hunt BJ, Lyons G. Thromboelastography should be available in every labour ward. Int J Obstet Anesth 2005; 14:324-325

41. Ballem PJ, Buskard N, Wittmann BK, et al. ITP in pregnancy: Use of the bleeding time as an indicator for treatment. Blut 1989;59:132-135

42. Gill KK, Kelton JG. Management of idiopathic thrombocytopenic purpura in pregnancy. Semin Hematol 2000;37:275-289

43. Kelton JG. Management of the pregnant patient with idiopathic thrombocytopenic purpura. Ann Intern Med 1983;99:796-800

44. Burrows RF, Kelton JG. Fetal thrombocytopenia and its relation to maternal thrombocytopenia. N Engl J Med 1993;329:1463-1466

45. Christianens GC, Nieuwenhuis HK, Bussel JB. Comparison of platelet counts in first and second newborns of mothers with immune thrombocytopenic purpura. Obstet Gynecol 1997;90:546-552

46. Samuels P, Bussel JB, Braitman LE, et al. Estimation of the risk of thrombocytopenia in the offspring of pregnant women with presumed immune thrombocytopenic purpura. N Engl J Med 1990;323:229-235

47. Koyama S, Tomimatusu T, Kanagawa T, et al. Reliable predictors of neonatal immune thrombocytopenia in pregnant women with idiopathic thrombocytopenic purpura. Am J Hematol 2012;87:15-21

48. Burrows RF, Kelton JG. Low fetal risks in pregnancies associated with idiopathic thrombocytopenic purpura. Am J Obstet Gynecol 1990;163:1147-1150

# 15. Drugs in ITP: mechanisms of action

Immune thrombocytopenia (ITP) is an autoimmune disorder characterised by the production of platelet-reactive autoantibodies which induce platelet clearance, resulting in thrombocytopenia. Platelet clearance appears to occur mainly, though not exclusively [1-4], via phagocytosis in the mononuclear phagocytic system (MPS). As platelet clearance may occur via different mechanisms, patient therapy will be adversely affected depending on the mechanism of platelet destruction. Herein, we discuss five different drug classes used to initiate platelet recovery in ITP and explore their mechanisms of action.

## 15.1. Steroids

A first-line treatment regimen for ITP is non-specific immunosuppression by oral corticosteroids, primarily prednisone or methylprednisolone.

Steroid treatment in ITP results in increased platelet survival by decreasing production of anti-platelet antibodies by B cells and decreasing the clearance of opsonized platelets by phagocytic cells such as macrophages. However, the exact mechanisms involved remain unclear. Steroid therapy can induce remissions in more than 60% of patients, but relapse of thrombocytopenia is common when the dose is tapered off, and only one-third of patients will experience long-term responses [5]. In many centres in the United States, steroids are often used in pediatric ITP patients who fail to respond to initial therapy with IVIg [6]. In one recent study, ITP patients with IgA levels higher than median had a significantly higher chance of failing steroid therapy. Patients in the same study demonstrating a low IgM level, failed to respond to steroid therapy in comparison to patients with a normal IgM level; the authors suggest that patients with immune dysregulation may be more resistant to steroid therapy [7].

Steroids have a potent immunosuppressive effect [8, 9].

This is achieved not only by blocking the synthesis of pro-inflammatory cytokines but also by blocking their systemic effects. Steroids inhibit the synthesis of certain cytokine receptors such as the IL-2 receptor [10]. At high stress-induced levels, steroids act to dampen and reduce the immune response at all levels, including preventing the further driving of cytokine activation, the priming of lymphocytes by antigen presenting cells and reducing the responsiveness of already activated cells [11]. Specifically, steroids have a uniform inhibitory effect on the synthesis, release and efficacy of the pro-inflammatory cytokines IL-1, IL-2, IL-6, IL-8, IL-11, IL-12, IFN-$\gamma$ and TNF-$\alpha$ [12], and they can also inhibit cytokine effects of IL-2, IL-4, IL-7 and IL-15 in target cells [10].

Steroids mainly exert their anti-inflammatory effects through binding to the glucocorticoid receptor (GR) which is expressed in a variety of tissues; these are referred to as genomic effects. As an example, in T cells, dexamethasone enters target cells by passive diffusion across the cell membrane where it binds the ligand-binding domain of the GR initiating dimerization and translocation of the GR to the nucleus, where it binds to genomic DNA at specific DNA hormone response elements in the promoter control regions of target genes and alters the rate of gene transcription. This in turn initiates the transcription of factors that result in decreased cellular proliferation, decreased proinflammatory cytokine synthesis and inhibition of the effects of cytokines (reviewed in [11]). Macrophages, which also express GR, are thought to be generally affected in a similar manner.

It has been shown that steroids can rapidly (<30 min) inhibit phagocytosis and superoxide anion production in murine peritoneal macrophages [13]. In line with this potential mechanism, a recent study has shown that ITP patients with antibodies directed to the platelet GPIIb/IIIa antigen, which likely induce platelet clearance via phagocytosis, respond significantly better to dexamethasone than patients with antibodies to GPIb$\alpha$, which can induce platelet clearance via a phagocytosis independent mechanism [14]. Another study showed that ITP patients treated with high dose dexamethasone demonstrated a decreased ratio of inhibitory Fc$\gamma$ receptor (Fc$\gamma$R) to activating Fc$\gamma$R on monocytes, compared with untreated patients, suggesting that the ability of dexamethasone to increase inhibitory FcγR expression and/or decrease activating FcR expression may contribute to its mechanism of action [15].

Rapid inhibition of phagocytosis is an example of non-genomic steroid effects, which are acute and often occur within minutes. In other examples, Hafezi-Moghadam et al. showed that steroids activate endothelial nitric oxide synthase (NOS) resulting in vasorelaxation, which explains some of the rapid cardioprotective effects of steroids [16]. Similarly, nongenomic neuroprotective effects were detected following high-dose steroid therapy in a cerebral ischemia model, due to activation of one of the NOS enzymes (eNOS), resulting in acute neuroprotective effects through an increase in cerebral blood flow [17]. Moreover, rapid clinical improvement (occurring within minutes) of allergic and anaphylactic reactions and spinal trauma have been reported due to acute (and local) treatment with high steroid doses [18]. However, the precise molecular mechanisms that underlie all nongenomic steroid-induced immunosuppressive effects remain to be defined, and taking into account recent data discussed here, the effects of steroids in ITP may be more complicated than originally thought.

## 15.2. Intravenous immunoglobulin (IVIg)

☞ Chapter 16. "Mechanism of action of high dose intravenous immunoglobulin in ITP".

## 15.3. Anti-D

Polyclonal anti-D (a type of IVIg) consists of IgG selectively taken from the plasma of RhD negative donors immunized to the D antigen. It has been used to treat ITP in both children and adults [21, 43-45] and has also been used to treat HIV-associated thrombocytopenia [46, 47]. Salama and coworkers theorized that the success of anti-D in treating ITP was due to competitive inhibition of the MPS by sensitized red blood cells (RBC) [20, 21], and other reports have also suggested that anti-D functions by MPS blockade [44, 46, 48, 49]. Thus MPS blockade has classically been considered to be a primary mechanism of action of anti-D. Further evidence to support this as a potential mechanism derives from studies showing that anti-D is ineffective in thrombocytopenic patients who are RhD antigen negative [50, 51]. Additional evidence to support the theory of anti-D functioning by MPS blockade is the observation that patients with chronic ITP after splenectomy (the spleen being the primary site of the MPS) had nominal or no response to anti-D treatment [45, 46], although one study found that two splenectomized ITP patients did respond to anti-D [52].

Using the murine model of ITP, we have found that RBC-specific antibodies successfully increased platelet counts in association with downregulation of the activating FcγRIIIA on splenic macrophages [53], suggesting that anti-RBC antibodies downmodulate the expression of the activating FcγRIIIA on phagocytic cells. If anti-D and IVIg have the ability to ameliorate thrombocytopenia by different mechanisms (i.e. downmodulation and/or blockade of activating FcγR vs. functioning through the inhibitory FcγRIIB) it might be expected that patients who are refractory to one treatment might respond to the other. Indeed, Bussel et al. found no relation in the response of ITP patients to anti-D and IVIg [54], suggesting that although anti-D and IVIg both exhibit a common ability to inhibit MPS function, they may act by different mechanisms.

The ability of anti-D to induce cytokine modulation has been well documented. Many groups have demonstrated increases in IL-6, IL-10, TGF-β, TNF-α, MCP-1 and GM-CSF in patients receiving anti-D [34, 55-57]. Cooper et al. found that 2 hours post treatment, anti-D induced the production of IL-6, IL-10, TNF-α and MCP-1, while at 2 hours after IVIg treatment only IL-10 was increased [34]; the authors suggested that these treatments may ameliorate thrombocytopenia via different mechanisms. Semple et al. found that anti-D treatment resulted in significant increases in the anti-inflammatory compound IL-1 receptor antagonist (IL-1Ra), as well as increases in IL-6, GM-CSF, MCP-1α, TNF-α and MCP-1 [56]. This same group later demonstrated that anti-D sensitized RBC induced the production of IL-1Ra by monocytes and granulocytes *in vitro*, which correlated with a decrease in phagocytosis [58]. Although anti-D does regulate the production of numerous cytokines in patients with ITP, their role in the therapeutic activity of anti-D is still unclear.

A recent study found that ITP patients with IgA levels higher than median had a significantly higher chance of failing anti-D therapy [7]. In addition, patients in the same study demonstrating a low IgM level, failed to respond to anti-D therapy more than patients with a normal IgM level. The authors speculate that patients with immune dysregulation may be more resistant to anti-D therapy.

In 2010, the Food and Drug Administration added a "black box" warning to anti-D for treatment of ITP, to warn against complications related to severe hemolysis. Numerous reports of hemolysis due to anti-D have been reported [59-61]. It is of interest to note that 2 reports examining the administration of anti-D via subcutaneous injection found that ITP patients responded well and showed no sign of hemolysis in the study [62, 63]. From a mechanistic point of view, it could be speculated that subcutaneous injection of anti-D results in a slow release into the venous circulation, resulting in undetectable hemolysis, or that pathogenic (i.e. hemolytic) antibodies in the anti-D preparation are somehow removed during passage from the subcutis to the peripheral blood. Thus the subcutaneous route could prove to be a safer delivery method for anti-D administration in ITP patients. A promising new anti-D preparation is Rozrolimupab (Sym001), composed of 25 genetically unique recombinant monoclonal antibodies specific for the D antigen. Although not yet in use for ITP patients, phase II clinical trials using healthy donors found no serious adverse events [64].

## 15.4. Rituximab (anti-CD20)

Rituximab is a human/murine chimeric monoclonal antibody that specifically depletes B cells from the blood, lymph nodes and bone marrow by targeting CD20, which is expressed on the surface of premature and mature B lymphocytes [65]. CD20 antibodies are classified as Class I (Rituximab-like), which stabilize CD20 in lipid rafts and induce complement dependent cytotoxicity (CDC), but only weakly induce apoptosis *in vitro*, and Class II, which do not localize CD20 into lipid rafts and only weakly induce CDC, but appear to induce higher levels of apoptosis [66].

Rituximab was first developed for the treatment of haematological malignancies and is indicated for the treatment of non-Hodgkin lymphoma and to treat patients with chronic lymphocytic leukaemia. Rituximab is currently used to treat ITP patients that had been refractory to other treatment regimens [67, 68]. The rationale for its use in chronic ITP rested on the attempt to eliminate autoreactive B-cell clones, and indeed a reduction in peripheral B cells was observed. In a follow-up study [69], this same group theorized that the acute response observed in some ITP patients undergoing rituximab therapy could be due to the opsonization of B cells, resulting in a blockade of the MPS, a mechanism similar to the theory of FcR blockade by opsonized red cells following anti-D treatment, while the depletion of B cells and subsequent decrease in antiplatelet antibody helped to explain the late and sustained response. However, a long-term study by Cooper et al. demonstrated that the recovery of B cells in ITP patients treated with rituximab did not result in relapse in those patients who achieved a complete recovery [70]. In addition, a recent study found that patients who did not respond to rituximab nonetheless had complete B cell depletion in peripheral blood and a significant reduction in splenic B cells; the authors suggest that rituximab-induced B cell depletion is not correlated with its therapeutic effects [71]. Thus the relationship between the prophylactic effects of rituximab and B cell depletion is unclear. Only after examining the mechanism of action in more detail do we realize that there is more than mere B cell depletion involved. Insights into the mechanism of rituximab action in ITP indicate that significant changes occur in T cells in patients who respond to rituximab [72]. The response to rituximab-induced B cell depletion was associated with a normalization of the T helper cell-1/2 (Th1/Th2) ratio, normalized expression of the apoptotic cell marker Fas ligand on Th1 and Th2 cells, and an indication of potential normalization of the T cell repertoire, thus reverting some of the abnormalities of T cells in patients that respond to treatment.

A subclass of T cells known as regulatory T cells (Treg) can suppress activation of the immune system and potentially function to inhibit autoimmunity. It has been demonstrated that Tregs are reduced and abnormal in patients with ITP [73, 74]. Work from Stasi and colleagues [75] has revealed new insights on the effect of rituximab on Tregs in ITP: responding patients demonstrated restored numbers and function of Tregs after treatment with rituximab, suggesting that this B cell-targeted therapy can in turn modulate the defects seen with Treg cells and may be a contributing mechanism by which this drug functions.

Another Class I CD20 antibody that is in clinical trials for treating chronic ITP is a fully humanized monoclonal termed veltuzumab. In dose-finding phase I/II clinical trials in patients with low-grade NHL, it demonstrated a substantial rate of complete responses in concurrence with shorter and more tolerable infusions compared with rituximab [76].

## 15.5. Drugs that stimulate platelet production

☞ also Chapter 4.

Antibodies from ITP patients have been shown to inhibit the production of platelets by megakaryocytes [77, 78], an event that could contribute to the thrombocytopenia observed in ITP. Thrombopoietin is a glycoprotein hormone that stimulates the proliferation of both the early and late stages of megakaryocyte maturation. Initial clinical testing using recombinant thrombopoietin failed due to an immune response to the recombinant thrombopoietin itself, including the endogenous thrombopoietin, resulting in secondary thrombocytopenia and bleeding [79]. This setback initiated research into agonists of the thrombopoietin receptor (c-MPL) that did not display sequence homology to endogenous thrombopoeitin. Several thrombopoeitin mimetic drugs that successfully stimulate the *in vivo* production of platelets, including romiplostim (Nplate™), eltrombopag (Revolade™) and avatrombopag (Doptelet™), have proven to be promising therapeutic agents for ITP. Romiplostim, eltrombopag and avatrombopag bind to and cause activation of the thrombopoietin receptor.

### Romiplostim

Romiplostim is a fusion protein analogue of thrombopoietin, which binds the extracellular region of the thrombopoietin receptor at the normal thrombopoietin binding site. It is comprised of two covalently-linked IgG-Fc domains, each expressing multiple thrombopoietin receptor binding sequences. It was initially used in a randomized trial in 48 healthy adults and induced a dose-dependent increase in platelet counts [80]. Multiple clinical trials have demonstrated that romiplostim can successfully increase platelet counts in ITP patients, although platelet counts return to prior low baseline counts within 2 weeks of discontinuation of the drug as they do not affect the underlying rate of platelet destruction [81-84].

### Eltrombopag

Eltrombopag is a synthetic thrombopoeitin receptor agonist that binds the receptor in the transmembrane spanning region. A prospective Phase I clinical study was initiated to study the safety, pharmacokinetics, pharmacodynamics and safety in healthy volunteers, and showed a consistent and safe increase in platelet counts at 8 days post repeated dosing [85]. Additional trials with ITP patients have shown that greater than 80% of patients showed significant increases in platelet count, with the median nearing the normal platelet range [86, 87].

### Avatrombopag

Avatrombopag is an orally-administered small molecule thrombopoietin receptor agonist. It was the third thrombopoietin receptor agonist approved for the treatment of immune thrombocytopenia and the first approved to treat periprocedural thrombocytopenia in patients with chronic liver disease (thereby providing an alternative to blood transfusions for these patients). Unlike eltrombopag, avatrombopag does not require a 4 hr food-restricted window around its use and it has not been associated with hepatotoxicity in ITP patients or portal vein thrombosis in patients with chronic liver disease [97]. In ITP patients it can often be dosed less frequently than once daily. It is overall well-tolerated with a side-effect profile similar to placebo in randomized clinical trials.

While it is clear that platelet counts generally return to thrombocytopenic levels after patients are tapered off these drugs, one study reported the interesting finding that ITP patients undergoing successful treatment with thrombopoietic agents also demonstrated improved activity of regulatory T cells (Treg) [88]. The authors speculated that thrombopoietic agent treatment may improve

Treg function by enhanced release of TGF-β1 as a result of greater platelet turnover.

On the horizon, another TPO receptor agonist, E5501 (AKR-501) has shown promise in increasing platelet counts in ITP patients [89].

While the results of these thrombopoeitin receptor agonist drugs are encouraging, the long-term effects of megakaryocyte stimulation are currently unknown, but may include reticulin formation in the bone marrow of a low percentage of patients, although this appears to be reversible and is also found in healthy subjects [90]. Additional reports have also found thromboembolic complications in some patients, possibly arising from an excessive increase in platelet counts [91].

## 15.6. Conclusion

In addition to the drugs discussed here, there are other treatments for ITP including splenectomy, and other classes of immunosuppressants. For example, a clinical trial using the Syk inhibitor fostamatinib demonstrated that inhibition of the activity of the tyrosine kinase Syk resulted in improved platelet counts in ITP patients [92]. Another Syk inhibitor, P505-15, which shows promise in treating animal models of rheumatoid arthritis [93], may one day also be a new treatment for ITP. Treatment of ITP patients with a monoclonal antibody to the leukocyte antigen CD52, alemtuzumab, has also been successful [94-96]. Further research using animal models will undoubtedly help to delineate the precise, potentially overlapping, mechanisms of action of the drugs discussed here as well as other treatments.

### References


1. Li Z, Nardi MA, Li YS, et al. C-terminal ADAMTS-18 fragment induces oxidative platelet fragmentation, dissolves platelet aggregates, and protects against carotid artery occlusion and cerebral stroke. Blood 2009;113:6051-6060.

2. Nieswandt B, Bergmeier W, Rackebrandt K, et al. Identification of critical antigen-specific mechanisms in the development of immune thrombocytopenic purpura in mice. Blood 2000;96:2520-2527.

3. Olsson B, Andersson PO, Jernas M, et al. T-cell-mediated cytotoxicity toward platelets in chronic idiopathic thrombocytopenic purpura. Nat Med 2003;9: 1123-1124.

4. Webster ML, Sayeh E, Crow M, et al. Relative efficacy of intravenous immunoglobulin G in ameliorating thrombocytopenia induced by antiplatelet GPIIbIIIa versus GPIbalpha antibodies. Blood 2006;108:943-946.

5. Guidelines for the investigation and management of idiopathic thrombocytopenic purpura in adults, children and in pregnancy. Br J Haematol 2003;120(4):574-596.

6. Pels SG. Current therapies in primary immune thrombocytopenia. Semin Thromb Hemost 2011;37:621-630.

7. Arnason JE, Campigotto F, Neuberg D, Bussel JB. Abnormalities in IgA and IgM are associated with treatment-resistant ITP. Blood 2012;119:5016-5020.

8. Elenkov IJ, Chrousos GP. Stress hormones, proinflammatory and antiinflammatory cytokines, and autoimmunity. Ann N Y Acad Sci 2002;966:290-303.

9. Wilckens T. Glucocorticoids and immune function: physiological relevance and pathogenic potential of hormonal dysfunction. Trends Pharmacol Sci 1995;16:193-197.

10. Bianchi M, Meng C, Ivashkiv LB. Inhibition of IL-2-induced Jak-STAT signaling by glucocorticoids. Proc Natl Acad Sci USA 2000;97:9573-9578.

11. Cole TJ. Glucocorticoid action and the development of selective glucocorticoid receptor ligands. Biotechnol Annu Rev 2006;12:269-300.

12. Webster JI, Tonelli L, Sternberg EM. Neuroendocrine regulation of immunity. Annu Rev Immunol 2002; 20:125-163.

13. Long F, Wang YX, Liu L, et al. Rapid nongenomic inhibitory effects of glucocorticoids on phagocytosis and superoxide anion production by macrophages. Steroids 2005;70:55-61.

14. Zeng Q, Zhu L, Tao L, et al. Relative efficacy of steroid therapy in immune thrombocytopenia mediated by anti-platelet GPIIbIIIa versus GPIbalpha antibodies. Am J Hematol. 2011;Epub ahead of print.

15. Liu XG, Ma SH, Sun JZ, et al. High-dose dexamethasone shifts the balance of stimulatory and inhibitory Fcgamma receptors on monocytes in patients with primary immune thrombocytopenia. Blood 2011;117: 2061-2069.

16. Hafezi-Moghadam A, Simoncini T, et al. Acute cardiovascular protective effects of corticosteroids are mediated by non-transcriptional activation of endothelial nitric oxide synthase. Nat Med 2002;8:473-479.

17. Limbourg FP, Huang Z, Plumier JC, et al. Rapid nontranscriptional activation of endothelial nitric oxide synthase mediates increased cerebral blood flow and stroke protection by corticosteroids. J Clin Invest 2002; 110:1729-1738.

18. Buttgereit F, Straub RH, Wehling M, Burmester GR. Glucocorticoids in the treatment of rheumatic diseases: an update on the mechanisms of action. Arthritis Rheum 2004;50:3408-3417.

19. Imbach P, Barandun S, d'Apuzzo V, et al. High-dose intravenous gammaglobulin for idiopathic thrombocytopenic purpura in childhood. Lancet 1981;1:1228-1231.

20. Salama A, Mueller-Eckhardt C, Kiefel V. Effect of intravenous immunoglobulin in immune thrombocytopenia. Lancet 1983;2:193-195.

21. Salama A, Kiefel V, Amberg R, Mueller-Eckhardt C. Treatment of autoimmune thrombocytopenic purpura with rhesus antibodies (anti-Rh0(D)]. Blut 1984;49:29-35.

22. Fehr J, Hofmann V, Kappeler U. Transient reversal of thrombocytopenia in idiopathic thrombocytopenic purpura by high-dose intravenous gamma globulin. N Engl J Med 1982;306:1254-1258.

23. Crow AR, Song S, Semple JW, et al. IVIg inhibits reticuloendothelial system function and ameliorates murine passive-immune thrombocytopenia independent of anti-idiotype reactivity. Br J Haematol 2001;115: 679-686.

24. Siragam V, Brinc D, Crow AR, et al. Can antibodies with specificity for soluble antigens mimic the therapeutic effects of intravenous IgG in the treatment of autoimmune disease? J Clin Invest 2005;115:155-160.

25. Burdach SE, Evers KG, Geursen RG. Treatment of acute idiopathic thrombocytopenic purpura of childhood with intravenous immunoglobulin G: comparative efficacy of 7S and 5S preparations. J Pediatr 1986;109: 770-775.

26. Tovo PA, Miniero R, Fiandino G, et al. Fc-depleted vs intact intravenous immunoglobulin in chronic ITP. J Pediatr 1984;105:676-677.

27. Samuelsson A, Towers TL, Ravetch JV. Anti-inflammatory activity of IVIG mediated through the inhibitory Fc receptor. Science 2001;291:484-486.

28. Crow AR, Song S, Freedman J, et al. IVIg-mediated amelioration of murine ITP via Fc{gamma}RIIB is independent of SHIP1, SHP-1, and Btk activity. Blood 2003; 102:558-560.

29. Bazin R, Lemieux R, Tremblay T. Reversal of immune thrombocytopenia in mice by cross-linking human immunoglobulin G with a high-affinity monoclonal antibody. Br J Haematol 2006;135:97-100.

30. Leontyev D, Katsman Y, Branch DR. Mouse background and IVIG dosage are critical in establishing the role of inhibitory Fcgamma receptor for the amelioration of experimental ITP. Blood 2012;119:5261-5264.

31. Shimomura M, Hasegawa S, Seki Y, et al. Intravenous immunoglobulin does not increase FcgammaRIIB expression levels on monocytes in children with immune thrombocytopenia. Clin Exp Immunol 2012;169:33-37.

32. Bayary J, Dasgupta S, Misra N, et al. Intravenous immunoglobulin in autoimmune disorders: An insight into the immunoregulatory mechanisms. Int Immunopharmacol 2006;6:528-534.

33. Crow AR, Song S, Semple JW, et al. A role for IL-1 receptor antagonist or other cytokines in the acute therapeutic effects of IVIg? Blood 2007;109:155-158.

34. Cooper N, Heddle NM, Haas M, et al. Intravenous (IV) anti-D and IV immunoglobulin achieve acute platelet increases by different mechanisms: modulation of cytokine and platelet responses to IV anti-D by FcgammaRIIa and FcgammaRIIIa polymorphisms. Br J Haematol 2004;124:511-518.

35. Sewell WA, North ME, Cambronero R, et al. In vivo modulation of cytokine synthesis by intravenous immunoglobulin. Clin Exp Immunol 1999;116:509-515.

36. Aukrust P, Froland SS, Liabakk NB, et al. Release of cytokines, soluble cytokine receptors, and interleukin-1 receptor antagonist after intravenous immunoglobulin administration in vivo. Blood 1994;84:2136-2143.

37. Crow AR, Lazarus A.H. Role of Fc Receptors in the Pathogenesis and Treatment of Idiopathic Thrombocytopenic Purpura. J Pediatr Hematol Oncol 2003;25: S14-S18.

38. Berchtold P, Dale GL, Tani P, McMillan R. Inhibition of autoantibody binding to platelet glycoprotein IIb/IIIa by anti-idiotypic antibodies in intravenous gammaglobulin. Blood 1989;74:2414-2417.

39. Crow AR, Suppa SJ, Chen X, et al. The neonatal Fc receptor (FcRn) is not required for IVIg or anti-CD44 monoclonal antibody-mediated amelioration of murine immune thrombocytopenia. Blood 2011;118:6403-6406.

40. Siragam V, Crow AR, Brinc D, et al. Intravenous immunoglobulin ameliorates ITP via activating Fcgamma receptors on dendritic cells. Nat Med 2006;12:688-692.

41. Marjon KD, Marnell LL, Mold C, Du Clos TW. Macrophages activated by C-reactive protein through Fc gamma RI transfer suppression of immune thrombocytopenia. J Immunol 2009;182:1397-1403.

42. Huang HS, Sun DS, Lien TS, Chang HH. Dendritic cells modulate platelet activity in IVIg-mediated amelioration of ITP in mice. Blood 2010;116:5002-5009.

43. Andrew M, Blanchette VS, Adams M, et al. A multicenter study of the treatment of childhood chronic idiopathic thrombocytopenic purpura with anti-D. J Pediatr 1992;120(4 Pt 1):522-527.

44. Becker T, Kuenzlen E, Salama A, et al. Treatment of childhood idiopathic thrombocytopenic purpura with Rhesus antibodies (anti-D). Eur J Pediatr 1986;145:166-169.

45. Salama A, Kiefel V, Mueller-Eckhardt C. Effect of IgG anti-Rho(D) in adult patients with chronic autoimmune thrombocytopenia. Am J Hematol 1986;22:241-250.

46. Bussel JB, Graziano JN, Kimberly RP, et al. Intravenous anti-D treatment of immune thrombocytopenic purpura: analysis of efficacy, toxicity, and mechanism of effect. Blood 1991;77:1884-1893.

47. Scaradavou A, Woo B, Woloski BM, et al. Intravenous anti-D treatment of immune thrombocytopenic purpura: experience in 272 patients. Blood 1997;89: 2689-2700.

48. Ware RE, Zimmerman SA. Anti-D: mechanisms of action. Semin Hematol 1998;35(1 Suppl 1):14-22.

49. Ambriz-Fernandez R, Martinez-Murillo C, Quintana-Gonzalez S, et al. Fc receptor blockade in patients with refractory chronic immune thrombocytopenic purpura with anti-D IgG. Arch Med Res 2002;33:536-540.

50. Bussel JB, Graziano JN, Kimberly RP. Anti-D Ig for treatment of immune thrombocytopenic purpura (letter). Blood 1991;78:2157-2158.

51. Oksenhendler E, Bierling P, Brossard Y, et al. Anti-RH immunoglobulin therapy for human immunodeficiency virus-related immune thrombocytopenic purpura. Blood 1988;71:1499-1502.

52. Ramadan KM, El-Agnaf M. Efficacy and response to intravenous anti-D immunoglobulin in chronic idiopathic thrombocytopenic purpura. Clin Lab Haematol 2005;27:267-269.

53. Song S, Crow AR, Siragam V, et al. Monoclonal antibodies that mimic the action of anti-D in the amelioration of murine ITP act by a mechanism distinct from that of IVIg. Blood 2005;105:1546-1548.

54. Bussel JB, Kaufmann CP, Ware RE, Woloski BM. Do the acute platelet responses of patients with immune thrombocytopenic purpura (ITP) to IV anti-D and to IV gammaglobulin predict response to subsequent splenectomy? Am J Hematol 2001;67:27-33.

55. Branch DR, Shabani F, Lund N, Denomme GA. Antenatal administration of Rh-immune globulin causes significant increases in the immunomodulatory cytokines transforming growth factor-beta and prostaglandin E2. Transfusion 2006;46:1316-1322.

56. Semple JW, Allen D, Rutherford M, et al. Anti-D (WinRho SD) treatment of children with chronic autoimmune thrombocytopenic purpura stimulates transient cytokine/chemokine production. Am J Hematol 2002;69:225-227.

57. Malinowska I, Obitko-Pludowska A, Buescher ES, et al. Release of cytokines and soluble cytokine receptors after intravenous anti-D treatment in children with chronic thrombocytopenic purpura. Hematol J 2001; 2:242-249.

58. Coopamah MD, Freedman J, Semple JW. Anti-D initially stimulates an Fc-dependent leukocyte oxidative burst and subsequently suppresses erythrophagocytosis via interleukin-1 receptor antagonist. Blood 2003;102: 2862-2867.

59. Gaines AR. Disseminated intravascular coagulation associated with acute hemoglobinemia or hemoglobinuria following Rh(0)(D) immune globulin intravenous administration for immune thrombocytopenic purpura. Blood 2005;106:1532-1537.

60. Imbach P, Kuhne T. Sequelae of treatment of ITP with anti-D (Rho) immunoglobulin. Lancet 2000;356: 447-448.

61. Long M, Kalish LA, Neufeld EJ, Grace RF. Trends in anti-D immune globulin for childhood immune thrombocytopenia: usage, response rates, and adverse effects. Am J Hematol 2012;87:315-317.

62. Kjaersgaard M, Edslev PW, Hasle H. Subcutaneous anti-D treatment of idiopathic thrombocytopenic purpura in children. Pediatr Blood Cancer 2009;53(7):1315-1317.

63. Trebo MM, Frey E, Gadner H, Minkov M. Subcutaneous anti-D globulin application is a safe treatment option of immune thrombocytopenia in children. Ann Hematol 2010;89:415-418.

64. Stasi R. Rozrolimupab, symphobodies against rhesus D, for the potential prevention of hemolytic disease of the newborn and the treatment of idiopathic thrombocytopenic purpura. Curr Opin Mol Ther 2010;12:734-740.

65. Reff ME, Carner K, Chambers KS, et al. Depletion of B cells in vivo by a chimeric mouse human monoclonal antibody to CD20. Blood 1994;83:435-445.

66. Rezvani AR, Maloney DG. Rituximab resistance. Best Pract Res Clin Haematol. 2011;24(2):203-216.

67. Patel VL, Mahevas M, Lee SY, et al. Outcomes 5 years after response to rituximab therapy in children and adults with immune thrombocytopenia. Blood 2012; 119:5989-5995.

68. Stasi R, Pagano A, Stipa E, Amadori S. Rituximab chimeric anti-CD20 monoclonal antibody treatment for adults with chronic idiopathic thrombocytopenic purpura. Blood 2001;98:952-957.

69. Stasi R, Stipa E, Forte V, et al. Variable patterns of response to rituximab treatment in adults with chronic idiopathic thrombocytopenic purpura. Blood 2002;99: 3872-3873.

70. Cooper N, Stasi R, Cunningham-Rundles S, et al. The efficacy and safety of B-cell depletion with anti-CD20 monoclonal antibody in adults with chronic immune thrombocytopenic purpura. Br J Haematol 2004;125: 232-239.

71. Audia S, Samson M, Guy J, et al. Immunologic effects of rituximab on the human spleen in immune thrombocytopenia. Blood 2011;118:4394-4400.

72. Stasi R, Del Poeta G, Stipa E, et al. Response to B-cell depleting therapy with rituximab reverts the abnormalities of T-cell subsets in patients with idiopathic thrombocytopenic purpura. Blood 2007;110:2924-2930.

73. Liu B, Zhao H, Poon MC, et al. Abnormality of CD4(+)CD25(+) regulatory T cells in idiopathic thrombocytopenic purpura. Eur J Haematol 2007;78:139-143.

74. Sakakura M, Wada H, Tawara I, et al. Reduced Cd4+ Cd25+ T cells in patients with idiopathic thrombocytopenic purpura. Thromb Res 2007;120:187-193.

75. Stasi R, Cooper N, Del Poeta G, et al. Analysis of regulatory T-cell changes in patients with idiopathic thrombocytopenic purpura receiving B cell-depleting therapy with rituximab. Blood 2008;112:1147-1150.

76. Milani C, Castillo J. Veltuzumab, an anti-CD20 mAb for the treatment of non-Hodgkin's lymphoma, chronic lymphocytic leukemia and immune thrombocytopenic purpura. Curr Opin Mol Ther 2009;11:200-207.

77. Chang M, Nakagawa PA, Williams SA, et al. Immune thrombocytopenic purpura (ITP) plasma and purified ITP monoclonal autoantibodies inhibit megakaryocytopoiesis in vitro. Blood 2003;102:887-895.

78. Houwerzijl EJ, Blom NR, van der Want JJ, et al. Ultrastructural study shows morphologic features of apoptosis and para-apoptosis in megakaryocytes from patients with idiopathic thrombocytopenic purpura. Blood 2004;103:500-506.

79. Li J, Yang C, Xia Y, et al. Thrombocytopenia caused by the development of antibodies to thrombopoietin. Blood 2001;98:3241-3248.

80. Wang B, Nichol JL, Sullivan JT. Pharmacodynamics and pharmacokinetics of AMG 531, a novel thrombopoietin receptor ligand. Clin Pharmacol Ther 2004;7 6:628-638.

81. Bussel JB, Kuter DJ, George JN, et al. AMG 531, a thrombopoiesis-stimulating protein, for chronic ITP. N Engl J Med 2006;355:1672-1681.

82. Bussel JB, Kuter DJ, Pullarkat V, et al. Safety and efficacy of long-term treatment with romiplostim in thrombocytopenic patients with chronic ITP. Blood 2009;113: 2161-2171.

83. Newland A, Caulier MT, Kappers-Klunne M, et al. An open-label, unit dose-finding study of AMG 531, a novel thrombopoiesis-stimulating peptibody, in patients with immune thrombocytopenic purpura. Br J Haematol 2006;135:547-553.

84. Kuter DJ. Romiplostim. Cancer Treat Res 2011;157: 267-288.

85. Jenkins JM, Williams D, Deng Y, et al. Phase 1 clinical study of eltrombopag, an oral, nonpeptide thrombopoietin receptor agonist. Blood 2007;109:4739-4741.

86. Bussel JB, Cheng G, Saleh MN, et al. Eltrombopag for the treatment of chronic idiopathic thrombocytopenic purpura. N Engl J Med 2007;357:2237-2247.

87. Bussel JB, Pinheiro MP. Eltrombopag. Cancer Treat Res 2011;157:289-303.

88. Bao W, Bussel JB, Heck S, et al. Improved regulatory T-cell activity in patients with chronic immune thrombocytopenia treated with thrombopoietic agents. Blood 2010;116:4639-4645.

89. Cohn CS, Bussel JB. Romiplostim: a second-generation thrombopoietin agonist. Drugs Today (Barc) 2009; 45:175-188.

90. Kuter DJ, Mufti GJ, Bain BJ, et al. Evaluation of bone marrow reticulin formation in chronic immune thrombocytopenia patients treated with romiplostim. Blood 2009;114:3748-3756.

91. Kuter DJ, Rummel M, Boccia R, et al. Romiplostim or standard of care in patients with immune thrombocytopenia. N Engl J Med 2010;363:1889-1899.

92. Podolanczuk A, Lazarus AH, Crow AR, et al. Of mice and men: an open-label pilot study for treatment of immune thrombocytopenic purpura by an inhibitor of Syk. Blood 2009;113:3154-3160.

93. Coffey G, DeGuzman F, Inagaki M, et al. Specific inhibition of spleen tyrosine kinase suppresses leukocyte immune function and inflammation in animal models of rheumatoid arthritis. J Pharmacol Exp Ther 2012;340: 350-359.

94. Gomez-Almaguer D, Solano-Genesta M, Tarin-Arzaga L, et al. Low-dose rituximab and alemtuzumab combination therapy for patients with steroid-refractory autoimmune cytopenias. Blood 2010;116:4783-4785.

95. Lim SH, Hale G, Marcus RE, et al. CAMPATH-1 monoclonal antibody therapy in severe refractory autoimmune thrombocytopenic purpura. Br J Haematol 1993;84:542-544.

96. Marsh JC, Gordon-Smith EC. CAMPATH-1H in the treatment of autoimmune cytopenias. Cytotherapy 2001;3:189-195.

97. Cheloff AZ, Al-Samkari H. Avatrombopag for the treatment of immune thrombocytopenia and thrombocytopenia of chronic liver disease. J Blood Med. 2019; 10:313-321.

# 16. Mechanism of action of high dose intravenous immunoglobulin in ITP

## 16.1. Introduction

Intravenous immunoglobulin (IVIg) was originally used as a replacement product for those deficient in immunoglobulin G (IgG). However, following the first report of the treatment of an autoimmune disease (immune thrombocytopenia) with IVIg by Imbach et al. [1] its use has greatly expanded. This expansion has led to concerns regarding potential IVIg shortages as IVIg is sourced from human blood and plasma donations. The broad anti-inflammatory activity of IVIg as well as the desire for a replacement therapy has spurred significant research into IVIg's mechanism in autoimmunity. There is evidence for multiple mechanisms by which IVIg can mediate anti-inflammatory effects, each of which may play a lesser or greater role in a particular autoimmune condition. Because of the presence of multiple potential mechanisms, determining which mechanisms are critical for IVIg activity has been controversial. Additionally, there is an incomplete knowledge on the basic pathophysiology of autoimmune diseases such as immune thrombocytopenia (ITP), making determining IVIg's mechanism in these diseases more difficult. For example, there is currently no established way to determine which ITP patients will benefit from IVIg and which will not. In theory, such a test could be established if both IVIg's mechanism(s) and ITP pathophysiology were sufficiently understood.

IVIg anti-inflammatory activity has been implicated in autoimmune and inflammatory diseases where autoantibodies and Fc receptors play a pivotal role in the autoimmune pathophysiology. In many of these diseases IgG autoantibodies exert their inflammatory effects through activating Fcγ receptors (FcγRs), a well-established class of immune cell surface receptors that interact with the Fc domain of IgG. There are five known activating FcγRs in humans that can be partitioned as either high or low affinity receptors. Such receptors are known as "activating" in part because they carry an immunoreceptor tyrosine-based activation motif (ITAM) either directly on their intracellular tail (FcγRIIA and FcγRIIC) or by association with the ITAM-bearing FcR-γ chain signaling subunit (FcγRI and Fcγ). One exception is FcγRIIIB, which is glycosylphosphatidylinositol-linked and apparently lacks any intracellular signaling motifs; how Fcγmediates its effects is not well understood. FcγRI is considered high affinity as it binds non-complexed (i.e. monomeric) IgG under experimental conditions, while FcγRIIA, FcγRIIC, FcγRIIIA, and FcγRIIIB are known as low affinity receptors and are considered to mostly bind high avidity (complexed) IgG.

FcγRIIC is present in approximately twenty-five percent of individuals (otherwise encoding a stop codon). FcγRIIA and Fcγare found in humans but not mice while a different FcγR (FcγRIV) exists in mice but not humans. There is also an Fc receptor known as an inhibitory receptor (FcγRIIB) which exists in both mice and humans and is considered inhibitory due to its ability to recruit phosphatases SHIP1 and SHP-1 to its immunoreceptor tyrosine-based inhibitory motif (ITIM) to ostensibly antagonize activating FcγR signaling. Despite being considered inhibitory, FcγRIIB can nevertheless mediate clearance of soluble immune complexes in the liver [2]. Conversely while FcγRIIIA is well known as an activating receptor, it also can mediate inhibitory signalling through an alternative monophosphorylation configuration at its ITAM [3]. There exists also a number of FcγR allelic variants which impact FcγR affinity and function, and IgG itself additionally possesses complexity through multiple IgG subclasses, allotypes, and glycosylation profiles – these concepts have been reviewed extensively elsewhere (reviews by Vidarsson 2014 and Bruhns 2015) [4, 5].

To understand the mechanisms of IVIg in ameliorating autoimmune disease activity, animal models have been critically important. A passive model of ITP has been favoured for understanding IVIg action, partly due to the simplicity of the model and the extensive use of IVIg in human ITP where it is of clear benefit. This model evaluates antibody-mediated platelet clearance by the passive injection of an anti-platelet antibody, which may be immediately preceded or followed (e.g. after 24 hours) by an intervention such as IVIg. Platelet counts are typically measured daily and up to several days. Thus this model evaluates the mechanisms of IVIg that lead to rapid amelioration of antibody-mediated platelet clearance. However as platelet clearance mediated by antibodies is generally regarded as the predominating effector mechanism of thrombocytopenia in human ITP, the passive ITP model has retained validity as a method to study ITP and has been used as a preclinical model for numerous drug candidates. There is also an immune active model of murine ITP where the thrombocytopenia can be mediated by humoral immunity and/or T cell mediated immunity. In this active ITP model, IVIg anti-inflammatory activity was evident when the thrombocytopenia was caused by humoral immunity but not by T cell-dependent active ITP [6]. In part through animal models of ITP and other autoimmune diseases, a substantial number of potential mechanisms have been identified (☞ Figure 16.1). Below we review the major mechanisms of IVIg described for the potential amelioration of ITP.

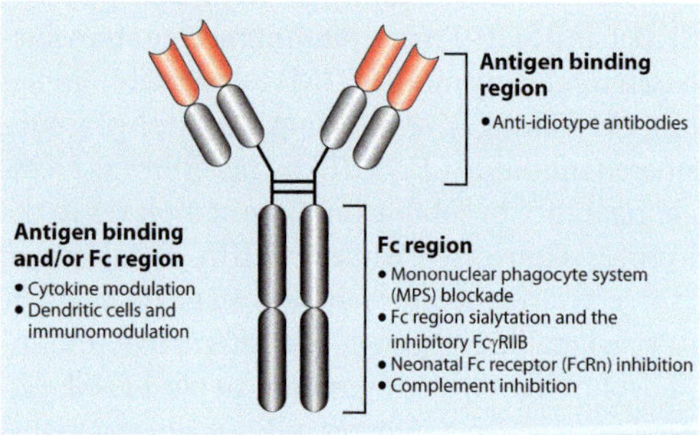


***Figure 16.1:*** Potential mechanisms of IVIg-mediated disease amelioration and the antibody region responsible. The anti-idiotype antibody mechanism is attributed to the antigen binding region of IgG in IVIg, while mechanisms of mononuclear phagocyte system blockade, Fc sialylated IgG, FcRn inhibition, and complement inhibition are attributed to the Fc region. Mechanisms of cytokine modulation and dendritic cell modulation/immunomodulation may be attributable to either the antigen binding and/or the Fc region.

## 16.2. Mononuclear phagocyte system (MPS) blockade

In ITP, the sites of platelet clearance are largely considered to be the spleen and liver which are organs that also host the mononuclear phagocyte system (MPS, previously referred to as the reticuloendothelial system). The spleen predominates as the site of platelet clearance in ITP, supported by a recent meta-analysis of platelet clearance scintigraphy studies showing a 65.7 % (±13.7) splenic pattern, 13.2 % (±10.8) hepatic pattern, and 17.6 % (±11.6) mixed pattern of platelet clearance across n=2,317 ITP patients [7]. Splenic platelet clearance is thought to be mediated by autoantibodies (particularly those against glycoprotein (GP) IIb/IIIa) directing platelets to macrophage FcγRs [8, 9]. Thus the majority of ITP patients may have an FcγR-mediated platelet clearance mechanism. However other mechanisms may be additionally involved in hepatic platelet clearance such as anti-GPIb autoantibody-mediated platelet desialylation [10].

Because clinically relevant increases in platelet counts can be observed rapidly after IVIg administration (potentially within 24 hours) [1, 11, 129, this may signal that IVIg is interfering with the clearance of platelets. Given that FcγRs likely mediate platelet clearance in the majority of ITP patients, an obvious hypothesis of IVIg function is that the substantial quantity of IgG in IVIg may saturate FcγRs and block them or inhibit their function (☞ Figure 16.2).

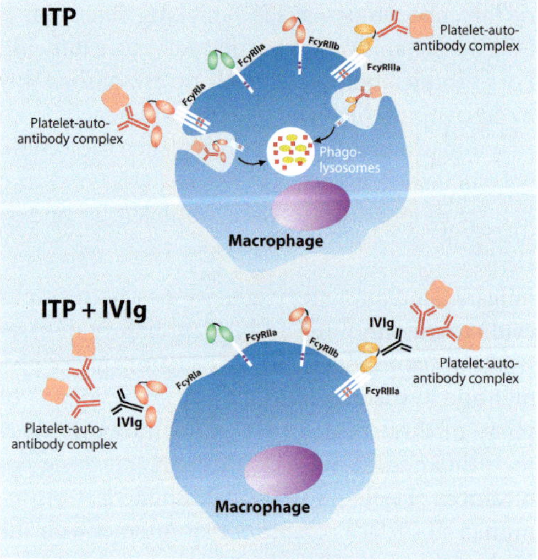


***Figure 16.2:*** Potential IVIg-mediated blockade of the mononuclear phagocyte system/FcγRs. In ITP, macrophages may clear antibody-opsonized platelets through FcγR-mediated phagocytosis (top). IVIg may saturate or block FcγRs (potentially saturating the FcγRs by monomeric IgG or IVIg-formed immune complexes), preventing FcγR-mediated platelet clearance (bottom).

Early direct experiments that MPS blockade by IVIg could rescue antibody-opsonized cells from phagocytosis were performed by Fehr and colleagues [13] who demonstrated that in patients with ITP who were not splenectomised, IVIg treatment decreased *in vivo* clearance of antibody-opsonized red blood cells (RBCs). Newland et al. (1994) [14] similarly showed that the half life of anti-D-opsonized RBCs was increased in ITP patients after infusion of IVIg; in contrast, the half life of heat-damaged RBCs was not increased, supporting the conception that IVIg inhibition of phagocytosis is targeted towards the FcγR pathway. Several other studies have confirmed reduced clearance of anti-D-opsonized RBCs after IVIg administration [15, 16], an effect which occurs rapidly but wanes over the course of approximately two weeks [16]. IVIg has also been shown to directly inhibit human monocyte-derived macrophage phagocytosis of anti-RhD-opsonized human RBCs *in vitro* [17]. These studies show clear support for MPS blockade occurring in humans after IVIg administration, but formal demonstration of this blockade being causative for platelet increases, and a mechanistic consensus for how MPS blockade occurs are both lacking.

Regarding the mechanism of MPS blockade by IVIg, there is debate about the contribution of monomeric vs oligomeric IgG. IVIg is primarily monomeric, but as much as 2-20 % of IgG in IVIg can exist as dimers, and this percentage increases with product age [18, 19] as well as increased donor pool size and IgG concentration [20]. Monomeric IgG is generally considered a poor ligand for FcγRs with only "high affinity" FcγRs showing significant binding, while complexed IgG with high avidity may bind both "high" and "low affinity" FcγRs. It should be noted that studies supporting high and low affinity concepts are often performed with IgG concentrations in the microgram range (e.g. 10-15 µg/mL [21] which is several orders of magnitude lower than the concentration of IgG in human peripheral blood (7-18 mg/mL total IgG [22] which can be further increased to 40 mg/mL following IVIg infusion) [15]. This may be important because monomeric IgG interactions with "low affinity" FcγRs such as human FcγRIIIA can unexpectedly result in an inhibitory ITAM (ITAMi) configuration that recruits the phosphatase SHP-1 and inhibits phagocytosis [3]. Thus infusion of a large quantity of monomeric IgG in IVIg may antagonize FcγRs by providing substantial irrelevant ligand that saturates them or may promote an ITAMi configuration that may reduce the agonistic signaling of FcγRs for platelet immune complexes.

Dimeric IgG on the other hand should have higher avidity for FcγRs and thus may be superior at inhibiting Fcγrelative to monomeric IgG. However a lack of consensus exists on the involvement of dimers. There is evidence that IgG dimers have enhanced therapeutic efficacy relative to monomeric IVIg in the murine passive ITP model [18, 23]. Addition of an antibody to crosslink human IgG (thus theoretically forming an up to three-molecule complex) enhances IVIg function in the passive ITP model [24], supporting that small oligomers can modulate IVIg's activity. One study in support of IgG dimers by Teeling et al showed that IgG dimers in IVIg are required for amelioration of murine passive ITP [18], while another study by Tremblay et al showed that IVIg-formed dimers and immune complexes are dispensable for the effects of IVIg in the passive ITP model [25]. A lack of consensus has left IgG dimers in the IVIg product generally regarded as not required for IVIg's function, but whether dimers form with a patient's endogenous IgG after IVIg injection is an open question.

Another possibility is that given the large number of donor IgG that is pooled into IVIg, there may be appreciable amounts of anti-self antibodies due to antigenic variation between individuals and the relatively high prevalence (nearly 25 %) of healthy individuals seropositive for autoantibodies [26]. These anti-self antibodies may form immune complexes with cells or particulate antigens in the blood, potentially generating immune complexes to inhibit FcγRs in the MPS. There is some precedent for this mechanism being able to ameliorate ITP, as antibodies to soluble antigens (albumin and transferrin) are able to ameliorate murine passive ITP [27]. However to our knowledge no studies have formally demonstrated such immune complexes forming after IVIg infusion in humans. It is worth considering that differences between murine and human antigens may make this mechanism much more significant in animal models.

Inhibition of the MPS through FcγRs is almost certainly an Fc-dependent mechanism, and there is evidence in human ITP that the Fc region is responsible for much of IVIg's therapeutic function. Infusion of IVIg Fc fragments produced therapeutic responses in children with ITP, with all children but one (of twelve) showing rapid platelet count increases [28]. Two studies evaluating an Fc-null IVIg product (one F(ab')2, other unspecified) in children have been reported [29, 30], with 3/9 and 3/10 patients in the two studies responding to the Fc-null version. In contrast, 8/9 and 9/10 patients responded to the intact IVIg product. While some appeared to respond to the Fc-null product (approximately 30 %), the response rate was decidedly higher when intact IVIg was used. Further it should be considered that the frequent spontaneous remission of ITP in children [31] may confound the apparent low responses to the Fc-deactivated IVIg. However there may also be bona fide F(ab')2-mediated mechanisms that mediated disease amelioration in the few that responded.

Together, there is evidence that IVIg inhibits FcγRs from in vitro systems and animal models, and data from human ITP patients shows inhibition of the MPS system and apparent requirement (at least in children) of the IgG Fc region for the majority of IVIg's beneficial effects. These data can compose a cogent hypothesis for IVIg's function in ITP based on MPS blockade, but where a consensus lacks is on the mechanism of MPS inhibition, and on data directly linking MPS blockade to platelet count increases in humans.

## 16.3. Anti-idiotype antibodies

Anti-idiotype antibodies can be functionally defined as antibodies whose antigen binding regions target the novel sequences/structures (termed idiotope) in the variable region of other antibodies. Anti-idiotype interactions therefore form antibody-antibody dimers (in the case of IgG) [32] at the antigen binding region, leading to the neutralization of antigen binding capacity. These dimers can be visualized by electron microscopy, with IgG3 being overrepresented in dimer formation potentially due to increased hinge region flexibility [33]. The wide variety of anti-idiotype antibodies that have been reported supports that anti-idiotype antibody formation is quite common [34]. In antibody-mediated autoimmune disease, the anti-idiotype hypothesis suggests that anti-idiotype antibodies present within IVIg are able to neutralize autoantibodies (e.g. anti-GPIIb/IIIa autoantibodies in ITP) by anti-idiotype interactions.

Early work demonstrated that IVIg contains antibodies capable of neutralizing the activity of autoantibodies against GPIIb/IIIa [35], where autoantibody titres against GPIIb/IIIa were decreased after incubation of ITP patient serum with IVIg. However a separate study failed to confirm this finding and found IVIg to be ineffective in preventing autoantibody binding in patients with ITP with no changes in autoantibody levels in patients acutely responding to IVIg [36]. Additional evidence for IVIg-mediated anti-idiotypic interactions in human primary ITP is relatively limited. In ITP associated with human immunodeficiency virus 1, circulating immune complexes appeared to be composed of anti-GPIIb/IIIa autoantibodies complexed primarily with IgM anti-idiotype antibodies [37] presumably leading to anti-GPIIb/IIIa antibody neutralization. In murine and rat models of passive ITP, studies from two different groups have shown that anti-idiotype antibodies were not necessary for disease amelioration [38, 39]. Thus at least in ITP, potential anti-idiotype antibodies are likely not required for the effects of IVIg.

It is important to note that IVIg has efficacy in a large number of different autoimmune diseases and inflammatory states, and there is evidence that anti-idiotype interactions may be more important in neuroinflammatory diseases. IgG dimer formation post IVIg treatment in chronic inflammatory demyelinating polyradiculoneuropathy (CIDP) and the miller fisher syndrome variant of Guillain-Barre syndrome (GBS) was shown in one study to correlate with better treatment outcomes, and remonomerized IgG dimers isolated from patients showed reactivity to peripheral nerve tissue gangliosides [40]. Other studies have also independently observed anti-idiotype antibodies against neuroinflammatory anti-ganglioside antibodies [41, 42], and the formation of IgG dimers after IVIg infusion in GBS patients [43]. Interestingly, antibodies in the serum from patients who spontaneously resolved GBS were shown to be able to block autoantibodies from GBS patients with active disease by an F(ab')2-dependent mechanism [44], supporting the possibility of anti-idiotype antibodies as a form of natural autoimmune disease suppression. Together, while anti-idiotype interactions are not likely required for IVIg-mediated amelioration in ITP, there is evidence of this mechanism potentially playing a role in neuroinflammatory diseases.

## 16.4. IgG Fc region sialylation and the inhibitory Fc receptor (FcγRIIB)

The heavy chain of IgG possesses an N-linked glycan moiety at a conserved asparagine residue within the Fc region (asparagine 291 in human IgG1) that is critical for FcγR binding [4]. The core Fc glycan consists of *N*-acetylglucosamine and mannose residues, which can be modified to produce a variety of IgG glycoforms [45] which influence inflammatory activities [46] including FcR and complement binding [45, 47].

In IVIg, a typical IgG glycoform distribution shows approximately 94 % core fucosylation, 56 % terminal galactose, 14 % bisecting *N*-acetylglucosamine, and 16 % terminal sialic acid [48]. The sialylation hypothesis of IVIg function proposes that the fraction of IgG bearing terminal Fc sialylation is responsible for much of IVIg's anti-inflammatory properties (☞ Figure 16.3) [49-53]. In this mechanism, sialylation of the IgG Fc glycan enables binding to specific ICAM-3 grabbing non-integrin-related 1 (SIGN-R1) in mice, or its human orthologue dendritic cell-specific intercellular adhesion molecule-3-grabbing non-integrin (DC-SIGN) expressed on dendritic cells (DCs) and/or macrophages [49, 54, 55]. This binding was suggested to lead to increased IL-33 production, which activates and expands basophils to produce IL-4, driving FcγRIIB upregulation on macrophages, particularly in the spleen [49]. FcγRIIB upregulation may then drive an anti-inflammatory and anti-phagocytic signal reducing platelet clearance, as FcγRIIB can reduce the magnitude of FcγR mediated phagocytosis in cell lines [56].

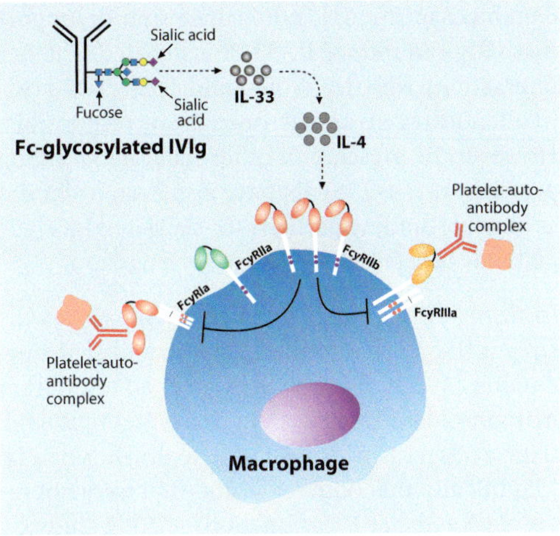


***Figure 16.3:*** Potential IVIg-mediated upregulation of FcγRIIB by Fc-sialylated IgG. The sialylated IgG fraction in IVIg has been hypothesized to interact with dendritic cell-specific intercellular adhesion molecule-3-grabbing non-integrin (DC-SIGN), leading to the sequential induction of IL-33 and IL-4 which then upregulates splenic macrophage FcγRIIB. Upregulated FcγRIIB could then ostensibly antagonize the signaling mediated by activating Fcγand reduce platelet clearance.

While a sophisticated mechanism, there is a lack of consensus on several aspects of the sialylated IVIg/FcγRIIB hypothesis. A 2019 study by Temming et al found that a number of human IgG1 sialic acid glycovariants, including both Fab- and Fc-sialylated IgG, were unable to bind to DC-SIGN.57 supporting previous observations by Yu et al. [58]. DC-SIGN-positive human splenic cells or monocyte-derived DCs have also been shown to not express IL-33 when exposed to IVIg [59]. However IVIg has been observed to significantly increase IL-33 in patients with inflammatory myopathies [59] and GBS, although IL-33 levels did not correlate with improved outcomes in GBS patients [60]. A study covering patients with varying autoimmune/inflammatory (including ITP) or immune deficiency conditions that received high dose IVIg did increase blood IL-4, IL-13, and IL-33 after infusion, but no increase in FcγRIIB was observed on circulating monocytes or myeloid DCs [61]. *In vitro*, myeloid DCs isolated from healthy individuals then cultured with IVIg showed no changes in FcγRIIB expression, while culturing with IL-4 or IL-13 actually decreased FcγRIIB expression.61 Finally, macrophages incubated with IVIg *in vitro* secreted IL-33 but through a DC-SIGN-independent mechanism [61]. While these studies support that IVIg can induce IL-33, it is debated whether interactions with DC-SIGN and DC-SIGN positive dendritic cells or macrophages are responsible. However the presence of other sialic acid binding proteins such as L-SIGN have also been proposed as possible binding partners for sialylated IgG [62] and may be a target for future investigation.

In this sialylation-dependent mechanism, downstream IL-33 is basophil expansion and IL-4 production [49]. A study by Schwab et al. found that neuraminidase-treated IVIg (enzyme removing sialic acids) was no longer able to ameliorate ITP [55] but also that both IL-33 and IL-4 were not required for intact IVIg function. A 2019 study by Galeotti et al found that IVIg can activate basophils to produce IL-4, albeit through an Fab-dependent mechanism via interaction with surface-bound IgE, rather than sialylated IgG [63]. Furthermore, IL-33 did not lead to basophil activation [63]. Lewis et al. have also recently observed that IL-4 was not required at least in a murine model of ITP [64], in line with previous work by Crow et al. [65].

Finally, FcγRIIB was hypothesized to play an important role in IVIg's mechanism. Although an initial study by Samuelsson et al in 2001 showed that FcγRIIB was required for IVIg function in murine ITP [66], multiple studies have followed showing that this is not necessarily the case. Mouse strain selection can influence the apparent requirement of FcγRIIB, with C57BL/6 and BALB/c mice not requiring FcγRIIB [24, 67, 68] while B6;129S mice appear to be sensitive to FcγRIIB knockout [68]. Further, a study by Crow et al. showed that in a model where FcγRIIB is required, that the SHIP1 and SHP-1 phosphatases (recruited to the ITIM of FcγRIIB) are not required individually for IVIg function [69], complicating the apparent FcγRIIB-required mechanism.

Together, with other studies showing no requirement of IVIg sialylation in a murine ITP [70] and collagen antibody-induced arthritis models [71], as well as differential requirement for FcγRIIB between mouse strains in ITP [67, 68], this leads us to believe that sialylated IVIg mediating anti-inflammatory effects downstream DC-SIGN eventually leading to modulated FcγRIIB expression is unlikely to be the primary mechanism of IVIg in ITP. These inconsistencies have been suggested by Washburn et al to be due to the varying methods used to generate and isolate sialylated IgG [51]. For those who are interested, readers are referred to reviews which discuss the sialylation hypothesis from a positive perspective [46, 72] as well some which discuss the pitfalls [73, 74].

## 16.5. Cytokine modulation

Cytokines are important soluble regulators of the immune system. One important concept of autoimmune disease is that there is often a pro-inflammatory cytokine state present in the affected tissues or peripheral blood, which persists due to the inability of homeostatic mediators to "resolve" the inflammation.

Broadly in ITP, there exists a cytokine polarization towards a T helper (Th) 1 cytokine response [75-77] and Th17 response [77, 78]. The imbalanced levels of these cytokines could provoke disordered T-cell function which can contribute to the loss of immune tolerance.

Because a dysregulated and pro-inflammatory cytokine state exists in patients with ITP, several authors have looked for modulation of cytokines after treatment with IVIg. The first pieces of evidence suggesting that IVIg can modulate cytokine levels came from *in vivo* studies performed during the 1990s [79-81]. Aukrust et al. observed an increase in interleukin (IL)-6, IL-8, tumor necrosis factor (TNF)-α, and IL-1 receptor antagonist one hour after the administration of IVIg in patients with primary hypogammaglobulinemia [79]. Cooper et al. conducted a study in ITP patients to evaluate the cytokines response to the administration of IVIg [82], observing an increase in IL-10 levels two hours post-treatment as well as increased monocyte chemotactic protein-1 (MCP-1) levels on day seven after treatment, but no changes were detected for IL-6 and TNF-α levels.

Studies in animal models have also been performed to evaluate the relationship between IVIg, cytokine modulation, and the amelioration of ITP. Our laboratory has previously observed that IVIg is able to ameliorate ITP in mice lacking specific cytokines/receptors (IL-1R, IL-4, IL-10, IL-12β, TNF-α, IFN-γR, MIP-1α), demonstrating IL-4 and other cytokines are dispensable for the amelioration of the disease [65]. Additionally, in the same study, we also found that IVIg controlled ITP in mice deficient for the common cytokine receptor γ chain (an immune signaling component required for signal transduction through the receptors for IL-2, IL-4, IL-7, IL-9, IL-15, and IL-21). Although these cytokines were not required for IVIg function, high amounts of IL-4 are produced in wild type BALB/cJ and C57BL/6J mice in response to the treatment of ITP with IVIg [83]; as previously described, IL-4 is a component of the IgG Fc sialylation/FcγRIIB theory [49]. However these cytokines (Il-4, IL-33) are not required for IVIg function. A study conducted in an ITP mouse model by Aubin and colleagues showed that IVIg did not modulate the mRNA expression of 84 cytokines, chemokines or their receptors involved in the inflammatory response associated with ITP [84].

To clarify contradictions regarding IL-4 and IVIg, Lewis and colleagues evaluated the activity of IVIg in IL-4R knock-out mice after the passive induction of ITP [64]. They found mice developed ITP similar to wild-type mice and IVIg was able to control the disease in both groups of animals, demonstrating IL-4 was not necessary to ameliorate the ITP. Another cytokine, GM-CSF (which is increased following IVIg infusion in mice) was also not required as IVIg functioned in GM-CSF knockout mice. IL-11 however, another cytokine increased in mice following IVIg administration, had a more intriguing role. Treatment of wild-type thrombocytopenic mice with recombinant human IL-11 led to increases in platelet numbers in the passive ITP model, and wild type mice administered an anti-IL-11 antibody showed a significant reduction in the ability of IVIg to ameliorate the ITP. However IL-11Rα-/- mice with ITP responded to IVIg similarly to wild-type mice, which may indicate that IL-11 may be mediating its effects through a receptor other than IL-11Rγ [64]. The contribution of IL-11 still requires more evaluation.

Together, there has not been any particular cytokine or set of cytokines clearly identified as required for IVIg's mechanism in ITP amelioration. There are many factors that can complicate the true contribution of cytokines upon IVIg treatment in ITP. For example, the time of cytokine analysis, the particular biological source used for the analysis (e.g. blood or tissue/cell fractions), and assessment of mRNA (as an indirect measurement) may confound conclusions. Further investigations into the involvement of IL-11 in IVIg's mechanism are warranted.

## 16.6. Neonatal Fc receptor (FcRn)

The long half-life of IgG in circulation is largely due to the activity of the neonatal Fc receptor (FcRn) which binds internalized IgG and protects it from intracellular degradation, allowing it to be trafficked out of the cell [85]. Because IVIg is given at a very high dosage, it has been hypothesized that it may saturate the binding capacity of FcRn, leading to clearance of antibodies that fail to engage FcRn (including autoantibodies, ☞ Figure 16.4).

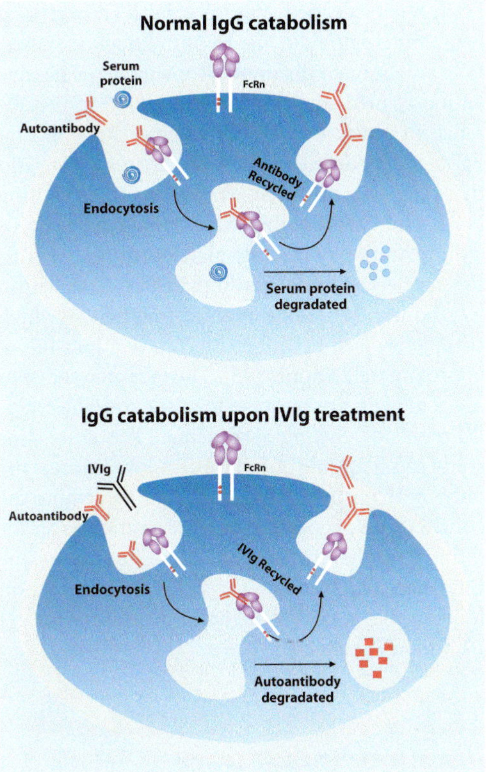


***Figure 16.4:*** Potential IVIg-mediated saturation of FcRn. FcRn reduces IgG catabolism following internalization of the IgG by binding to the internalized IgG at low endosomal pH. FcRn-bound IgG is then recycled to the surface and released (top). IVIg may saturate the binding capacity of FcRn with substantial exogenous IgG, leading to the accelerated catabolism of antibodies that fail to engage FcRn (including autoantibodies).

IVIg has been shown to accelerate the clearance of pathogenic antibodies [86] and there is precedent that specific inhibition of FcRn can lead to ITP amelioration, as emergent FcRn inhibiting therapies appear effective in ITP [87-90]. Thus a strategy of FcRn inhibition is viable to ameliorate human ITP.

Early support for the hypothesis of FcRn inhibition in ITP came from studies observing that IVIg increased the clearance of anti-platelet antibodies in the murine passive ITP model [39, 91, 92]. This is partially consistent with other autoimmune models such as autoimmune skin blistering diseases, where there is evidence for FcRn involvement in IVIg's action [86]. However to directly address the hypothesis of the contribution of FcRn activity to IVIg effects in ITP, we used two different models of FcRn genetically deficient mice, both FcRn -/- and beta 2 microglobulin -/-. In both knockout cases, IVIg ameliorated thrombocytopenia in the passive antibody-mediated murine ITP model in the absence of FcRn activity [93], demonstrating that FcRn-independent mechanisms are occurring and that IVIg does not likely work by solely inhibiting FcRn. One caveat of this study is that passive bolus administration of the anti-platelet antibody in this ITP model can lead to nadir platelet counts within two hours [94], while F(ab')2 fragments (which completely lack FcRn binding) have a half-life of approximately 6 hours [95]. Thus the effects due to a lack of FcRn are expected to occur after the establishment of thrombocytopenia. Therefore this study can help rule out that FcRn inhibition is the only mechanism but was unable to determine the contribution of potential FcRn saturation as an additional mechanism of IVIg action. Regardless, the total non-requirement for FcRn in IVIg action leads us to not favour the FcRn hypothesis for explaining IVIg effects.

## 16.7. Dendritic cells (DCs) and immunomodulation

Professional antigen presenting cells such as dendritic cells (DCs) play a central role in priming and controlling adaptive immune responses. Additionally, DCs can also induce immune tolerance (e.g. towards CD4+ and CD8+ T cells) depending on the DC maturation status. ITP, like many autoimmune conditions, has a recognized and critical T cell component involved in disease pathogenesis [96, 97]. Thus modulation of DCs by IVIg may lead to a pro-tolerogenic immune response and/or decrease B and T cell effector functions.

Early work showing that modulation of DCs can directly control platelet clearance comes from a study by Siragam et al. (2006) [98], where it was demonstrated that adoptive transfer of IVIg-primed CD11c+ DC, but not CD11c- cells could recapitulate the ameliorative effects of IVIg in the passive ITP model. Anthony et al obtained similar results with adoptively transferred IVIg-treated splenocytes [54], and such effects may be downstream DC FcγR signaling [98]. Because the passive murine ITP model is a model of antibody-mediated platelet clearance, presumably the transfer of IVIg-primed DCs was sufficient to inhibit MPS FcγR function. However the mechanism behind the effect of IVIg on DCs is not well understood and a number of effects of IVIg on DCs have been described.

Exposure of DCs to IVIg in vitro inhibits DC maturation and alters the pattern of DC cytokine production, including up-regulation of anti-inflammatory cytokines such as IL-10, and downregulation of proinflammatory cytokines such as IL-12 [99]. A recent study indicated that such production of anti-inflammatory cytokines may potentially be due to IVIg-induced autophagy in DCs through an F(ab')2-dependent mechanism [100]. As mentioned previously, sialylated IgG in IVIg may interact with DC-SIGN on human DCs leading to a sequence of cytokine production and FcγRIIB upregulation [49, 54], although this theory has been debated. Other targets on murine DCs for sialylated IgG have also been identified, such as the dendritic cell immunoreceptor (DCIR), where there exists evidence that DCIR ligation leads to induction of regulatory T cells [101].

In addition to potential altered cytokine expression, IVIg can modulate the antigen-presenting molecules (MHC-II) and co-stimulatory molecules on DCs, possibly resulting in abrogated T-cell activation and proliferation (reviewed in Crow, Brinc and Lazarus 2009 and Kaufman 2015) [102, 103]. Incubation of DCs with IVIg modulates expression of the CD1 family of proteins (important in presenting lipid antigens to T cells), up-regulating CD1d and decreasing CD1a, CD1b, and CD1c through a mechanism involving FcγRIIA [104]. A DC phenotype favorable to regulatory T cell (Treg) expansion is observed after IVIg treatment including an upregulation of tolerizing DCs in the spleen [105], and several studies have demonstrated expansion of Tregs in response to IVIg [103, 106]. Secretion of prostaglandin E2 ($PGE_2$) by DCs following IVIg infusion may be a mechanism of Treg expansion in both mice and humans [107], and human plasma $PGE_2$ concentrations correlate with expansion of Tregs following IVIg infusion [108]. Because prostaglandin E1 ($PGE_1$) and $PGE_2$ are inhibitory against macrophage phagocytosis [109, 110] there is the additional theoretical possibility that $PGE_1$ and $PGE_2$ expression by DCs may directly reduce platelet clearance. There is also evidence that IVIg may directly influence T cells potentially through an F(ab')2-mediated mechanism, including promoting CD4+ T cells towards a Treg phenotype [111] as well as inhibition of Th17 T cell expansion and cytokine production [112].

Together, the multitude of apparent effects of IVIg on DCs and ability to modulate T cells make these series of mechanisms complex. Studies evaluating requirement and sufficiency of these mediators (such as $PGE_2$) should be performed to determine the contribution of these mechanisms to ITP disease amelioration. Effects on T cells and increased Treg expansion may be unlikely to explain the immediate acute effects of IVIg but may contribute to potential longer-term modulation of the immune system, although mediators such as $PGE_1$ and $PGE_2$ may reduce platelet clearance by inhibiting phagocyte function. More studies are needed to evaluate the contribution of DCs and T cell modulation to the effects of IVIg on amelioration of ITP.

## 16.8. Current and emerging IVIg alternatives and mimetics for use in ITP

Unfortunately, IVIg suffers from several important limitations including hemolysis and other side effects, risks related to blood borne pathogens, and high cost [113]. However probably chief among IVIg's limitations is the significant issue of supply shortages. IVIg is a human blood product, and its manufacturing requires a constant supply of human plasma and blood donors. With IVIg being approved for an increasing number of autoimmune and inflammatory diseases as well as its increased off-label use, it is unclear whether IVIg is a sustainable strategy to manage these diseases. One strategy to address these problems associated with IVIg is to replace its use in autoimmune and inflammatory diseases with suitable IVIg mimetics or alternatives. A summary of potential IVIg mimetics and alternatives currently being developed are presented in Table 16.1.

One common strategy to develop an IVIg alternative/mimetic is to multimerize the Fc region of IgG to form recombinant Fc (rFc) multimers. GL-2045 is a human IgG1 rFc multimer linked by the hinge region of human IgG2. This compound ameliorated rodent models of ITP to similar efficacies as IVIg [114, 115] and is currently being assessed for safety in a phase I clinical trial with healthy adults (NCT03275740). Similarly, CSL730, a rFc trimer engineered from three human IgG1 Fc fragments, was effective in animal ITP models and is also being evaluated for safety in a phase I clinical trial (NCT04446000) [116]. A variety of hexameric rFc multimers have also been investigated in preclinical ITP models. The first of these compounds to be developed was HexaGard, an IgG1 Fc hexamer fused to the human IgM μ-tailpiece, which exhibited high avidity to all activating FcγRs [117, 118]. CSL777, a comparable hexameric compound, demonstrated efficacy in ameliorating murine models of various autoimmune diseases including ITP [88, 119]. Other hexameric rFc variants include an Fc-fusion compound from human IgG1 and IgG4 Fc fragments bound by the human IgM μ-tailpiece [120], which showed effective FcγR blockade and inhibition of phagocytosis in preclinical ITP models [120]. It is also worth noting that, like IVIg, some rFc multimers can also inhibit the complement pathway. In ITP, binding of autoantibodies to platelets likely activates the complement pathway and approximately 50 % of ITP patients exhibit deposition of C3 and C4 on their platelet surfaces [121, 122]. GL-2045 was found to inhibit the classical complement pathway by binding to C1q and reducing the formation of membrane attack complexes [123], while CSL777 prevented C2 cleavage, preventing the activation of downstream complement molecules [119]. A specific inhibitor of complement component C1s

| Mechanism of Action | Drug/agent type | Drug/agent name | Developmental Stage |
|---|---|---|---|
| FcγR/MPS inhibition | FcγRIII-blocking antibody | GMA161 | Stopped |
| | Anti-CD44 antibody | n.a. | Preclinical |
| | Syk inhibitors | Fostamatinib | Approved for use in ITP* |
| | BTK inhibitors | Rilzabrutinib | Phase 3 (NCT04562766) |
| | Recombinant Fc Multimers | GL-2045 | Phase 1 (NCT03275740) |
| | | CSL730 | Phase 1 (NCT04446000) |
| | | HexaGard™ | Unknown |
| | | CSL777 | Preclinical |
| | | Hexameric-Fc | Preclinical |
| FcRn blockade | Mutated IgG Fc fragment | Efgartigimod | Phase 3 (NCT04687072) |
| | Monoclonal anti-FcRn antibodies | M281 | Phase 2 for myasthenia gravis (NCT03772587), HDFN (NCT03842189), and WAIHA (NCT04119050) |
| | | Rozanolixizumab | Phase 3 (NCT02718716) |
| | | SYNT001 | Phase 2 (NCT03075878) |
| Complement inhibition | Complement inhibitors | Sutimlimab | Phase 2 (NCT04669600) |
| Sialylated IgG | Hyper-sialylated IgG | M254 | Phase 1/2 (NCT03866577) |
| T cell modulation | T cell targeting therapies | Letolizumab | Phase 1/2 (NCT02273960) |

***Table 16.1:*** Current and emerging **IVIg mimetics and alternatives for use in ITP**. **n.a.**: not applicable, **MPS**: mononuclear phagocyte system, **HDFN**: hemolytic disease of the fetus and newborn, **WAIHA**: warm autoimmune hemolytic anemia.
* Fostamatinib is currently approved for use by the United States' Food and Drug Administration, Health Canada, and European Medicines Agency, in their respective jurisdictions.

(sutimlimab) is being evaluated for efficacy of persistent/chronic ITP in a phase II clinical trial (NCT04669600). Results from the phase I trial reported rapid increases (within 24 hours) in platelet counts increasing to seven days, with an overall response in 42 % of chronic, highly refractory ITP patients [116].

Given the evidence for inhibition of platelet clearance by IVIg, therapies blocking this process may also be suitable IVIg alternatives. A humanized, deglycosylated variant of the monoclonal antibody 3G8 (termed GMA161), which targets and blocks the IgG binding site of human FcγRIII, showed clinically significant increases in platelet counts in a group of refractory ITP patients [124]. Unfortunately, GMA161 led to adverse events that halted further development; such adverse events were explored to be potentially due to FcγR crosslinking [125]. Monoclonal antibodies against the CD44 protein, which were recently shown to unexpectedly engage macrophage FcγRs and mediate FcγR inhibition have shown equivalent potency to IVIg but at a 3 log fold lower dosage in murine ITP models and could therefore be a candidate as an IVIg alternative [94]. Inhibitors of FcγR signaling such as fostamatinib, a small molecule inhibitor of spleen tyrosine kinase (required for signaling in the FcγR pathway) is effective for some ITP patients [116, 124]. Finally, rilzabrutinib, an inhibitor of bruton tyrosine kinase (BTK) hypothesized to inhibit platelet clearance, has also shown potential in a phase I/II clinical trial in chronic ITP patients (NCT04562766) [116].

Inhibition of FcRn is another novel therapeutic approach for ITP with several FcRn inhibitors under development. Efgartigimod, a human IgG Fc fragment mutated at five amino acid residues to improve FcRn affinity [126, 127] is currently being investigated in a phase III clinical trial in ITP (NCT 04687072) based on previous data demonstrating clinically relevant improvements in platelet count in 46-58 % of patients (NCT03102593) [87]. Nipocalimab (M281) is a deglycosylated IgG1 anti-FcRn monoclonal antibody that exhibited therapeutic efficacy in murine models of ITP [128] and demonstrated a reduction of serum IgG by 80 % at the highest tested dose in a phase I clinical trial in healthy volunteers (NCT02828046) [129]. Rozanolixizumab, a human IgG4 anti-FcRn antibody for the treatment of ITP [89] reported positive results from a phase II clinical trial (NCT02718716) and was well-tolerated and induced clinically relevant improvement in platelet count in 66.7 % of patients with a 24-69 % decrease in serum IgG levels [90].

Several other therapies for ITP are being investigated (☞ Table 16.1, also reviewed recently by Audia et al. [116]), which if successful, may lead to the reduction in the utilization of IVIg. One potential therapy to keep an eye on, because of the mechanistic controversy in the literature, is the hypersialylated IVIg product M254 by Momenta Pharmaceuticals. M254 is currently being evaluated in a phase I/II clinical trial (NCT03866577) to evaluate safety in healthy individuals and initial efficacy in ITP patients. Thus far, M254 safety appears similar to unmodified IVIg [130]. It will be very interesting to follow the results of M254 and whether it indeed does have a substantially increased anti-inflammatory activity relative to unmodified IVIg, theoretically effective at one tenth the dose as demonstrated by Washburn et al. [51].

## 16.9. Other mechanisms and conclusions

IVIg is extraordinary in the number of mechanisms of action that have been described. In the above sections we have discussed mechanisms that have received extensive research focus in ITP. Because IVIg is used in numerous autoimmune and inflammatory disorders, it perhaps may not be surprising that different mechanisms are emphasised to greater or lesser extents for different diseases. For example in neuroinflammatory disorders such as Guillain-Barre syndrome (GBS), myasthenia gravis, and chronic inflammatory demyelinating polyneuropathy (CIDP), complement inhibition by IVIg may be a critical mechanism [124], whereas MPS blockade may be less important. Other mechanisms include the ability of IVIg to affect programmed cell death or apoptosis, increased peripheral blood mononuclear cell autophagy [100], and reduced antigen presentation by B cells (through an FcγRIIB-independent mechanism) [131]. The total number of identified mechanisms for IVIg function has made identifying the contribution of any particular one difficult. Some mechanisms probably inhibit the same pathway of disease and may therefore be functionally redundant – for example MPS blockade, FcRn inhibition, and anti-idiotype antibodies may all lead to the reduction of antibody-mediated platelet clearance in ITP. This problem is also apparent in knockout systems – these systems can show that a particular mechanism is not required, but it does not rule out that the mechanism in question can contribute to disease amelioration. Studies evaluating the contribution of a particular mechanism in the presence of multiple other (potentially redundant) mechanisms are difficult to design. Many hypotheses put forward to explain IVIg activity in ITP have risen and fallen in favor, leaving generally no consensus towards a single mechanism as being responsible. This lack of consensus may suggest IVIg is able to ameliorate human ITP through multiple, potentially therapeutically redundant mechanisms, and that the "holy grail" of mechanisms that will reconcile existing controversies may not exist. Probably the largest consensus for IVIg's mechanism in ITP is that it leads to reduced platelet clearance and IVIg's effect is primarily mediated by the Fc region – a rather unsatisfying conclusion, given the several decades of mechanistic research. The push to replace IVIg in the management of autoimmune and inflammatory disorders with alternatives will hopefully alleviate many of the problems associated with IVIg use and give rise to a superior product for patients.

### References

1. Imbach P, Barandun S, d'Apuzzo V, et al. High-dose intravenous gammaglobulin for idiopathic thrombocytopenic purpura in childhood. Lancet (London, England). 1981;1(8232):1228-1231.

2. Ganesan LP, Kim J, Wu Y, et al. FcγRIIb on liver sinusoidal endothelium clears small immune complexes. J Immunol. 2012;189(10):4981-4988.

3. Aloulou M, Ben Mkaddem S, Biarnes-Pelicot M, et al. IgG1 and IVIg induce inhibitory ITAM signaling

through FcγRIII controlling inflammatory responses. Blood. 2012;119(13):3084-3096.

4. Vidarsson G, Dekkers G, Rispens T. IgG subclasses and allotypes: from structure to effector functions. Front Immunol. 2014;5:520.

5. Bruhns P, Jonsson F. Mouse and human FcR effector functions. Immunol Rev. 2015;268(1):25-51.

6. Chow L, Aslam R, Speck ER, et al. A murine model of severe immune thrombocytopenia is induced by antibody- and CD8+ T cell-mediated responses that are differentially sensitive to therapy. Blood. 2010;115(6): 1247-1253.

7. Amini SN, Nelson VS, Sobels A, Schoones JW, Zwaginga JJ, Schipperus MR. Autologous platelet scintigraphy and clinical outcome of splenectomy in immune thrombocytopenia: A systematic review and meta-analysis. Crit Rev Oncol Hematol. 2020;153:103040.

8. Norris PAA, Segel GB, Burack WR, et al. FcgammaRI and FcgammaRIII on splenic macrophages mediate phagocytosis of anti-glycoprotein IIb/IIIa autoantibody-opsonized platelets in immune thrombocytopenia. Haematologica. 2021;106(1):250-254.

9. Zufferey A, Kapur R, Semple JW. Pathogenesis and Therapeutic Mechanisms in Immune Thrombocytopenia (ITP). J Clin Med. 2017;6(2).

10. Li J, van der Wal DE, Zhu G, et al. Desialylation is a mechanism of Fc-independent platelet clearance and a therapeutic target in immune thrombocytopenia. Nat Commun. 2015;6:7737.

11. Carcao M, Silva M, David M, et al. IVMP+IVIG raises platelet counts faster than IVIG alone: results of a randomized, blinded trial in childhood ITP. Blood Adv. 2020;4(7):1492-1500.

12. Khan AM, Mydra H, Nevarez A. Clinical Practice Updates in the Management Of Immune Thrombocytopenia. P T. 2017;42(12):756-763.

13. Fehr J, Hofmann V, Kappeler U. Transient reversal of thrombocytopenia in idiopathic thrombocytopenic purpura by high-dose intravenous gamma globulin. N Engl J Med. 1982;306(21):1254-1258.

14. Newland AC, Macey MG. Immune thrombocytopenia and Fc receptor-mediated phagocyte function. Ann Hematol. 1994;69(2):61-67.

15. Budde U, Auch D, Niese D, Schäfer G, Reske SN, Schmidt RE. Reticuloendothelial system Fc-receptor function in patients with immune thrombocytopenia after treatment with high dose intravenous immunoglobulin. Scand J Haematol. 1986;37(2):125-129.

16. Bussel JB, Kimberly RP, Inman RD, et al. Intravenous gammaglobulin treatment of chronic idiopathic thrombocytopenic purpura. Blood. 1983;62(2):480-486.

17. Nagelkerke SQ, Dekkers G, Kustiawan I, et al. Inhibition of FcγR-mediated phagocytosis by IVIg is independent of IgG-Fc sialylation and FcγRIIb in human macrophages. Blood. 2014;124(25):3709-3718.

18. Teeling JL, Jansen-Hendriks T, Kuijpers TW, et al. Therapeutic efficacy of intravenous immunoglobulin preparations depends on the immunoglobulin G dimers: studies in experimental immune thrombocytopenia. Blood. 2001;98(4):1095-1099.

19. Dolman C, Thorpe SJ, Thorpe R. Enhanced efficacy of anti-D immunoglobulin for treating ITP is not explained by higher immunoglobulin polymer content. Biologicals. 2001;29(2):75-79.

20. Durandy A, Kaveri S V, Kuijpers TW, et al. Intravenous immunoglobulins—understanding properties and mechanisms. Clin Exp Immunol. 2009;158 Suppl(Suppl 1):2-13.

21. Bruhns P, Iannascoli B, England P, et al. Specificity and affinity of human Fcgamma receptors and their polymorphic variants for human IgG subclasses. Blood. 2009;113(16):3716-3725.

22. Gonzalez-Quintela A, Alende R, Gude F, et al. Serum levels of immunoglobulins (IgG, IgA, IgM) in a general adult population and their relationship with alcohol consumption, smoking and common metabolic abnormalities. Clin Exp Immunol. 2008;151(1):42-50.

23. Machino Y, Suzuki E, Higurashi S, et al. Chemically dimerized intravenous immunoglobulin has potent ameliorating activity in a mouse immune thrombocytopenic purpura model. Biochem Biophys Res Commun. 2012;418(4):748-753.

24. Bazin R, Lemieux R, Tremblay T. Reversal of immune thrombocytopenia in mice by cross-linking human immunoglobulin G with a high-affinity monoclonal antibody. Br J Haematol. 2006;135(1):97-100.

25. Tremblay T, Paré I, Bazin R. Immunoglobulin G dimers and immune complexes are dispensable for the therapeutic efficacy of intravenous immune globulin in murine immune thrombocytopenia. Transfusion. 2013; 53(2):261-269.

26. Haller-Kikkatalo K, Alnek K, Metspalu A, et al. Demographic associations for autoantibodies in disease-free individuals of a European population. Sci Rep. 2017; 7:44846.

27. Siragam V, Brinc D, Crow ARAR, Song S, Freedman J, Lazarus AHAH. Can antibodies with specificity for soluble antigens mimic the therapeutic effects of intravenous IgG in the treatment of autoimmune disease? J Clin Invest. 2005;115(1):155-160.

28. Debré M, Bonnet MC, Fridman WH, et al. Infusion of Fc gamma fragments for treatment of children with

acute immune thrombocytopenic purpura. Lancet (London, England). 1993;342(8877):945-949.

29. Tovo PA, Miniero R, Fiandino G, Saracco P, Messina M. Fc-depleted vs intact intravenous immunoglobulin in chronic ITP. J Pediatr. 1984;105(4):676-677.

30. Burdach SE, Evers KG, Geursen RG. Treatment of acute idiopathic thrombocytopenic purpura of childhood with intravenous immunoglobulin G: comparative efficacy of 7S and 5S preparations. J Pediatr. 1986;109 (5):770-775.

31. Despotovic JM, Grimes AB. Pediatric ITP: is it different from adult ITP? Hematol Am Soc Hematol Educ Progr. 2018;2018(1):405-411.

32. Fields BA, Goldbaum FA, Ysern X, Poljak RJ, Mariuzza RA. Molecular basis of antigen mimicry by an anti-idiotope. Nature. 1995;374(6524):739-742.

33. Roux KH, Tankersley DL. A view of the human idiotypic repertoire. Electron microscopic and immunologic analyses of spontaneous idiotype-anti-idiotype dimers in pooled human IgG. J Immunol. 1990;144(4): 1387-1395.

34. Berger M, McCallus DE, Lin CS-Y. Rapid and reversible responses to IVIG in autoimmune neuromuscular diseases suggest mechanisms of action involving competition with functionally important autoantibodies. J Peripher Nerv Syst. 2013;18(4):275-296.

35. Berchtold P, Dale GL, Tani P, McMillan R. Inhibition of autoantibody binding to platelet glycoprotein IIb/IIIa by anti-idiotypic antibodies in intravenous gammaglobulin. Blood. 1989;74(7):2414-2417.

36. Barbano G, Saleh MN, Mori PG, LoBuglio AF, Shaw DR. Effect of intravenous gammaglobulin on circulating and platelet-bound antibody in immune thrombocytopenia. Blood. 1989;73(3):662-665.

37. Nardi M, Karpatkin S. Antiidiotype antibody against platelet anti-GPIIIa contributes to the regulation of thrombocytopenia in HIV-1-ITP patients. J Exp Med. 2000;191(12):2093-2100.

38. Crow AR, Song S, Semple JW, Freedman J, Lazarus AH. IVIg inhibits reticuloendothelial system function and ameliorates murine passive-immune thrombocytopenia independent of anti-idiotype reactivity. Br J Haematol. 2001;115(3):679-686.

39. Hansen RJ, Balthasar JP. Effects of intravenous immunoglobulin on platelet count and antiplatelet antibody disposition in a rat model of immune thrombocytopenia. Blood. 2002;100(6):2087-2093.

40. Ritter C, Bobylev I, Lehmann HC. Chronic inflammatory demyelinating polyneuropathy (CIDP): change of serum IgG dimer levels during treatment with intravenous immunoglobulins. J Neuroinflammation. 2015;12: 148.

41. Lopez PH, Irazoqui FJ, Nores GA. Normal human plasma contains antibodies that specifically block neuropathy-associated human anti-GM1 IgG-antibodies. J Neuroimmunol. 2000;105(2):179-183.

42. Jacobs BC, O'Hanlon GM, Bullens RWM, Veitch J, Plomp JJ, Willison HJ. Immunoglobulins inhibit pathophysiological effects of anti-GQ1b-positive sera at motor nerve terminals through inhibition of antibody binding. Brain. 2003;126(Pt 10):2220-2234.

43. Svacina MKR, Röth P, Bobylev I, Sprenger A, Zhang G, Sheikh KA, Lehmann HC. Changes of Serum IgG Dimer Levels after Treatment with IVIg in Guillain-Barré Syndrome. J Neuroimmune Pharmacol. 2019;14 (4):642-648.

44. Lundkvist I, van Doorn PA, Vermeulen M, Brand A. Spontaneous recovery from the Guillain-Barré syndrome is associated with anti-idiotypic antibodies recognizing a cross-reactive idiotype on anti-neuroblastoma cell line antibodies. Clin Immunol Immunopathol. 1993; 67(3 Pt 1):192-198.

45. Dekkers G, Treffers L, Plomp R, et al. Decoding the Human Immunoglobulin G-Glycan Repertoire Reveals a Spectrum of Fc-Receptor- and Complement-Mediated-Effector Activities. Front Immunol. 2017;8:877.

46. Schwab I, Nimmerjahn F. Intravenous immunoglobulin therapy: How does IgG modulate the immune system? Nat Rev Immunol. 2013;13(3):176-189.

47. Quast I, Keller CW, Maurer MA, et al. Sialylation of IgG Fc domain impairs complement-dependent cytotoxicity. J Clin Invest. 2015;125(11):4160-4170.

48. Fokkink WJR, Falck D, Santbergen TCM, Huizinga R, Wuhrer M, Jacobs BC. Comparison of Fc N-Glycosylation of Pharmaceutical Products of Intravenous Immunoglobulin G. PLoS One. 2015;10(10):e0139828.

49. Anthony RM, Kobayashi T, Wermeling F, Ravetch J V. Intravenous gammaglobulin suppresses inflammation through a novel T(H)2 pathway. Nature. 2011;475 (7354):110-113.

50. Kaneko Y, Nimmerjahn F, Ravetch J V. Anti-inflammatory activity of immunoglobulin G resulting from Fc sialylation. Science. 2006;313(5787):670-673.

51. Washburn N, Schwab I, Ortiz D, et al. Controlled tetra-Fc sialylation of IVIg results in a drug candidate with consistent enhanced anti-inflammatory activity. Proc Natl Acad Sci U S A. 2015;112(11):E1297-306.

52. Pagan JD, Kitaoka M, Anthony RM. Engineered Sialylation of Pathogenic Antibodies In Vivo Attenuates Autoimmune Disease. Cell. 2018;172(3):564-577.e13.

53. Schwab I, Mihai S, Seeling M, Kasperkiewicz M, Ludwig RJ, Nimmerjahn F. Broad requirement for terminal sialic acid residues and FcγRIIB for the preventive and

therapeutic activity of intravenous immunoglobulins in vivo. Eur J Immunol. 2014;44(5):1444-1453.

54. Anthony RM, Wermeling F, Karlsson MCI, Ravetch J V. Identification of a receptor required for the anti-inflammatory activity of IVIG. Proc Natl Acad Sci U S A. 2008;105(50):19571-19578.

55. Schwab I, Biburger M, Krönke G, Schett G, Nimmerjahn F. IVIg-mediated amelioration of ITP in mice is dependent on sialic acid and SIGNR1. Eur J Immunol. 2012;42(4):826-830.

56. Hunter S, Indik ZK, Kim MK, Cauley MD, Park JG, Schreiber AD. Inhibition of Fcgamma receptor-mediated phagocytosis by a nonphagocytic Fcgamma receptor. Blood. 1998;91(5):1762-1768.

57. Temming AR, Dekkers G, van de Bovenkamp FS, et al. Human DC-SIGN and CD23 do not interact with human IgG. Sci Rep. 2019;9(1):9995.

58. Yu X, Vasiljevic S, Mitchell DA, Crispin M, Scanlan CN. Dissecting the molecular mechanism of IVIg therapy: the interaction between serum IgG and DC-SIGN is independent of antibody glycoform or Fc domain. J Mol Biol. 2013;425(8):1253-1258.

59. Sharma M, Schoindre Y, Hegde P, et al. Intravenous immunoglobulin-induced IL-33 is insufficient to mediate basophil expansion in autoimmune patients. Sci Rep. 2014;4:5672.

60. Maddur MS, Stephen-Victor E, Das M, et al. Regulatory T cell frequency, but not plasma IL-33 levels, represents potential immunological biomarker to predict clinical response to intravenous immunoglobulin therapy. J Neuroinflammation. 2017;14(1):58.

61. Tjon ASW, van Gent R, Jaadar H, et al. Intravenous immunoglobulin treatment in humans suppresses dendritic cell function via stimulation of IL-4 and IL-13 production. J Immunol. 2014;192(12):5625-5634.

62. Tjon ASW, van Gent R, Geijtenbeek TB, Kwekkeboom J. Differences in Anti-Inflammatory Actions of Intravenous Immunoglobulin between Mice and Men: More than Meets the Eye. Front Immunol. 2015;6:197.

63. Galeotti C, Stephen-Victor E, Karnam A, et al. Intravenous immunoglobulin induces IL-4 in human basophils by signaling through surface-bound IgE. J Allergy Clin Immunol. 2019;144(2):524-535.e8.

64. Lewis BJB, Leontyev D, Neschadim A, Blacquiere M, Branch DR. GM-CSF and IL-4 are not involved in IVIG-mediated amelioration of ITP in mice: a role for IL-11 cannot be ruled out. Clin Exp Immunol. 2018;193(3): 293-301.

65. Crow AR, Song S, Semple JW, Freedman J, Lazarus AH. A role for IL-1 receptor antagonist or other cytokines in the acute therapeutic effects of IVIg? Blood. 2007;109(1):155-158.

66. Samuelsson A, Towers TL, Ravetch J V. Anti-inflammatory activity of IVIG mediated through the inhibitory Fc receptor. Science. 2001;291(5503):484-486.

67. Leontyev D, Katsman Y, Branch DR. Mouse background and IVIG dosage are critical in establishing the role of inhibitory Fcγ receptor for the amelioration of experimental ITP. Blood. 2012;119(22):5261-5264.

68. Crow AR, Amash A, Lazarus AH. CD44 antibody-mediated amelioration of murine immune thrombocytopenia (ITP): mouse background determines the effect of FcgammaRIIb genetic disruption. Transfusion. 2015;55(6 Pt 2):1492-1500.

69. Crow AR, Song S, Freedman J, et al. IVIg-mediated amelioration of murine ITP via FcgammaRIIB is independent of SHIP1, SHP-1, and Btk activity. Blood. 2003;102(2):558-560.

70. Leontyev D, Katsman Y, Ma X-Z, Miescher S, Käsermann F, Branch DR. Sialylation-independent mechanism involved in the amelioration of murine immune thrombocytopenia using intravenous gammaglobulin. Transfusion. 2012;52(8):1799-1805.

71. Campbell IK, Miescher S, Branch DR, et al. Therapeutic effect of IVIG on inflammatory arthritis in mice is dependent on the Fc portion and independent of sialylation or basophils. J Immunol. 2014;192(11):5031-5038.

72. Anthony RM, Ravetch J V. A Novel Role for the IgG Fc Glycan: The Anti-inflammatory Activity of Sialylated IgG Fcs. J Clin Immunol. 2010;30(S1):9-14.

73. von Gunten S, Shoenfeld Y, Blank M, et al. IVIG pluripotency and the concept of Fc-sialylation: challenges to the scientist. Nat Rev Immunol. 2014;14(5): 349-349.

74. Crow AR, Lazarus AH. Mechanistic properties of intravenous immunoglobulin in murine immune thrombocytopenia: support for FcγRIIB falls by the wayside. Semin Hematol. 2016;53:S20-S22.

75. Semple JW, Milev Y, Cosgrave D, et al. Differences in serum cytokine levels in acute and chronic autoimmune thrombocytopenic purpura: relationship to platelet phenotype and antiplatelet T-cell reactivity. Blood. 1996;87 (10):4245-4254.

76. Panitsas FP, Theodoropoulou M, Kouraklis A, et al. Adult chronic idiopathic thrombocytopenic purpura (ITP) is the manifestation of a type-1 polarized immune response. Blood. 2004;103(7):2645-2647.

77. Zhang J, Ma D, Zhu X, Qu X, Ji C, Hou M. Elevated profile of Th17, Th1 and Tc1 cells in patients with immune thrombocytopenic purpura. Haematologica. 2009;94(9):1326-1329.

78. Wei Y, Hou M. T cells in the pathogenesis of immune thrombocytopenia. Semin Hematol. 2016;53 Suppl 1: S13-5.

79. Aukrust P, Frøland SS, Liabakk NB, et al. Release of cytokines, soluble cytokine receptors, and interleukin-1 receptor antagonist after intravenous immunoglobulin administration in vivo. Blood. 1994;84(7):2136-2143.

80. Skull S, Kemp A. Treatment of hypogammaglobulinaemia with intravenous immunoglobulin, 1973-93. Arch Dis Child. 1996;74(6):527-530.

81. Sewell WA, North ME, Cambronero R, Webster AD, Farrant J. In vivo modulation of cytokine synthesis by intravenous immunoglobulin. Clin Exp Immunol. 1999; 116(3):509-515.

82. Cooper N, Heddle NM, Haas M, et al. Intravenous (IV) anti-D and IV immunoglobulin achieve acute platelet increases by different mechanisms: modulation of cytokine and platelet responses to IV anti-D by FcgammaRIIa and FcgammaRIIIa polymorphisms. Br J Haematol. 2004;124(4):511-518.

83. Leontyev D, Neschadim A, Branch DR. Cytokine profiles in mouse models of experimental immune thrombocytopenia reveal a lack of inflammation and differences in response to intravenous immunoglobulin depending on the mouse strain. Transfusion. 2014;54(11): 2871-2879.

84. Aubin E, Lemieux R, Bazin R. Absence of cytokine modulation following therapeutic infusion of intravenous immunoglobulin or anti-red blood cell antibodies in a mouse model of immune thrombocytopenic purpura. Br J Haematol. 2007;136(6):837-843.

85. Roopenian DC, Akilesh S. FcRn: the neonatal Fc receptor comes of age. Nat Rev Immunol. 2007;7(9):715-725.

86. Li N, Zhao M, Hilario-Vargas J, et al. Complete FcRn dependence for intravenous Ig therapy in autoimmune skin blistering diseases. J Clin Invest. 2005;115(12):3440-3450.

87. Newland AC, Sánchez-González B, Rejto L, et al. Phase 2 study of efgartigimod, a novel FcRn antagonist, in adult patients with primary immune thrombocytopenia. Am J Hematol. 2020;95(2):178-187.

88. Zuercher AW, Spirig R, Baz Morelli A, Rowe T, Käsermann F. Next-generation Fc receptor-targeting biologics for autoimmune diseases. Autoimmun Rev. 2019;18(10):102366.

89. Kiessling P, Lledo-Garcia R, Watanabe S, et al. The FcRn inhibitor rozanolixizumab reduces human serum IgG concentration: A randomized phase 1 study. Sci Transl Med. 2017;9(414).

90. Robak T, Kazmierczak M, Jarque I, et al. Phase 2 multiple-dose study of an FcRn inhibitor, rozanolixizumab, in patients with primary immune thrombocytopenia. Blood Adv. 2020;4(17):4136-4146.

91. Deng R, Balthasar JP. Pharmacokinetic/pharmacodynamic modeling of IVIG effects in a murine model of immune thrombocytopenia. J Pharm Sci. 2007;96(6): 1625-1637.

92. Hansen RJ, Balthasar JP. Intravenous immunoglobulin mediates an increase in anti-platelet antibody clearance via the FcRn receptor. Thromb Haemost. 2002;88 (6):898-899.

93. Crow AR, Suppa SJ, Chen X, Mott PJ, Lazarus AH. The neonatal Fc receptor (FcRn) is not required for IVIg or anti-CD44 monoclonal antibody-mediated amelioration of murine immune thrombocytopenia. Blood. 2011; 118(24):6403-6406.

94. Norris PAA, Kaur G, Khan R, Zhu G, Ni H, Lazarus AH. Anti-inflammatory activity of CD44 antibodies in murine immune thrombocytopenia is mediated by Fcγ receptor inhibition. Blood. 2021;137(15):2114-2124.

95. Molthoff CF, Pinedo HM, Schlüper HM, Nijman HW, Boven E. Comparison of the pharmacokinetics, biodistribution and dosimetry of monoclonal antibodies OC125, OV-TL 3, and 139H2 as IgG and F(ab')2 fragments in experimental ovarian cancer. Br J Cancer. 1992; 65(5):677-683.

96. Semple JW, Freedman J. Increased antiplatelet T helper lymphocyte reactivity in patients with autoimmune thrombocytopenia. Blood. 1991;78(10):2619-2625.

97. Olsson B, Andersson P-O, Jernas M, et al. T-cell-mediated cytotoxicity toward platelets in chronic idiopathic thrombocytopenic purpura. Nat Med. 2003;9(9): 1123-1124.

98. Siragam V, Crow ARAR, Brinc D, Song S, Freedman J, Lazarus AHAH. Intravenous immunoglobulin ameliorates ITP via activating Fc gamma receptors on dendritic cells. Nat Med. 2006;12(6):688-692.

99. Bayry J, Lacroix-Desmazes S, Carbonneil C, et al. Inhibition of maturation and function of dendritic cells by intravenous immunoglobulin. Blood. 2003;101(2):758-765.

100. Das M, Karnam A, Stephen-Victor E, et al. Intravenous immunoglobulin mediates anti-inflammatory effects in peripheral blood mononuclear cells by inducing autophagy. Cell Death Dis. 2020;11(1):50.

101. Massoud AH, Yona M, Xue D, et al. Dendritic cell immunoreceptor: a novel receptor for intravenous immunoglobulin mediates induction of regulatory T cells. J Allergy Clin Immunol. 2014;133(3):853-63.e5.

102. Crow AR, Brinc D, Lazarus AH. New insight into the mechanism of action of IVIg: the role of dendritic cells. J Thromb Haemost. 2009;7:245-248.

103. Kaufman GN, Massoud AH, Dembele M, Yona M, Piccirillo CA, Mazer BD. Induction of Regulatory T Cells by Intravenous Immunoglobulin: A Bridge between Adaptive and Innate Immunity. Front Immunol. 2015; 6:469.

104. Smed-Sörensen A, Moll M, Cheng T-Y, et al. IgG regulates the CD1 expression profile and lipid antigen-presenting function in human dendritic cells via FcgammaRIIa. Blood. 2008;111(10):5037-5046.

105. Kapur R, Aslam R, Kim M, et al. Thymic-derived tolerizing dendritic cells are upregulated in the spleen upon treatment with intravenous immunoglobulin in a murine model of immune thrombocytopenia. Platelets. 2017;28(5):521-524.

106. Massoud AH, Kaufman GN, Xue D, et al. Peripherally Generated Foxp3(+) Regulatory T Cells Mediate the Immunomodulatory Effects of IVIg in Allergic Airways Disease. J Immunol. 2017;198(7):2760-2771.

107. Trinath J, Hegde P, Sharma M, et al. Intravenous immunoglobulin expands regulatory T cells via induction of cyclooxygenase-2-dependent prostaglandin E2 in human dendritic cells. Blood. 2013;122(8):1419-1427.

108. Maddur MS, Trinath J, Rabin M, et al. Intravenous immunoglobulin-mediated expansion of regulatory T cells in autoimmune patients is associated with increased prostaglandin E2 levels in the circulation. Cell Mol Immunol. 2015;12(5):650-652.

109. Oropeza-Rendon RL, Bauer HC, Fischer H. Effect of prostaglandin E1 on the level of cAMP in bone marrow macrophages. Inhibition of phagocytosis and cell shape changes. J Immunopharmacol. 1980;2(1):133-147.

110. Aronoff DM, Canetti C, Peters-Golden M. Prostaglandin E2 inhibits alveolar macrophage phagocytosis through an E-prostanoid 2 receptor-mediated increase in intracellular cyclic AMP. J Immunol. 2004;173(1): 559-565.

111. Kessel A, Ammuri H, Peri R, et al. Intravenous immunoglobulin therapy affects T regulatory cells by increasing their suppressive function. J Immunol. 2007; 179(8):5571-5575.

112. Maddur MS, Vani J, Hegde P, Lacroix-Desmazes S, Kaveri S V, Bayry J. Inhibition of differentiation, amplification, and function of human TH17 cells by intravenous immunoglobulin. J Allergy Clin Immunol. 2011; 127(3):823-827.

113. Fitzpatrick EA, Wang J, Strome SE. Engineering of Fc Multimers as a Protein Therapy for Autoimmune Disease. Front Immunol. 2020;11:496.

114. Zhang X, Owens J, Olsen HS, et al. A recombinant human IgG1 Fc multimer designed to mimic the active fraction of IVIG in autoimmunity. JCI insight. 2019; 4(2).

115. Jain A, Olsen HS, Vyzasatya R, et al. Fully recombinant IgG2a Fc multimers (stradomers) effectively treat collagen-induced arthritis and prevent idiopathic thrombocytopenic purpura in mice. Arthritis Res Ther. 2012;14(4):R192.

116. Audia S, Bonnotte B. Emerging Therapies in Immune Thrombocytopenia. J Clin Med. 2021;10(5).

117. Mekhaiel DNA, Czajkowsky DM, Andersen JT, et al. Polymeric human Fc-fusion proteins with modified effector functions. Sci Rep. 2011;1:124.

118. Czajkowsky DM, Andersen JT, Fuchs A, et al. Developing the IVIG biomimetic, Hexa-Fc, for drug and vaccine applications. Sci Rep. 2015;5(1):9526.

119. Spirig R, Campbell IK, Koernig S, et al. rIgG1 Fc Hexamer Inhibits Antibody-Mediated Autoimmune Disease via Effects on Complement and FcγRs. J Immunol. 2018;200(8):2542-2553.

120. Qureshi OS, Rowley TF, Junker F, et al. Multivalent Fcγ-receptor engagement by a hexameric Fc-fusion protein triggers Fcγ-receptor internalisation and modulation of Fcγ-receptor functions. Sci Rep. 2017;7(1):17049.

121. Najaoui A, Bakchoul T, Stoy J, et al. Autoantibody-mediated complement activation on platelets is a common finding in patients with immune thrombocytopenic purpura (ITP). Eur J Haematol. 2012;88(2):167-174.

122. Peerschke EIB, Andemariam B, Yin W, Bussel JB. Complement activation on platelets correlates with a decrease in circulating immature platelets in patients with immune thrombocytopenic purpura. Br J Haematol. 2010;148(4):638-645.

123. Zhou H, Olsen H, So E, et al. A fully recombinant human IgG1 Fc multimer (GL-2045) inhibits complement-mediated cytotoxicity and induces iC3b. Blood Adv. 2017;1(8):504-515.

124. Norris PAA, Kaur G, Lazarus AH. New insights into IVIg mechanisms and alternatives in autoimmune and inflammatory diseases. Curr Opin Hematol. 2020;27(6): 392-398.

125. Yu X, Menard M, Prechl JJ, Bhakta V, Sheffield WPP, Lazarus AHH. Monovalent Fc receptor blockade by an anti-Fcgamma receptor/albumin fusion protein ameliorates murine ITP with abrogated toxicity. Blood. 2016;127(1):132-138.

126. Ulrichts P, Cousin T, Dreier T, de Haard H, Leupin N. Argx-113, a Novel Fc-Based Approach for Antibody-Induced Pathologies Such As Primary Immune Thrombocytopenia. Blood. 2016;128(22):4919.

127. Ulrichts P, Guglietta A, Dreier T, et al. Neonatal Fc receptor antagonist efgartigimod safely and sustainably reduces IgGs in humans. J Clin Invest. 2018;128(10): 4372-4386.

128. Ling LE, Roy S, Daly T, et al. M281: A Therapeutic Anti-FcRn Blocking Antibody for Rapid Clearance of IgG and IgG Autoantibodies in Immune Cytopenias and Other Auto/Allo-Immune Disease. Blood. 2015;126 (23):3472.

129. Ling LE, Hillson JL, Tiessen RG, et al. M281, an Anti-FcRn Antibody: Pharmacodynamics, Pharmacokinetics, and Safety Across the Full Range of IgG Reduction in a First-in-Human Study. Clin Pharmacol Ther. 2019;105(4):1031-1039.

130. Arroyo S, Tiessen RG, Denney WS, et al. Hyper-Sialylated IgG M254, an Innovative Therapeutic Candidate, Evaluated in Healthy Volunteers and in Patients with Immune Thrombocytopenia Purpura: Safety, Tolerability, Pharmacokinetics, and Pharmacodynamics. Blood. 2019;134(Supplement_1):1090.

131. Paquin Proulx D, Aubin E, Lemieux R, Bazin R. Inhibition of B cell-mediated antigen presentation by intravenous immunoglobulins (IVIg). Clin Immunol. 2010;135(3):422-429.

# 17. Immune thrombocytopenia – the patients' perspective

In 1995 the UK ITP Support Association was founded by Shirley Watson whose son has ITP. The American Platelet Disorder Support Association (PDSA) started 1997 as an internet platform for patients to exchange information on ITP. More self-support groups in other countries commenced their activities in the late 1990s and early 2000s. The objective of all these groups is to provide support, education, and communication to people with ITP and other platelet disorders. This reflects both dissatisfaction with the conventional medical system and a new self-understanding of the patients role in coping with their disease. What has happened?

- Platelet Disorder Support Association (USA) www.pdsa.org
- ITP Foundation (USA) www.itpfoundation.org
- ITP-Selbsthilfe (D) www.morbus-werlhof.de
- ITP at the Netherlands Haemophilia Association (NL) www.itp-pv.nl
- ITP at The Swedish Hemophilia Society (S) www.fbis.se
- The ITP Support Association (UK) www.itpsupport.org.uk

***Table 17.1:*** List of self-support groups.

ITP is a rare disorder. With an annual incidence rate of <1 in 10.000 it formally qualifies as an orphan disease and this is how many patients feel – orphaned. Because of the rarity of their disorder they usually see physicians who have limited personal experience from only a handful of cases. To address this need for guidance, the American Society of Hematology convened an expert panel which published its recommendations in the *1996 ASH guideline* [1]. A British guideline followed in 2003 [2]. The advent of new therapies prompted reevaluation of those older recommendations and within the last years several updates have been published, the internationally most relevant being the *International Consensus Report* [3] and the new *2011 ASH guideline* [4]. These academic publications primarily address physicians' educational needs and view on the disease. Many patients feel that they do not adequately reflect the impact of disease and treatments on their daily lifestyle activities, occupation, and families.

## 17.1. Patients "hate steroids"

According to the old and new guidelines [1-4] corticosteroids is the standard 1st-line treatment for newly-diagnosed ITP in adults. Patient surveys show that between 90 and 100% of patients have received corticosteroids at some time during their disease [5-7]. These guidelines put much emphasis on side effects such as hypertension, hyperglycemia, cataracts, and osteoporosis [1]. Instead the side effects most commonly reported by patients are weight gain, increased appetite, changes in personality, mood, or emotions, "moon face" or puffy cheeks, and problems with sleeping [7, 8]. Patients rank treatment-bother with corticosteroids higher than with any other ITP therapy [7-9]. More patients treated with corticosteroids stop or reduce treatment due to side effects than with any other type of therapy [5, 7].

Corticosteroid toxicities are dose and duration dependent. Therefore the 1996 ASH guideline had recommended that $1^{st}$-line treatment should not last longer than 2-4 weeks if the patient does not respond adequately. Toxicities during $1^{st}$-line therapy ("newly-diagnosed ITP" according to the International Working Group terminology, 10) are acceptable because in this initial phase fear from bleeding is more prevalent [11]. The situation changes with longer disease and treatment duration ( "persistent" and "chronic" phase according to [10]). Patients who fail splenectomy and further treatment lines are often placed on long-term steroids as long as this achieves some increase in platelet counts. There are patients with months and years of steroid-therapy merely to keep platelets in a "safe" range. The argument for this is the theoretical risk of severe bleeding when platelet counts are low. In children it has been shown that occurrence of bleeding is unrelated to management [12].

## 17.2. Rituximab

In 1998 there was the first report on rituximab in ITP. Initial results fuelled great expectations that rituximab could relieve patients from steroids. Since then there have been numerous case-reports and smaller studies but very little phase III data. The long-term success rate is not as high as expected and ranges between 20 and 30% [13]. Until today rituximab is not licensed for treatment of ITP, neither in Europe nor in any other country in the world. Nevertheless surveys show that it is frequently used [5-7]. Many patients request rituximab as an option to reduce or stop corticosteroids. Others choose this therapy to postpone or avoid splenectomy [14]. The side effect feared most by physicians are infections, including a very rare type of leukoencephalopathy [15, 16]. Instead, the most bothersome side effects reported by patients are fatigue, tiredness, infusion reactions, headaches, and dizziness. The tolerability seems to be a little better than of intravenous immunoglobulins (IVIg) or anti-D [7, 9]. The high cost, the off-label status and the limited long-term success rate are points of concern to patients especially in health care systems where they have to cover part of the costs themselves.

## 17.3. Patients try to avoid splenectomy

Although the authors of the 1996 ASH guideline admitted that all available evidence regarding splenectomy was low level and inadequate to make evidence-based recommendations on indications and timing, they did not abstain from proposing 2$^{nd}$-line splenectomy in all patients who "have had the diagnosis for 3 months, have experienced a transient or incomplete response to primary treatment, have a platelet count of <30,000, and are either bleeding *or not bleeding*". This recommendation has not changed in the 2011 ASH-guideline [4]. Consequently physicians must consider medico-legal consequences if they don't bring their patient to splenectomy and if this patient eventually develops bleeding.

Despite guidelines and expert recommendations patients shy away from surgery. Studies on new thrombopoetin receptor agonists in chronic ITP show that only a minority (~30%) of the patients included in these studies had undergone splenectomy before. Considering the good long-term success rate for splenectomy this fear might be perceived as irrational or overt emotional. What it really reflects is that all ITP-patients have been told from the first day of their disease to avoid all injuries if they don't want to "bleed to death". Patients perceive this permanent risk of bleeding as the worst emotional burden of the disease [11]. Minor procedures such as dental extractions or endoscopy require complex preparation and the major logistic effort in the run-up to therapeutic interventions causes anxieties. Patients worry that in an emergency they have to travel long distances to reach a doctor or a center experienced in ITP. This leaves the impression that their health is in a very labile status and that they should carefully weigh all benefits and risks of any new treatment and particularly of such an invasive procedure as splenectomy.

## 17.4. Patients and Thrombopoetin-Receptor Agonists (TRAs)

TRAs are a new class of agents that stimulate platelet production in chronic ITP. TRAs raise platelets to sufficient counts in almost 80% of patients. TRAs are well tolerated and significantly improve quality of life [17-19]. Three agents are currently available: romiplostim (Nplate™), eltrombopag (Promacta™, in EU: Revolade™) and avatrombopag (Doptelet™). The major difference is that romiplostim has to be given as a weekly subcutaneous injection while eltrombopag and avatrombopag are oral preparations for daily use. Eltrombopag has to be taken on an empty stomach. In contrast, avatrombopag can be administered orally without regard to food type. It is the experience of the author that some patients feel safer with weekly office visits and regular blood counts while others prefer regained independence with oral treatment. The need for taking eltrombopag on an empty stomach can pose a problem to some patients.

A therapeutic dilemma develops when women on TRAs want to become pregnant. With low platelets and risk of bleeding they usually refrain from becoming pregnant. With TRAs and normal platelet counts they may wish again to start a family. There is no experience on the safety of TRAs in pregnancy. Fetal harm cannot be excluded. The statement in the prescribing information, that TRAs should only be used during pregnancy "if the potential benefit to the mother justifies the potential risk to the fetus", is not really helpful. This leaves the decision to the woman whether to continue TRAs with potential harms to the fetus or to go back to steroids and IVIg which also have side effects and risks during pregnancy.

## 17.5. Other therapies

IVIg and anti-D (the latter not being licensed in Europe) are considered emergency treatments in adults. Commonly reported side effects are fatigue, tiredness, infusion reactions, headaches, and dizziness [7]. For the bleeding patient benefits usually outweigh side effects.

Other 3$^{rd}$ and X$^{th}$-line therapies e.g. azathioprin, cyclophosphamide, ciclosporin, mycophenolate, danazol, vinca alkaloids are used in refractory patients with continuing relevant bleedings. A survey shows that many patients experience side effects from these treatments [20]. In addition it is the author's experience that patients shrink back from taking cyclophosphamide or vinca alkaloids after they read in the drug information that antineoplastic drugs may cause thrombocytopenia.

## 17.6. The quagmire of modern medicine

As has been outlined before, the need for guidance in this rare disorder led to several guidelines, the first one being the 1996 ASH ITP-guideline [1]. This was and still is the most cited publication in the field. The authors conceded that most literature on ITP at that time was case series or small phase II studies and recommendations were mainly based on opinion rather than solid medical evidence. Nonetheless they propose a treatment sequence that might be perceived by many patients as stringent and bothersome. Quality of life assessments and patients' preferences did not play a major role at that time. The most recent guidelines from 2009 [3] and 2011 [4] have not really changed this unsatisfactory situation. In addition to all that and despite all academic guideline efforts, 20-25% of patients have the impression that their doctors do not know enough about ITP [21].

The 1996 guideline proposed platelet thresholds below which treatment had to be continued. The authors went so far to state that with low counts withholding treatment would be inappropriate "even at the patient's request". There were no data to support this at that time. 15 years later, the experts of the 2011 ASH guideline [4] admit that there is still no evidence that could allow determination of a minimum platelet count threshold or specific age at which a typical patient with ITP should be treated. Patients perceive this approach as restrictive since a mere lab value and not clinical symptoms force the physician to continue therapeutic efforts ad infinitum, a good few patients ending up with long-term steroids. They are no longer willing to accept this situation and self-support groups voiced their dissatisfaction with school medicine's mantra "steroids and splenectomy". The 2009 International Consensus Statement [3] acknowledged this conceding, that it would be acceptable to live with low platelet counts foregoing further toxic treatments, as long as patients have no or only very mild bleeding and near normal quality of life. Then in 2011 the ASH guideline turned the clock back again. The authors came to the conclusion that stopping treatment is acceptable only with >30.000 platelets which means that it is unacceptable with lower counts and that these patients have to proceed to additional treatment lines even if completely asymptomatic [4].

The advent of TRAs had the potential to change this situation. The studies submitted for licensure showed equal efficacy in both splenectomized and non-splenectomized patients [22-24]. This and the improved quality of life in non-splenectomized patients [17] fuelled hope that TRAs would soon replace splenectomy as 2$^{nd}$ line therapy. Eventually in the US and Europe TRAs were licensed only for patients who "have had an insufficient response to corticosteroids, immunoglobulins, or splenectomy". This means that splenectomy is required before insurances or public health will cover TRAs (except for patients with contraindications to splenectomy).

The authors of the International Consensus Report admitted that treatment is limited by financial resources and regulatory requirements. For these non-medical reasons they explicitly avoided to give preference to a particular 2$^{nd}$-line therapy but instead chose to list all treatment options alphabetically [3]. It has been without precedence that an international group of renowned experts authoring a consensus statement on a potentially

| Exemplary questions (list not complete) from PDSA publications and booklets (www.pdsa.org/products-a-publications/free-materials.html, accessed 7/2012) and from The Platelet, the quarterly journal of the UK ITP Support Association (www.itpsupport.org.uk/leaflets.htm, accessed 7/2012) | |
|---|---|
| **ITP diagnosis and treatment**<br>• What is ITP? How does it develop? How is its course (acute vs. chronic) and prognosis?<br>• Typical and atypical symptoms and when to seek medical help?<br>• Signs of serious injury or bleeding in children?<br>• What is a safe platelet count? When does it become dangerous?<br>• Available treatments, treatment goals and side effects (steroids, IVIg, anti-D, monoclonal antibodies, immunosuppressant drugs, splenectomy, platelet growth factors, etc.), $1^{st}$-line, $2^{nd}$-line treatment and sequencing<br>• Experimental therapies, participation in studies | |
| **ITP and other health issues**<br>• ITP and pregnancy<br>• Familial thrombocytopenia<br>• Dental care<br>• Surgery, anesthesia<br>• Thyroid disease<br>• Fatigue, mood changes, depression<br>• *H. pylori*, hepatitis, HIV<br>• Vaccinations (efficacy and safety, i.m. vaccinations)<br>• Common infections (cold and flu) while on immunosuppression.<br>• Drugs, supplements and foods that can affect platelet function<br>• Management of disorders that require anticoagulation (e.g. atrial fibrillation, thromboembolism, myocardial infarction, stroke)<br>• When to call the doctor, interaction with doctors, how to find an ITP specialist? | Covered by guidelines and academic literature |
| **ITP and daily living, occupation**<br>• Work performance and limitations, school attendance, and sports<br>• Social stigmatization from hematomas and bleeding<br>• Dietary changes (e.g. to minimize weight gain from steroids)<br>• Regular exercise<br>• Travelling with ITP, alert medical cards<br>• Effect of ITP on partnership and family<br>• Coping with unpredictability of the disease and constantly changing platelet counts<br>• Coping with anxiety and feeling depressed<br>• Coping with feeling helpless and dependent | |
| **Complementary and alternative medicines**<br>• CAMs (ayurvedic and traditional chinese medicine, herbal medicine, acupressure, acupuncture, Vitamin C, Vitamin K, collostrum, reiki, magnets, macrobiotic, diets, prayer, meditation, visualization, positive thinking, etc.)<br>• CAMs that should be avoided | |
| ETC<br>• Insurance issues, help with treatment costs<br>• Treatment for patients who cannot receive blood products | |

***Table 17.2:*** Common patient problems and questions.

life-threatening disorder abstained from ranking the available evidence to avoid financial frictions. The problems with coverage for off-label rituximab as splenectomy-sparing therapy, the restricted licensure of TRAs, and the constant pressure to undergo splenectomy have to many patients the smack that cost considerations exert more influence on treatment recommendations than medical evidence or patients' preferences. Indeed in the German survey 38% of patients had that impression [5]. This leaves both patient and physician in a quagmire. Can the patient still trust his physician to make Hippocratic decisions only to his benefit as a single individual? Can the physician still remain his patient's advocate while serving as a steward of society's resources? It is not surprising that many patients turn to complementary or alternative medicines (CAMs) outside the system of traditional and school medicine. Surveys show that almost half of the patients try CAMs at some time during their course of disease [5, 6, 9].

## 17.7. What patients really want

The burden of disease in ITP is high. Quality of life ranks lower than in cancer patients [25]. The internet platforms of PDSA, ITP-Support Association and other self-support groups give an impression of patients' daily problems and questions (☞ Table 17.2). They not only seek information on diagnosis and treatment but also on the impact of disease on lifestyle activities, occupation, relatives, and family planning. Only very recently quality of life has become an issue in medical research on ITP and this was mainly due to licensure requirements for the new TRAs [17-19]. Self-support groups were the first to address the impact of ITP on patients' lives, psychological and physical bother, fatigue, fears, anxieties, social activity, and workplace productivity [21, 26-29]. Many of these aspects of ITP have not been discussed in treatment guidelines and academic publications. This has to change.

## 17.8. Conclusions

Many patients perceive traditional ITP treatments as bothersome, particularly corticosteroids and splenectomy. The restricted licensure of new agents, problems with cost coverage, and the persistent recommendation of splenectomy have the smack that cost considerations may factor into treatment recommendations. While most patients state that they have a good relationship to their doctor and trust his recommendations, there is a major need for counseling on questions of daily living. Traditional academic medicine does not adequately address many of these problems. The gap is filled by patient self-help groups which provide support, education, and communication. Within the last decade ITP patients have begun to voice and lobby their perspectives on the disease. Patient representatives serve on scientific advisory boards and national regulatory committees. This new understanding of patients' role in coping with their disease is beginning to change our approach to ITP. It will hopefully soon find its way into treatment guidelines and academic medicine.

### References

1. George JN, Woolf SH, Raskob GE, et al. Idiopathic thrombocytopenic purpura: a practice guideline developed by explicit methods for the American Society of Hematology. Blood 1996;88:3-40

2. British Committee for Standards in Haematology General Haematology Task Force. Guidelines for the investigation and management of idiopathic thrombocytopenic purpura in adults, children and in pregnancy. Br J Haematol 2003;120:574-596

3. Provan D, Stasi R, Newland AC, et al. International consensus report on the investigation and management of primary immune thrombocytopenia. Blood 2019;115: 168-196

4. Neunert C, Lim W, Crother M, et al. The American Society of Hematology 2011 evidence-based practice guideline for immune thrombocytopenia. Blood 2011; 117:4190-4207

5. Matzdorff A, Arnold G. Treatment of chronic immune thrombocytopenic purpura: the patients' perspective. Eur J Haematol 2007;78:381-388

6. Matzdorff AC, Arnold G, Salama A, Ostermann H, Eberle S, Hummler S. Advances in ITP – Therapy and quality of life – a patient survey. Plos One 2011;6:e27350

7. Brown TM, Horblyuk RV, Grotzinger KM, Matzdorff AC, Pashos CL. Patient-Reported Treatment Burden of Chronic Immune Thrombocytopenia Therapies. BioMed Central 2012;22;12:2

8. Berti D, Moons P, Dobbels F, et al. Impact of corticosteroid-related symptoms in patients with immune thrombocytopenic purpura: results of a survey of 985 patients. Clin Ther 2008;30:1540-1552

9. PDSA Survey of Non-Traditional Treatments of ITP. www.pdsa.org/about-itp/surveys/non-traditional-treatments.html (accessed 7/2012)

10. Rodeghiero F, Stasi R, Gernsheimer T, et al. Standardization of terminology, definitions and outcome criteria in immune thrombocytopenic purpura (ITP) of adults and children: Report from an International Working Group. Blood 2009;113:2386-2393

11. The ITP Support Association's Survey of Treatment for ITP, Spring 2000.
www.itpsupport.org.uk/survey2000.htm (accessed 7/2012)

12. Neunert CE, Buchanan GR, Imbach P, et al. Severe hemorrhage in children with newly diagnosed immune thrombocytopenic purpura. Blood 2008;112:4003-4008

13. Patel V, Mahévas M, Lee SY, et al. Outcomes 5 years after response to rituximab therapy in children and adults with immune thrombocytopenia. Blood 2012; 119:5989-5995

14. Cooper N, Evangelista ML, Amadori S, Stasi R. Should rituximab be used before or after splenectomy in patients with immune thrombocytopenic purpura. Curr Opin Hematol 2007;14:642-646

15. Arnold DM, Dentali F, Crowther MA, et al. Systematic Review: Efficacy and Safety of Rituximab for Adults with Idiopathic Thrombocytopenic Purpura. Ann Intern Med 2007;146:25-33

16. Carson KR, Evens AM, Richey EA, et al. Progressive multifocal leukoencephalopathy after rituximab therapy in HIV-negative patients: a report of 57 cases from the Research on Adverse Drug Events and Reports project. Blood 2009;113:4834-4840

17. Kuter DJ, Mathias SD, Rummel M, et al. Health-related quality of life in nonsplenectomized immune thrombocytopenia patients receiving romiplostim or medical standard of care. Am J Hematol 2012;87:558-561

18. Mathias SD, Bussel JB, George JN, et al. A disease-specific measure of health-related quality of life in adults with chronic immune thrombocytopenic purpura: psychometric testing in an open-label clinical trial. Clin Ther 2007;29:950-962

19. George JN, Mathias SD, Go RS, et al. Improved quality of life for romiplostim-treated patients with chronic immune thrombocytopenic purpura: results from two randomized, placebo-controlled trials. Br J Haematol 2009;144:409-415

20. Survey of Non-Traditional Treatments of ITP. www.pdsa.org/about-itp/surveys/non-traditional-treatments.html (accessed 7/2012)

21. Lifestyle Survey 2007 for adults and children with ITP. www.itpsupport.org.uk/survey2007.htm (accessed 7/2012)

22. Bussel JB, Cheng G, Saleh MN, et al. Eltrombopag for the treatment of chronic idiopathic thrombocytpenic purpura. N Engl J Med 2007;357:2237-2247

23. Kuter DJ, Bussel JB, Lyons RM, et al. Efficacy of romiplostim in patients with chronic immune thrombocytopenic purpura: a double-blind randomised controlled trial. Lancet 2008;371:395-403

24. Olney HJ, Fogarty PF, Tarantino MD, et al. Efficacy of Eltrombopag In Splenectomized Versus Nonsplenectomized Patients with Chronic ITP In the RAISE Study. Blood 2010;116(Suppl.):1041, Abstr. #2512

25. McMillan R, Bussel JB, George JN, et al. Self-reported health-related quality of life in adults with chronic immune thrombocytopenic purpura. Am J Hematol 2008; 83:150–154

26. "The Impact of ITP" Questionnaire. www.pdsa.org/about-itp/surveys.html (accessed 7/2012)

27. Snyder CF, Mathias SD, Cella D, et al. Health-related quality of life of immune thrombocytopenic purpura patients: results from a web-based survey. Curr Med Res Opin 2008;24:2767-2776

28. ITP and Fatigue Survey in Autumn 2009
www.itpsupport.org.uk/survey2009.htm

29. Tarantino MD, Mathias SD, Snyder CF, et al. Impact of ITP on physician visits and workplace productivity. Curr Med Res Opin. 2010;26:319-328.

# 18. Quality of Life as a treatment endpoint for patients with ITP

## 18.1. Introduction

The impact of immune thrombocytopenia (ITP) on quality of life is complex. While all patients with ITP experience low platelet counts, there is significant variation in the correlation with symptoms with the degree of thrombocytopenia. At a given platelet count, some patients may be totally asymptomatic, some experience increased post-traumatic bruising, while others may have spontaneous bleeding ranging from mild (e.g. gum bleeding) to life threatening (e.g. intracranial hemorrhage, ICH).

> The degree of symptoms has a strong impact on a patient's quality of life but there is also significant variation between individuals. Physical bruising may lead to social limitations for one individual (e.g. change clothing to cover bruising, change activities) due to psychosocial distress but have less impact on another individual with similar symptoms.

While the management of ITP has evolved significantly over the last 20 years with new insights into pathophysiology and novel therapies emerging, perhaps the most important change has been a shift toward focussing on patient reported outcomes (PROs) to guide therapeutic decision making. Focussing on PROs is a significant change to previous ITP therapy response assessments which were primarily based on platelet counts and bleeding symptoms. As many ITP symptoms are only subjectively experienced (e.g. fatigue), the use of patient self-report is crucial for understanding disease impact.

> The primary PRO used in ITP is *Health Related Quality of Life* (HRQoL). HRQoL is an assessment of an individual's perceived well-being and includes evaluation of physical health, psychological health, and social health. HRQoL is increasingly used to guide therapeutic decision making and is reflected in recent international guidelines [1, 2].

Assessment of HRQoL has also been increasingly incorporated in the licensing and evaluation of new and emerging therapies ITP therapies including Thrombopoietin Receptor-Agonists (TPO-RAs) [20]. In this chapter, we will review the HR QoL in ITP, including assessment methods, the impact of symptoms and the effect of treatments.

## 18.2. Assessment of Health Related Quality of Life in ITP

Capturing a patient's illness experience as it relates to quality of life, necessitates using well-developed, validated and reliable instruments. The development of tools for assessing HRQoL needs to include consultation with patients and then once developed tools need to be validated with the target patient group. Ideally, HRQoL tools should be reliable (i.e. provide consistent results for a patient with a stable health status) and responsive (i.e. able to detect a change in a patient's health status).

The most well utilized tools for measuring patient HRQoL in ITP are questionnaires (patient-reported outcome measures or PROMs) that generate scores which can be tracked over time. There are unique differences in ITP by age, while the disease in children generally has a sudden onset but a good prognosis, ITP in adults often presents gradually, but tends to be chronic in nature. Thus, PROMs are age specific and may be generic (i.e. a tool used in many diseases) or ITP-specific (i.e. a tool designed to be used in ITP). Research focussed on tools to effectively measure HRQoL is critical to understand not only the impact of ITP symptoms but also how ITP therapies affect patients.

### 18.2.1. HRQoL in Adults

In adult patients with ITP, the most commonly used PROMs for evaluating quality of life have been the 36-Item Short-Form Health Survey (SF-36) and the ITP-Patient Assessment Questionnaire (ITP-PAQ). A short summary of these tools is detailed below.

### SF-36

The SF-36 is a generic tool that has been used to assess HRQoL in a range of adult patient groups with chronic disease but has also undergone validation and reliability assessment in adults with ITP [12]. The SF-36 provides a score (0-100 points) by measuring eight domains of quality of life including: physical functioning (PF), role physical (RP), bodily pain (BP), general pain (GP), vitality (V), social functioning (SF), role emotional (RE) and mental health (MH).

### ITP-PAQ™

The ITP-PAQ™ was developed to assess HRQoL in adult patients with ITP. It was designed using a combination of data from existing questionnaires, expert clinical opinion and input from ITP patient focus groups [13]. ITP-PAQ ask questions in the broad categories of Symptoms, Bother-Physical Health, Fatigue/Sleep, Activity, Fear, Psychological Health, Work, Social Activity, Women's Reproductive Health and Overall Quality of Life. It has been shown to be valid, reliable and responsive in adults with ITP [16].

## 18.2.2. HRQoL in Children

Assessing HRQoL in children is nuanced by the fact that the child's parent(s) and/or guardian(s) is often involved in completing assessment tools – in particular for younger children. Thus, validating tools for use in children requires involving the child and parent/guardian. The most frequently used PROMs to assess HRQoL in children with ITP are the Pediatric Quality of Life Inventory (PedsQL) and the Kids ITP Tools (KIT) questionnaire. Below is a brief description of these tools:

### PedsQL tool

The PedsQL tool is a well-established tool for use in both healthy and ill children. It does have several disease-specific modules but none specific for ITP [7]. The tool was developed using focus groups and includes parent-proxy report and child self-report to assess both parent and child perspectives. The PedsQL covers the domains of Physical Functioning, Emotional Functioning, Social Functioning, School Functioning.

### KIT questionnaire

The KIT questionnaire is the first ITP-specific HRQoL tool for children and has been shown to be valid and reliable. It was designed to be used in both clinic assessment and at home with child-self report, parent proxy-report and parent impact. The KIT questionnaire yields a score with potential range of 0 (worst) to 100 (best) [6].

## 18.3. ITP symptoms in HRQoL

The impact of ITP symptoms on HRQoL are complex and often interconnected with treatment responses and treatment-related side-effects. It is clear that for many individuals with ITP, HRQoL will vary with platelet count and response to therapy. However, the degree that symptoms will impact an individual is not uniform for any given platelet count and the benefit of treatment needs to be balanced with treatment related side-effects. To summarize these complex and dynamic interactions, Mathias et al proposed a conceptual model (☞ Figure 18.1) [13]. This model was developed using focus group data collected for the development of the ITP-PAQ and incorporating addition concepts from literature review and patient focus groups.

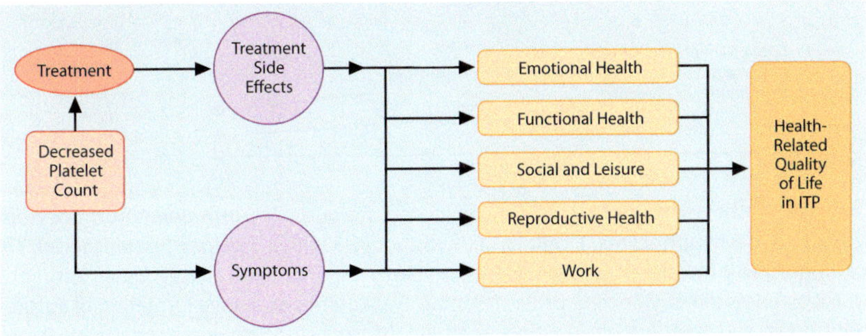


***Figure 18.1:*** Conceptual model for Health Related Quality of Life in ITP. Modified after Mathias SD et al. [13]

An additional consideration is how ITP influences HRQoL over time. Multiple studies have shown that the duration of ITP (i.e., acute, persistent, or chronic) has a bearing on HRQoL with patients in the persistent phase of their diagnosis reporting worse outcomes. In one study patients in the first year of their diagnosis had lower health scores in comparison to a group of patients who were diagnosed for over one year [16]. Another analysis showed that those with persistent ITP (i.e. 3-12 months from diagnosis) had lower outcomes that those who were diagnosed longer [12]. Whether this is due to patient adjustment to their diagnosis or achieving a stable therapy plan is unclear and additional research is needed to further understand the relationship between duration of ITP and HRQoL.

Two of the most extensively studied ITP symptoms that impact HRQoL are bleeding/bruising and fatigue. In the sections below, a summary is included focussed on HRQoL for these symptoms.

### 18.3.1. Bleeding and Bruising

People with ITP have increased bleeding and bruising tendency compared to individuals with normal platelet counts. While severe bleeding is rare, the fear of significant bleeding is much more common and reported in thirty percent of patients [14] and can impact on social functioning (e.g. activity restriction) and mental health (e.g. anxiety) leading to a reduced HRQoL. While not life threatening, the physical appearance of bruising is also impactful on self-esteem and can limit social engagements due to social embarrassment. In one study, an ITP patient encapsulated this sentiment in the statement, "*I find myself more reluctant about meeting new people because I have so many bruises so often*" [13].

Sex and gender also influence the experience of bleeding and bruising in ITP. Biologically, menstruation and child birth are unique hemostatic challenges for females of reproductive age with ITP. Heavy menstrual bleeding can require additional interventions (e.g. antifibrinolytic therapy) and can lead to anemia form acute blood loss or chronic iron deficiency. During pregnancy, patients with ITP may need additional monitoring and interventions. Increased bruising in an individual may also be perceived differently between men and women from a socio-cultural perspective. For example, a woman who is experiencing increased bruising may worry that people would perceive this as a sign of intimate partner violence [13].

Bleeding and bruising in children with ITP can lead to distress for the child and also their parent(s) and/or guardian(s). In one study, parental fear of

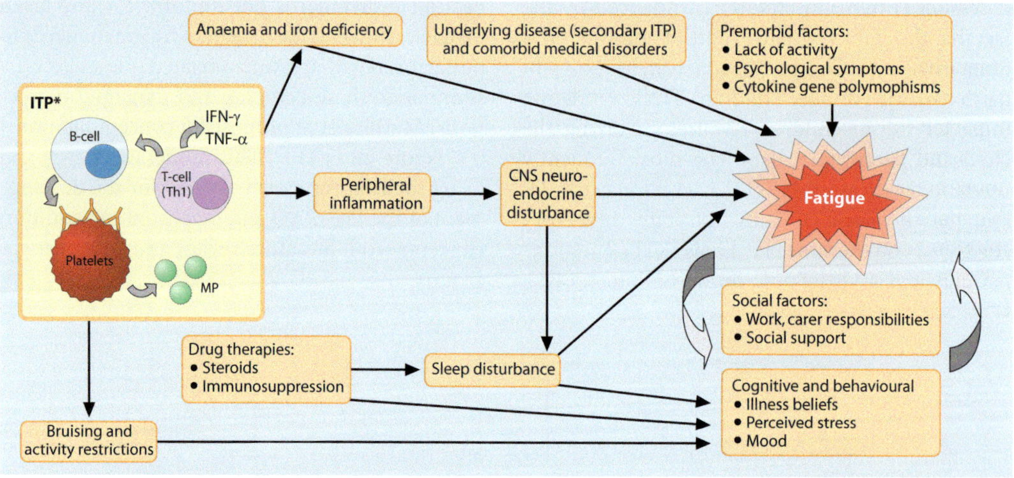


***Figure 18.2:*** Model of the pathogenesis of ITP-associated fatigue. ITP: immune thrombocytopenia, **B cell**: autoantibody producing B lymphocytes, **T cell**: Th1 (T lymphocytes with a T helper 1 polarization), **TNF-α**: tumour necrosis factor alpha, **IFN-γ**: interferon gamma, **MP**: microparticles, **CNS**: central nervous system.
* T cells can attack platelets directly, secrete pro-inflammatory cytokines and drive formation of autoreactive B cells. This results in antibody- and complement-mediated platelet destruction. Platelet microparticles are prothrombotic and able to activate the proinflammatory complement pathway. Modif. nach Hill and Newland [9].

their child bleeding was a significant concern and led to parental proxy HRQoL scores that were significantly lower than reported by their children [29]. Symptoms of bruising and bleeding may also lead parents to restrict activities (e.g. sports) on their own or at direction of their physician. As such, the frequency and significance of bleeding and bruising is a significant factor in decisions to start therapies for pediatric ITP patients [17].

### 18.3.2. Fatigue

In individuals with chronic disease, fatigue is commonly reported and can be one of the most distressing symptoms. While the causes for fatigue in ITP are not fully understood, they are likely multifactorial. For example, reduced platelets may lead to increased bleeding resulting in anemia and decreased oxygen delivery to tissues. Reduced activity due to risk of bleeding may also lead to suboptimal physical conditioning while treatment related side-effects (e.g. steroids) may lead to decreased sleep. A conceptual model for ITP impact on fatigue was proposed by Hill and Newland and is depicted below [9] (☞ Figure 18.2).

Fatigue affects both adults and children with ITP and has been reported to negatively impact HRQoL in both groups. Studies have shown that fatigue can lead to missed work and reduced school attendance [11] which can negatively impact individuals socially and financially. The experience of fatigue has been shown to vary over the ITP disease course with patients in the persistent phase most impacted in comparison to newly diagnosed ITP or chronic ITP [12]. In adolescents, newly diagnosed and persistent ITP reported higher fatigue than patients with chronic ITP [30]. While further study is needed, it is possible that an element of psychosocial adjustment may influence patient's experience over time.

## 18.4. Impact of treatments on HRQoL

ITP therapy may positively influence HRQoL when there is a response to treatment yet the benefits must also be balanced with negative impacts of treatment-related side effects. As such, patient experience with their previous treatments both in terms of platelet response and side effect profile should be considered when deciding on the best therapy. In some cases, close observation may be clinically appropriate from a bleeding perspective but the choice for observation alone must also take into account factors such as the logistics for obtaining additional bloodwork/appointments (time off work, transportation issues), risk for bleeding, and patient (and/or parent/caregiver) anxiety about not being treated during this period.

Medication administration considerations (i.e., intravenous vs oral; inpatient vs outpatient) and the impact on patient HRQoL must also be taken into account when deciding on therapy. For example, first-line therapies such as IVIg and anti-D require insertion of an IV and administration in a hospital setting while corticosteroids such as prednisone can be taken orally at home. The need for medical treatment in hospital may impact patients financially due to missed work or impact learning due to missed school.

Beyond first-line therapies, the financial costs of medical therapies are not insignificant and need to be considered [15]. Agents such as thrombopoietin-receptor agonists, fostamatinib and rituximab, if not covered by medical insurance, may be cost-prohibitive for many patients and even when there is coverage available, lifetime caps may be a cause of financial stress for patients and families. Studies on the impact of second-line agents on platelet count, bleeding and quality of life are ongoing and will help provide evidence for choice of second-line agents [4].

In the section below, we review common first-line and second-line treatments for ITP and the impact on HRQoL.

### 18.4.1. First-line agents

#### Corticosteroids

Corticosteroids (prednisone, prednisolone, dexamethasone, methylprednisone) are one of the most commonly prescribed treatments for ITP in both adults and children due to impact on platelet count. However, corticosteroids are also well-known to have a range of undesirable side effects including hypertension, hyperglycemia, weight gain, sleep and mood disturbances, gastrointestinal upset. For this reason, guidelines recommend treating with short courses of steroids when possible, to limit side-effects and avoid risks of immunosuppression with longer courses. Steroids can also negatively impact a patient's mental health and the recent ASH guidelines highlight the need to assess the impact of steroid treatment on a patients HRQoL [1].

The experience of steroid related side effects in ITP patients is well-described and is reported by a majority of individuals [14, 18]. Steroids have also been reported by patients as the most common cause of treatment related side effects and the concern for these side effects may influence a patient's decision to commence and adhere to treatment regimen [13]. In children with ITP, steroids can cause considerable behavioural changes (increased appetite, mood changes, sleep disturbances) that negatively impact HRQoL for the child and their parent(s)/caregiver(s). In one paediatric ITP study, which included mostly newly diagnosed ITP patients, there was no difference in self-reported HQRoL using the KIT questionnaire tool and parent proxy-scores were in fact worse with treatment (treatments included primarily prednisone or IVIg) [27].

#### Intravenous Immunoglobulin (IVIg)

Intravenous immunoglobulin increases platelet count by reducing macrophage mediated platelet clearance and patients who respond may experience a rise in platelet count lasting for approximately 4-6 weeks [22]. While side effects with IVIg are frequently mild and related infusion (e.g. nausea) these reactions can be severe (e.g. anaphylaxis). Headaches can also persist for several days following IVIg administration resulting missed school/work and negative impacts on HRQoL. Headaches may be severe enough to prolong hospitalization, require re-admission and/or necessitate neuroimaging to rule out intracranial haemorrhage. IVIg may also lead to hemolysis and rare but serious side effects include thrombosis and renal dysfunction. Given IVIg is a blood product there is also a potential risk for blood borne virus transmission. In children with mostly new-onset ITP, one study reported that treatment with IVIg did not improve HRQoL as measured through the KIT questionnaire [27].

### 18.4.2. Second-line therapies

#### Rituximab

Rituximab is a monoclonal antibody against CD20 leading to a reduction in B-cells and therefore antibody-mediated platelet destruction in patients with ITP. Rituximab has been used as a single agent and in combination with first line treatment [19]. The main side effects of rituximab include infusion reactions and risks of immunosuppression (e.g. infection due to reduced antibody production), with potential malignancy risk due decreased immune-surveillance. In clinical practice, rituximab can produce a sustained platelet response in patients for 6 months and even up to 12-18 months in some cases. While a sustained platelet response would likely be of benefit to a patient's HRQoL, studies focussed in this topic are limited.

#### Eltrombopag

Eltrombopag is a small molecule thrombopoietin receptor agonist medication that is formulated as a tablet and can be taken orally. Data from one randomized controlled trial, the RAISE trial, shows that Eltrombopag taken for a 6-month period was effective in raising platelet count and reducing bleeding events in adult patients [20]. In this same study, participants completed the SF-36 questionnaire for assessment of HRQoL and patients receiving Eltrombopag showed improvement in 5 of the 8 domains assessed (physical function, physical role, vitality, social function, and emotional role). The improvements in HQRoL were associated with rise in platelet count, reduction in bleeding symptoms and possibly improvements were also influenced by reduction in steroid usage.

More recently, the results of a longer-term assessment of Eltrombopag treatment (median medication duration 2.4 years; maximum 8.8 years) and impacts on HRQoL, the EXTEND trial, was published [23]. Four instruments were used to asses HRQoL, including the SF-36, and results showed improvement in HRQoL starting at 3 months and lasting up to 5 years. Patients on Eltrombopag also had an improvement in fatigue. Similarly, to the RAISE trial, there was an association between a response platelet count and improvement in HRQoL.

In children, Eltrombopag has been shown to improve platelet count, reduce bleeding symptoms and limit the need for emergency treatments in the PETIT trial [24 ]. In this study, the KIT questionnaire was used to assess HRQoL and no statistically significant difference was observed in HRQoL.

However, this study was not designed or powered to assess HRQoL and so further study is warranted.

### Romiplostim

Romiplostim is a thrombopoietin receptor agonist medication that is administered subcutaneously and has been shown to raise platelet count and reduce bleeding symptoms. In previous randomized controlled trials, HRQoL was assessed using the ITP-PAQ tool in splenectomised and non-splenectomised adult ITP patients [25]. Splenectomised patients showed significant improvements in HR QoL in the symptoms, bother, social activity and women's reproductive health scale, while non-splenectomised patients showed significant HR QoL improvement in activity scale. There was not reported improvement in fatigue in either group.

Paediatric studies of romiplostim have similarly demonstrated a rise platelet count and reduction in bleeding. While assessments of HRQoL on romiplostim are limited, one study reported a significant improvement in parental distress using the KIT questionnaire, however there was not a significant improvement in child reported HRQoL likely due to small sample size [26].

### Avatrombopag

Avatrombopag is a small molecule orally-administered at 20 mg/day. It was the third thrombopoietin receptor agonist approved for the treatment of immune thrombocytopenia and the first approved to treat periprocedural thrombocytopenia in patients with chronic liver disease (thereby providing an alternative to blood transfusions for these patients). Unlike eltrombopag, avatrombopag does not require a 4 hr food-restricted window around its use and it has not been associated with hepatotoxicity in ITP patients or portal vein thrombosis in patients with chronic liver disease. In ITP patients it can often be dosed less frequently than once daily. It is overall well-tolerated with a side-effect profile similar to placebo in randomized clinical trials [31].

### Splenectomy

Historically, splenectomy was recommended as a second line therapy in adult patients who were refractory to steroid therapy. However, with new effective agents (e.g. rituximab, TPO-RAs), the decision to pursue splenectomy is often delayed until after additional, less permanent, approaches are tried [10]. While approximately sixty percent of patients who undergo splenectomy will have a long-term response with improvement in platelet counts, there are a significant number of patients who will not respond. Unfortunately, the ability to predict those who will respond to splenectomy is limited as there are not currently universal methods available. As such the decision to perform an irreversible procedure with uncertain benefit can be a difficult decision. Further, complications post-splenectomy, both early (e.g. bleeding, infection) and late (e.g. thrombosis, infection), must also be weighed in the decision to pursue splenectomy [13]. The increased long-term risk of infection due to post-splenectomy is a significant stressor for some patients

## 18.5. Conclusion

In summary, the impact of ITP on an individual's HRQoL is both significant and multi-faceted, including the symptoms of the disease from bleeding and fatigue as well as the benefits and side effects of treatment. ITP specific tools for measuring HRQoL in adults and children have been developed and utilized to document patient experiences with ITP. With these tools, evaluations of ITP therapies are increasingly focused on HRQoL and have led to updated clinical recommendations. While there is more evidence to guide clinical decisions, further research is needed to evaluate the impact of both first-line and subsequent lines of therapy on HRQoL. As new therapies emerge, it is essential to continue to evaluate the impact of these treatments on PROMs, such as HRQoL, and not just the amount of bleeding or platelet count to ensure overall benefit to patients. At an individual patient level, continuing to incorporate PROMs including physical, psychosocial and lifestyle factors along with previous responses to therapy is imperative to optimize patient care.

## References

1. Neunert C, Terrell DR, Arnold DM, Buchanan G, Cines DB, Cooper N, Cuker A, Despotovic JM, George JN, Grace RF, Kühne T, Kuter DJ, Lim W, McCrae KR, Pruitt B, Shimanek H, Vesely SK. American Society of Hematology 2019 guidelines for immune thrombocytopenia. Blood Adv. 2019;3(23):3829-3866. Erratum in: Blood Adv. 2020;4(2):252.

2. Provan D, Arnold DM, Bussel JB, Chong BH, Cooper N, Gernsheimer T, Ghanima W, Godeau B, González-

López TJ, Grainger J, Hou M, Kruse C, McDonald V, Michel M, Newland AC, Pavord S, Rodeghiero F, Scully M, Tomiyama Y, Wong RS, Zaja F, Kuter DJ. Updated international consensus report on the investigation and management of primary immune thrombocytopenia. Blood Adv. 2019;3(22):3780-3817.

3. Trotter P, Hill QA. Immune thrombocytopenia: improving quality of life and patient outcomes. Patient Relat Outcome Meas. 2018;9:369-384.

4. Grace RF, Shimano KA, Bhat R, Neunert C, Bussel JB, Klaassen RJ, Lambert MP, Rothman JA, Breakey VR, Hege K, Bennett CM, Rose MJ, Haley KM, Buchanan GR, Geddis A, Lorenzana A, Jeng M, Pastore YD, Crary SE, Neier M, Neufeld EJ, Neu N, Forbes PW, Despotovic JM. Second-line treatments in children with immune thrombocytopenia: Effect on platelet count and patient-centered outcomes. Am J Hematol. 2019;94(7):741-750.

5. Kirsch M, Klaassen RJ, De Geest S, Matzdorff A, Ionova T, Dobbels F. Understanding the importance of using patient-reported outcome measures in patients with immune thrombocytopenia. Semin Hematol. 2013; 50 Suppl 1:S39-42.

6. Klaassen R, Blanchette V, Burke T et al. Quality of Life in Childhood Immune Thrombocytopenia: International Validation of the Kids' ITP Tools. Pediatr Blood Cancer. 2013;60:95-100.

7. Varni JW, Burwinkle TM, Seid M, Skarr D. The Peds QL 4.0 as a pediatric population health measure: feasibility, reliability, and validity. Ambul Pediatr 2003;3:329-41.

8. Klaassen et al. Validity, Reliability, and Responsiveness of a New Measure of Health-Related Quality of Life in Children with Immune Thrombocytopenic Purpura: The Kids' ITP Tools. J Pediatr 2007;150:510-5

9. Hill QA, Newland AC. Fatigue in immune thrombocytopenia. Br J Haematol. 2015 Jul;170(2):141-9.

10. Chaturvedi S, Arnold DM, McCrae KR; Splenectomy for immune thrombocytopenia: down but not out. Blood 2018;131(11):1172-1182.

11. Sarpatwari A, Bennett D, Logie JW, Shukla A, Beach KJ, Newland AC, Sanderson S, Provan D. Thromboembolic events among adult patients with primary immune thrombocytopenia in the United Kingdom General Practice Research Database. Haematologica 2010b; 95:1167-1175.

12. Efficace F, Mandelli F, Fazi P, Santoro C, Gaidano G, Cottone F, Borchiellini A, Carpenedo M, Simula MP, Di Giacomo V, Bergamaschi M, Vincelli ID, Rodeghiero F, Ruggeri M, Scaramucci L, Rambaldi A, Cascavilla N, Forghieri F, Petrungaro A, Ditonno P, Caocci G, Cirrincione S, Mazzucconi MG. Health-related quality of life and burden of fatigue in patients with primary immune thrombocytopenia by phase of disease. Am J Hematol. 2016;91(10):995-1001.

13. Mathias SD, Gao SK, Miller KL, et al. Impact of chronic Immune Thrombocytopenic Purpura (ITP) on health-related quality of life: a conceptual model starting with the patient perspective. Health Qual Life Outcomes. 2008;6:13.

14. Guidry JA, George JN, Vesely SK, Kennison SM, Terrell DR. Corticosteroid side-effects and risk for bleeding in immune thrombocytopenic purpura: patient and hematologist perspectives. Eur J Haematol. 2009;83(3): 175-182.

15. Ghanima W, Gernsheimer T, Kuter DJ. How I treat primary ITP in adult patients who are unresponsive to or dependent on corticosteroid treatment. Blood 2021; 137 (20):2736-2744.

16. Mathias SD, Bussel JB, George JN, et al. A disease-specific measure of health-related quality of life in adults with chronic immune thrombocytopenic purpura: psychometric testing in an open-label clinical trial. Clin Ther 2007;29:950-962.

17. Shimano KA, Neunert C, Bussel JB, Klaassen RJ, Bhat R, Pastore YD, Lambert MP, Bennett CM, Despotovic JM, Forbes P, Grace RF. Quality of life is an important indication for second-line treatment in children with immune thrombocytopenia. Pediatr Blood Cancer. 2021; 68(6): e29023.

18. Matzdorff A, Arnold G. Treatment of chronic immune thrombocytopenic purpura: the patients' perspective. Eur J Haematol. 2007;78(5):381-8.

19. Chugh S, Darvish-Kazem S, Lim W, Crowther MA, Ghanima W, Wang G, Heddle NM, Kelton JG, Arnold DM. Rituximab plus standard of care for treatment of primary immune thrombocytopenia: a systematic review and meta-analysis. Lancet Haematol. 2015;2(2): e75-81.

20. Cheng G, Saleh MN, Marcher C, et al. Eltrombopag for management of chronic immune thrombocytopenia (RAISE): a 6-month, randomised, phase 3 study. Lancet. 2011;377:393-402.

21. Cooper N, Cines DB. The child with immune thrombocytopenia: to treat or not to treat, is that still the question? Haematologica. 2019;104(11):2132-2134.

22. Rodeghiero F. First-line therapies for immune thrombocytopenic purpura: re-evaluating the need to treat. Eur J Haematol. 2008;80:19-26.

23. Khelif A, Saleh MN, Salama A, et al. Changes in health-related quality of life with long-term eltrombopag treatment in adults with persistent/chronic immune thrombocytopenia: Findings from the EXTEND study. Am J Hematol. 2019;94(2):200-208.

24. Grainger JD, Blanchette VS, Grotzinger KM, Roy A, Bussel JB. Health-related quality of life in children with chronic immune thrombocytopenia treated with eltrombopag in the PETIT study. Br J Haematol. 2019; 185(1):102-106.

25. George JN, Mathias SD, Go RS, Guo M, Henry DH, Lyons R, Redner RL, Rice L, Schipperus MR. Improved quality of life for romiplostim-treated patients with chronic immune thrombocytopenic purpura: results from two randomized, placebo-controlled trials. Br J Haematol. 2009;144(3):409-15.

26. Klaassen RJ, Mathias SD, Buchanan G, Bussel J, Deuson R, Young NL, Collier A, Bomgaars L, Blanchette V. Pilot study of the effect of romiplostim on child health-related quality of life (HRQoL) and parental burden in immune thrombocytopenia (ITP). Pediatr Blood Cancer. 2012; 58(3):395-8.

27. Grainger JD, Young NL, Blanchette VS, Klaassen RJ. Quality of life in immune thrombocytopenia following treatment. Arch Dis Child. 2013;98(11):895-7.

28. Grace RF, Klaassen RJ, Shimano KA, Lambert MP, Grimes A, Bussel JB, Breakey VR, Pastore YD, Black V, Overholt K, Bhat R, Forbes PW, Neunert C. Fatigue in children and adolescents with immune thrombocytopenia. Br J Haematol. 2020;191(1):98-106.

29. Flores A, Klaassen RJ, Buchanan GR, Neunert CE. Patterns and influences in health-related quality of life in children with immune thrombocytopenia: A study from the Dallas ITP Cohort. Pediatr Blood Cancer. 2017;64: e26405.

30. Grace RF. Standardized clinical assessment and management plans (SCAMPs): perspectives on a new method to understand treatment decisions and outcomes in immune thrombocytopenia. Semin Hematol. 2013;50 Suppl 1(01):S31-8.

31. Cheloff AZ, Al-Samkari H. Avatrombopag for the treatment of immune thrombocytopenia and thrombocytopenia of chronic liver disease. J Blood Med. 2019; 10:313-321.

# 19. Fatigue as a treatment end point in ITP

Fatigue is recognised as one of the most common and debilitating symptom in patients with chronic disease. It is a frequent symptom of autoimmune disorders and is commonly associated with the majority of patients with rheumatoid arthritis [40], systemic lupus erythematosus (SLE) [82] and primary biliary cirrhosis [9]. It is recognised as an important public health issue negatively impacting on the ability to work normally, and in the United States, it is estimated that fatigue cost employers $1364 billion annually in lost productive time [74].

Fatigue has been a common complaint among patients with immune thrombocytopenia (ITP) but has not always been taken seriously [34, 73]. Many patients feel that they have less energy when the platelet count is low [11, 38] although it is increasingly recognised that this association is not absolute. Since 2003, generic health-related quality of life measures have been applied in clinical studies of ITP which have usually involved trials of novel therapeutic agents. These have identified significant morbidity in patients with ITP, in particular fatigue, alongside a fear of bleeding and these have been found to have a negative impact on both social and work activities. An early survey of ITP patients in the UK and US, however, confirmed a clear association finding a prevalence of fatigue of 39 % and 22 %, respectively, which was higher than in normal subjects ($p < 0.0001$ for both) [64]. Although the causes are not well understood [38] fatigue has been shown to have a major impact on patients' health-related quality of life (HRQoL) [12].

## 19.1. How do we define fatigue

Historically, studies of physical illness have rarely addressed fatigue, possibly because it is a subjective complaint that is difficult to define and measure. This lack of a clear and widely accepted definition is illustrated by cancer-related fatigue, for which 24 different definitions have been put forward by experts [3]. It has also been associated with liver disease where it is postulated that an associated impact on neurotransmission in the brain is linked to the fatigue spectrum of symptoms [92].

> Fatigue can be typically defined as: extreme and persistent tiredness, weakness or exhaustion – mental, physical or both [16].

This is usually experienced in the absence of any excessive expenditure of energy as a cause and is often associated with decreased functioning, e.g. difficulty completing tasks.

## 19.2. How can we assess fatigue

Fatigue can be difficult to define as, in general, it is just a feeling of physical tiredness, often associated with the lack of energy and motivation that many of us occasionally experience. There are a number of scales that have been used to assess fatigue clinically and these usually take the form of a self-assessment fatigue scale or questionnaire [16]. Although it is preferable that whatever measure is used should be validated, reproducible and applicable to the patient population being studied but there are a variety of general measures available of differing complexity. They may be uni-dimensional (e.g. the Fatigue Severity Scale), multi-dimensional (e.g. the Visual Analogue Scale for Fatigue) or a more complex measure of outcome [e.g. Short Form-36 (SF-36)]. The variety of measures have been reviewed in detail by Trotter and Hill [94]. The Fatigue Impact Scale was developed to assess the symptoms of fatigue as part of an underlying health condition. It consists of 40 items that are designed to evaluate the impact of fatigue on three domains of daily life; cognitive, physical and psychosocial functioning [21]. Further variations of this scale have been developed including a more functional study consisting of only 8 items that can be used for sequential monitoring of changes in fatigue status; the Daily Fatigue Impact Scale or D-FIS [22].

While these generalised measurement tools may give some indication of the extent of the problem a more appropriate measure are those disease-specific tools that have been developed and validated in ITP patients. In general these assess overall health related quality of life (HRQoL) and include an evaluation of fatigue as one of the measures. The ITP Patient Assessment Questionnaire (ITP-PAQ) has demonstrated acceptable reliability and validity [57]. This assesses how ITP, or its treatment, impacted on the patient's fatigue status over the previous four weeks on a 5-point scale ranging from 'all the time' to 'never'. This tool was mainly used in clinical trials of romiplostim. The Functional Assessment of Chronic Illness Therapy (FACIT-F) questionnaire was originally designed for use in cancer but the reliability and validity of its fatigue subscale was also demonstrated in ITP patients [88]. This was primarily used in trials of Eltrombopag and consists of 13 questions related to fatigue, rated on a scale of 0 'not at all' to 4 'very much'.

There are also a number of scales that have been more specifically designed for children including the Hockenbury Fatigue Scale that was initially designed to measure fatigue in children with cancer from the perspectives of children, parents and staff [39]. Its usefulness has been assessed in a recent study in children and adolescents [29]. More disease specific assessments have been developed, particularly the Kids' ITP Tools (KIT) in Toronto [47], which was used in the pediatric eltrombopag studies (the PETIT study) [31].

## 19.3. How much of a problem is fatigue in ITP

Nearly 40 % of patients with ITP require no treatment and severe bleeding is restricted to a minority. However, bleeding manifestations and, more specifically, the platelet count is the problem that clinicians tend to concentrate on [24]. Whereas, fatigue is the most common symptom as reported by patients with ITP, regardless of their age [29, 56]. The Platelet Disorder Support Association (PDSA) has been keen to support the patient perspective regarding their perceived unmet needs and the physical and emotional burden of disease in an attempt to highlight the areas where healthcare providers treating the patients need to concentrate their efforts and guide their management. The PDSA highlighted the high incidence of fatigue among the adults participating in their study [50] (☞ Figure 19.1a+b) and the lack of importance that many clinicians attribute to it as a problem, concentrating on the platelet count and its impact [50].

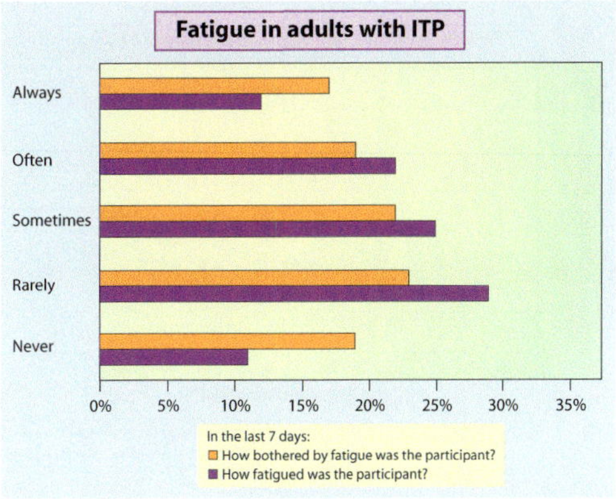


a

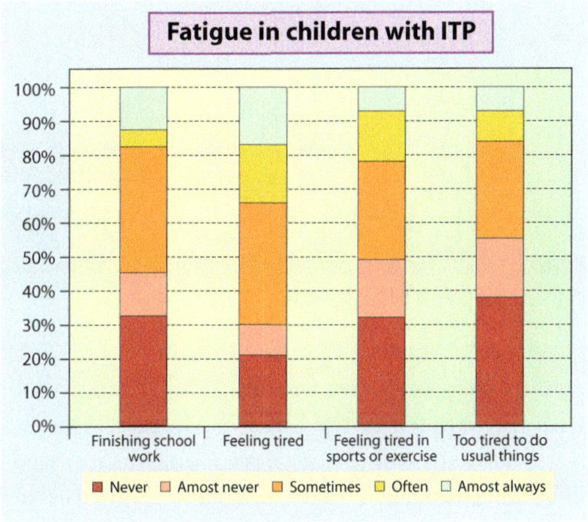


b

***Figure 19.1a+b:*** Fatigue in adults (**a**) and chilfren (**b**) with ITP. Modified after [51] with the permission of the publisher AME Publishing Company.

When the adult participants were asked to reflect on their fatigue levels over the previous 7 days, 89 % reported they were fatigued, and 81 % reported they were bothered by their fatigue. In many cases, it is the most severely debilitating symptom reported by patients living with ITP [12]. Unfortunately, many providers still undervalue the impact fatigue has on patients living with ITP [50] (☞ Figure 19.2). It is clear from patient preferences that they seek treatments that improve their wellbeing, are simple to take and have limited side effects [59].

These studies confirm the findings by Mathias et al in 2008 [56] which highlighted the degree to which fatigue affected patients with ITP in their small study. This was confirmed in a much larger quali-

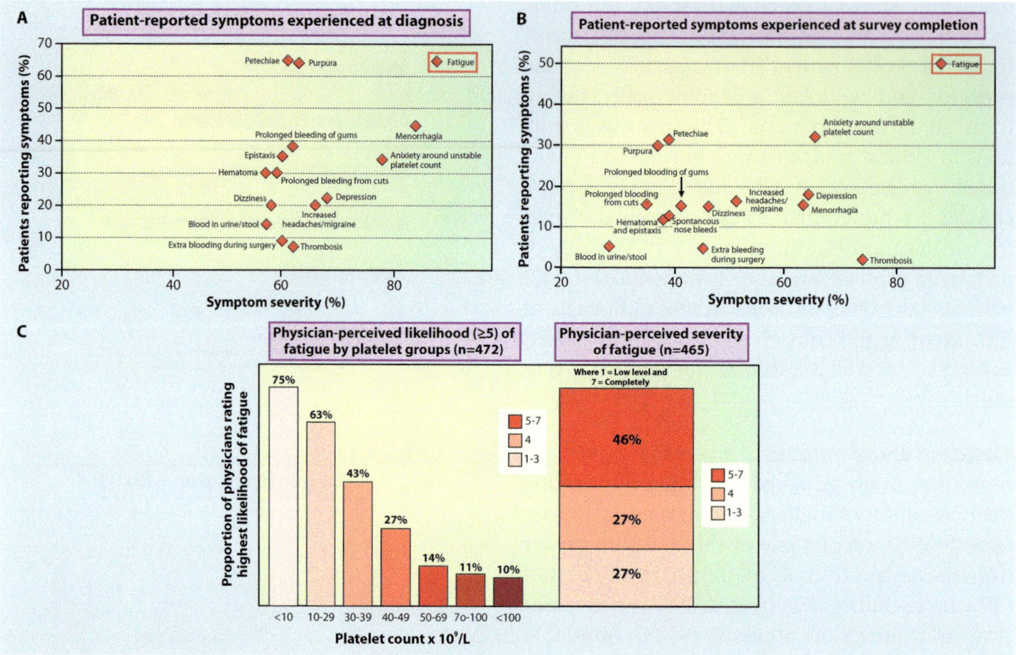


***Figure 19.2:*** Patient perception of symptoms and signs at diagnosis (**A**), time of survey completion (**B**) and physician perception of fatigue (**C**).

tative postal survey organised through the UK ITP Adult Registry (www.qmul.ac.uk/itpregistry/), with the support of the UK ITP Support Association (www.itpsupport.org). A 43-question, closed-field questionnaire was developed, addressing bruising and bleeding frequency, disease management, social engagement, work and school performance and recreational activities and was posted to members of the Association. Responses were received from 790 patients (696 adults, 94 children) with primary ITP (45 % response rate) [79]. 12.5 % of responders reported that they 'always' or 'often' missed work or school due to fatigue and these absences were not related to the severity of the disease. It is interesting and, perhaps, understandable that children were more likely than adults to experience frustration over restrictions in their activity that these symptoms caused (23.3 % vs. 9.5 % respectively; $p<0.001$). A later survey assessed 585 UK and 93 US patients with primary disease using the Fatigue Impact Scale (FIS) [64]. Significant fatigue (FIS ≥40) was found in 39 % (UK) and 22 % (US) of patients, significantly more than that expected in normal subjects.

A small study reported fatigue in 22 % (6/27) of children with ITP [5] and this was confirmed in a larger study in children and adolescents [29] and in the trial of eltrombopag in children [31]. The Grace study was an observational cohort of 120 children and adolescents receiving second-line therapies for ITP. Fatigue was assessed using the Hockenberry Fatigue Scale. A high level of fatigue was reported in both groups with 54 % (29/54) of children and 62 % (26/42) of adolescents reporting moderate-to-severe fatigue. There was no correlation between fatigue and age or gender. Adolescents with newly diagnosed and persistent ITP had higher mean fatigue scores than those with chronic ITP ($p=0.03$). Interestingly, fatigue significantly improved in children and adolescents by 1 month after starting second-line treatment, and this improvement persisted 12 months after starting treatment. Further analysis of this group confirmed QoL as the most frequent reason for paediatric patients to start second-line treatments and emphasised the importance of including QoL studies as part of normal therapeutic practice [87].

It is now customary to include HRQoL studies as part of ITP clinical trials and in two controlled trials of romiplostim in ITP (n=125), the baseline assessment of HRQoL by ITP-PAQ found that of 44 items evaluated, fatigue was among the five worst scores [25]. In the RAISE study of eltrombopag (n=197), the mean baseline FACIT-F score was lower in ITP patients than the general US population, suggesting a greater burden of fatigue [6, 10, 100]. Taken together, these studies provide evidence that fatigue occurs in a significant proportion of all patients with ITP.

Many of the studies associated with treatment effect have evaluated the patients at presentation, whereas the surveys based on the patient focus groups have assessed patients at varying times during their disease history and, often, not taking into account treatment history. It is not clear from these studies as to whether the fatigue is associated with the severity of the disease, the platelet count or treatment effect. In the large questionnaire based on the UK ITP Patients' Association, school or work absence due to fatigue did not significantly correlate with the platelet count (<20, 20-49 or >50 x $10^9$/L) at the last follow-up [79] although it is unclear how representative this was of the disease status. An assessment of 236 adult Chinese ITP patients using a version of the SF-36, the platelet count (<30, 30-100 or >100 x $10^9$/L) again was not a significant predictor of energy/vitality [102]. Whereas, the study of Newton et al. [64] found that 69 % of patients in the UK cohort and 50 % of those in the US cohort reported had less energy when their platelet count was low. Further analysis revealed that a platelet count <100 x $10^9$/L in patients with bleeding symptoms, and a platelet count <30 x $10^9$/L in patients without bleeding, were independent risk factors for fatigue. In a review of the HRQoL in adults in the romiplostim studies versus standard of care, over a 52 week period, overall treatment responders (platelet count ≥50 x $10^9$/L) had significantly less fatigue [52]. Similar improvements were seen in children and adolescents who showed rapid improvement in fatigue status following response to second line therapy, which was maintained over the ensuing 12 months of follow-up [29]. In conjunction with the I-WISh study a 10 item patient-reported outcome related measure was developed consisting of a psychometric evaluation of the ITP Life Quality Index (ILQI) that has been assessed for validity and reliability and can also be used in reviewing the patient during treatment and will be valuable in aiding patient-centric decision making [96].

Due to the uncertainty of the natural history of the disease and the response to treatments patients with ITP face many challenges. The disease burden and perceived disease risks both influence the physical, emotional, and social health of patients and families with ITP impacting negatively their overall health-related quality of life (HRQoL) which is exacerbated by the significant burden of fatigue [7, 23, 90, 106].

While many physicians focus primarily on low platelet counts as the best approach to manage their patients and avoid life-threatening bleeds, for many patients the platelet count is the last thing they are concerned with. In fact, patient respondents to the ITP World Impact Survey (I-WISh) stated that increasing energy levels is one of the top treatment goals [13]. The findings have been further validated in a Chinese sub-group of the I-WISh International survey with 90 % of patients considering that the ITP had a negative impact on their energy levels, working life/studies and daily tasks and capacity to exercise. It also highlighted the physicians lack of awareness of their patients fatigue and anxiety [98]. It has been an important development that the burden of fatigue has been recognised and its presence and management included in the recent international consensus guideline on ITP [72]. The guideline highlights the many tools available to assess quality of life, emphasising the degree of burden that reduced QoL is associated with, particularly fatigue [48, 94]. There is also an emphasis on the importance of patient-reported outcome measures (PROMs). PROM tools have been developed and validated using several different methodologies. The domains measured by each PROM and the time period over which a change can be detected vary and this needs to be taken into account when using a PROM outside of the geographical region in which it was developed, a validation of cultural and language changes are desirable. Consideration of which PROM tool to use should reflect the population being assessed and the time period in which to expect changes [72]. The guideline also agrees that, on balance, although the data can be contradictory fatigue improves with response to treatment in both adults and children. While fatigue assessment tools are important in assessing the impact of newer treatments and the change in patient well-being in trials their use should be considered as an adjunct to everyday treatment. This has been recognised with encouragement to include patient-reported outcome measures as part of routine assessment and was highlighted in the recent ASH guidelines [61].

## 19.4. Why does fatigue develop in ITP

ITP has a very heterogenous pathophysiology and our understanding of how the disease and its treatment affect the QoL and lead to fatigue is limited. ITP-related fatigue, and drug-induced toxicity from long-term use of steroids and other immunosuppressants are well known to impact the QoL [56] (☞ Table 19.1).

### Corticosteroids

Corticosteroids have multiple side effects that could contribute to fatigue, including sleep disturbance, a range of psychiatric reactions, fluid retention, acne, muscle weakness, proximal myopathy and susceptibility to infection. In a study of 986 adult ITP patients, 25/33 steroid-related symptoms, including fatigue, occurred more frequently in current corticosteroid users than patients who had not received steroids [4]. Fatigue was one of the most frequent and distressing symptoms in both groups. The severity of such symptoms and their importance to patients was not always appreciated by the treating clinicians and should become part of shared decision making in patient management [33]. In a further patient survey 17 % of patients said they would never take steroids again and 69 % would only take them if there were no other options [58].

### Immunosuppressive therapy

The side effects of immunosuppressive therapy, such as infection and anaemia, may also lead to fatigue, although the mechanisms of drug induced fatigue are not fully understood [107]. Azathioprine, a commonly used second-line treatment in ITP has also been associated with fatigue in patients [53]. In patients with primary refractory ITP receiving cyclosporine, fatigue was reported as a side effect in 2/12 [18] and 2/10 [45] cases. Rituxi-

| Treatment | HRQoL/Fatigue Impact | References |
|---|---|---|
| Steroids | Mood swings and fatigue | Guidry et al. 2009<br>Matzdorff et al. 2011 |
| | More impact in patients who have received steroids compared with those who haven't | Berti et al. 2008 |
| Immune Suppression | Increased fatigue seen with azathioprine (reported in Inflammatory Bowel Disease) | Zlott and Byrne 2010 |
| | and with cyclosporine | Kappers-Klunne and Van't Veer 2001<br>Emilia et al. 2002 |
| Rituximab | No change in HRQoL v Standard of Care | Kuter et al. 2012<br>Arnold et al. 2012 |
| | Increased fatigue when rituximab compared with rituximab plus dexamethasone; no significant impact from the dexamethasone | Gudbrandsdottir et al. 2013 |
| Splenectomy | No changes between pre and post surgery | Newton et al. 2011<br>Kuter et al. 2012 |
| | Some improvement in general health post-splenectomy | Suvajdzic et al. 2014 |
| TPO-RAs | No increase in fatigue in those receiving TPO-RAs versus placebo | Cuker 2010 |
| | Improvement in fatigue at 52 weeks in responders to romiplostim | Kuter et al. 2012 |
| | Improvement in fatigue in long-term f/u on eltrombopag in EXTEND study | Khelif et al. 2019 |

***Table 19.1:*** Impact of treatment on Health Related Quality of Life and fatigue.

mab was also shown to be associated with fatigue in a randomized control trial versus rituximab and dexamethasone. In this first-line study of primary ITP fatigue was the most frequently reported adverse event (ca. 40 %) and was not significantly more common with the addition of steroids [32]. In a further study that was placebo controlled 22 % (7/32) with primary ITP complained of fatigue after receiving rituximab compared with 8 % (2/26) receiving placebo [2].

As we have seen older evidence suggested an increase in fatigue when the platelet count drops below 30 x $10^9$/L [64], whereas newer studies suggest a much more complex relationship. The I-WISh study on the QoL of ITP patients recruited over 1500 patients, but no clear correlation was found between fatigue and platelet counts [13].

In some patients, ITP is secondary to a condition such as SLE that is itself associated with fatigue. There may be an associated disorder, such as hypothyroidism, or existing co-morbidities (e.g.anaemia) and these should be looked for during the initial work-up and treated as appropriately.

Sleep and mood disturbance are often associated with fatigue in chronic disease and daytime sleepiness has been independently associated with ITP-associated fatigue [64]. Lack of exercise may also predict development of chronic fatigue syndrome (CFS) and post-infectious fatigue [54] but these are only associations rather than causative. Social and behavioural predictors of fatigue in chronic disease include lack of social support [66, 82] and low self-belief in an ability to cope [75]. A variety of factors, including mood, illness belief, social support and ability to work, may be a consequence of fatigue but could also contribute to its development and it is likely that there is a dynamic interaction with fatigue both as cause and effect [37].

While the presence of other medical problems was an independent predictor of fatigue [64] in adults it is clear from the patient surveys that fatigue occurs without any other associated factors. This is particularly the case for young children with primary ITP, where it is more likely that there is an intrinsic explanation for fatigue as an underlying condition or associated co-morbidity is unusual. Whereas in adults, for the reasons already discussed, these are more frequent and are seen increasingly in the older populations. The findings in children and adolescents with ITP [29] support the concept that physiological fatigue is associated with ITP. A number of inflammatory mediators have been postulated to induce fatigue in autoimmune disease [105]. In the Grace et al. patient cohort, fatigue did not differ based on whether the ITP was primary, as in 85 % of the patients, or secondary to systemic immune dysregulation. It has been suggested that the destruction of antibody-coated platelets results in ongoing production of inflammatory cytokines and although altered cytokine patterns have been found in children with ITP, it remains to be seen whether there are specific cytokine changes that correlate with the presence of fatigue [15, 28, 51].

## 19.5. Cytokines and Immune dysregulation

In a number of chronic disorders it has been postulated that fatigue is driven by immune activation and the pro-inflammatory processes. ITP is a heterogenous disorder but its underlying process in the majority of cases involves immune dysregulation. A number of observations into its pathophysiology suggest a role for pro-inflammatory cytokines which we have previously reviewed [38] (☞ Figure 22.2). Cytokines, such as interleukin 6 (IL-6) have been shown to be raised in ITP and show a loose negative corelation with the platelet count [35, 97] and IL-6 is known to stimulate thrombopoiesis in stress conditions [44]. Interleukin 1b (IL-1B), IL-6 and tumour necrosis factor (TNF) are all normally produced in response to inflammation, which may be seen in the bone marrow in ITP. IL-6 has now been clearly found to be associated with fatigue in a number of systemic conditions and this may be reversed by the use of IL-6 inhibition [19, 36, 70]. While some degree of inflammation is considered as a potential contributor to fatigue, through the stimulation of cytokines, of which IL-6 is one, the underlying mechanisms remain poorly understood. It has been postulated that the multi-dimensional nature of central fatigue is the final common pathway that is seen in many systemic conditions that have an inflammatory component of which ITP is an example [43].

Cytokines are postulated to enter the central nervous system (CNS) through the blood brain barrier where they activate peripheral nerve afferents or recruit activated immune cells which then enter the CNS [20]. This leads to neuroinflammation by stimulating local inflammatory signalling pathways (e.g. nuclear factor kappa B, mitogen-activated protein kinases) and further cytokine production. This in turn alters neurotransmitter metabolism and affects endocrine pathways. These central effects stimulate corticotrophin releasing hormone [60] and suppress thyrotropin releasing hormone [42] leading to a combination of lethargy, decreased libido and sleep disturbance [1]. The central final common pathway explains why the same constellation of symptoms are seen in patients with a variety of conditions including cancer [60] and chronic disease [66, 82, 91].

We have also postulated that, in addition to the detection to the detection a raised inflammatory cytokine milieu, the incidence of an increased number of thromboembolic events (TE's) in the presence of a marked thrombocytopenia is further evidence of a pro-inflammatory environment in ITP. A study carried out through the UK ITP Registry study noted a non-significant trend towards a lower presenting platelet count in those who developed TE's [80]. This observation was supported from data from the Italian group who found that 21 % (9/43) of TE's occurred when the platelet count was $<50 \times 10^9/L$ and that patients who develop thrombosis had a significantly lower presenting platelet count than those who did not [78], suggesting thrombosis may be a marker of disease severity. It is recognised that platelets play an important role in thrombosis, inflammation and vascular injury. Activated platelets and platelet microparticles have an intrinsic capacity to activate the alternative and classical complement pathways on/near their surface, with measurable increases in soluble inflammatory mediators C3a and C5a [71]. This immune-mediated complement activation is found in ITP patients, in whom greater activation is associated with a lower platelet count supporting the presence of a pro-inflammatory and prothrombotic environment in ITP.

Genetic factors have been reported to be associated with ITP [84]. In particular, the behaviour of T-helper type 1 cells (Th1) and balance between Th1/Th2, which has been implicated in the regulation of many immune responses. A high Th1/Th2 ratio was reported in patients with chronic ITP [67]. Naive CD4+ T cells differentiate into several different Th cells, including Th1, Th2, Th17, and regulatory T (Treg) cells. Th cell functions are determined by their cytokine secretion patterns. Th1 cells secrete interleukin (IL)-2 and interferon-γ, whereas Th2 cells secrete IL-4, IL-5, IL-6 and/or IL-10. ITP has been documented to be associated with cytokine response and dysregulation [84, 86]. Many investigators have shown IFN-γ to be upregulated at both the mRNA and protein levels in chronic ITP patients [68, 103]. It was also reported that serum levels of IL-4 were decreased in patients with chronic disease [103].

Studies in children with acute and chronic ITP investigating the polymorphisms of interleukin (IL)-4 intron 3, IL-6 (-572 G/C), and IL-10 (-627 C/A) demonstrated significant differences in the RP1/RP2 genotype proportion ($p=0.04$) and the RP2 allelic frequency ($p=0.03$) of IL-4 intron 3 and the A/C genotype proportion ($p=0.01$) of IL-10 (-627) between children with chronic ITP and controls. The findings suggest that the IL-4 intron 3 and IL-10 (-627) polymorphisms contribute to the susceptibility of developing childhood chronic ITP [101].

More recent studies in adults with ITP showed a higher frequency of the IL-4Rα576 non-QQ genotype compared to healthy subjects ($p=0.04$). Patients with chronic ITP and the IFN-γ +874 non-AA genotype (high expression type) showed more severe thrombocytopenia than those with the AA genotype ($p<0.05$). This group also had a significantly higher Th1/Th2 ratio than control patients ($p<0.01$); this ratio was inversely correlated with platelet counts. Furthermore, patients with both IFN-γ +874 non-AA genotype (high expression type) and IFN-γR -611 non-AA genotype (high-function type) had a significantly higher Th1/Th2 ratio ($p<0.05$). These studies suggest that the cytokine polymorphisms affecting Th1/Th2 increase the susceptibility to, and severity of, chronic ITP [93].

Measurement of cytokine profiles is not always precise or reproducible on an individual basis and may be influenced by a variety of external factors including age [55], time of day of the studies and the genetic polymorphisms in the genes involved in the pro-inflammatory process [76, 83]. The state of the disease activity [68] and the type of treatment at the time of study may also have an impact [104]. The methods of analysis will need further refinement, however, the actual cytokine levels may be less important than the relative balance seen between the opposing cytokine activity [68]. Despite these variabilities sufficient studies have demonstrated changes in genetic polymorphisms, although not always consistent, and a significant positive correlation between fatigue and circulating levels of inflammatory makers, including IL-6, to suggest that these changes indicate an important step in the pathogenesis of fatigue.

## 19.6. How do we manage the ITP patient with fatigue

Fatigue can now be accepted as a common symptom of ITP and may affect nearly half of all patients to some degree [5, 79, 95]. Although the relationship between disease severity and fatigue is not clear at least one study showed a clear correlation in both UK and US cohorts [64] between energy levels and platelet count while others did not [79, 102]. The I-WISh study, which studied over 1500 patients found there was no clear correlation between the platelet count and the presence of fatigue [13]. However, if fatigue is associated with disease severity, effective targeted treatment would be expected to improve fatigue, although it is now clear that this is not always the case and the association between ITP, treatment and fatigue is more complicated [38].

Fatigue is one of the components of HRQoL and has been shown to be worse at 6 months than at presentation [102] and those with persistent disease are worse than those who are newly presenting or in chronic phase [17]. In a long term study over 52 weeks comparing treatment with romiplostim compared with medical standard of care (SOC) both groups showed improvement over the study period using the ITP-PAQ tool although over the 52 weeks those receiving romiplostim showed a statistically significant improvement compared with SOC [52]. The improvement was better for HRQoL than for fatigue in isolation [25] and among the patients a significant proportion of patients show an improvement in the platelet count but remained fatigued. Similar improvements in alleviating fatigue in long-term responders was also seen in the follow up of the EXTEND study using eltrombopag [46]. Although some of the non-improvement may just reflect a dilution of the treatment effect by the number of non-responders. It must be remembered, however, that the platelet count is purely a marker for a response of the ITP to treatment but is only, at best, a surrogate for overall clinical response. An increase in platelet count demonstrates a shift in the balance between platelet production and destruction but has no bearing on the underlying disease process [38, 94]. Thrombocytopenia alone is not the driver of fatigue but merely reflects the underlying immune dysregulation that is associated with the production of inflammatory cytokines that lead to fatigue. Only a complete or partial remission with reduction in disease activity, accompanied by regaining immune balance and a reduction in abnormal cytokine production, is likely to be associated with improvement in fatigue symptoms [85, 89].

There are no specific fatigue-directed drug-related therapies yet available although there have been a number of studies in a variety of conditions also associated with fatigue, including melatonin in solid organ cancer [99] and in Chronic Fatigue Syndrome a comparative study has suggested a role for amisulpride in reducing the perception of fatigue [8, 69]. A more recent study with agomelatine, a melatonin receptor agonist and serotonin-2C receptor antagonist, significantly reduced fatigue in a variety of neurological conditions, including CFS [77]. None of these approaches have received widespread acceptance and there has been little interest in their use in ITP, although preliminary studies with IL-6 inhibition have shown promising results [19]. Some of these approaches have been reviewed previously [ ]38.

Currently the only effective treatment in relieving fatigue in ITP appears to be therapy directed at a long term platelet response using the thrombopoietin receptor agonists. While the results from early studies have confirmed the safety and efficacy of the treatment [100] the impact on fatigue has been contradictory in both adults [25] and children [30]. However, long term follow up demonstrated clear improvement in fatigue with both romiplostim [52] and eltrombopag in the EXTEND study [46]. These results were seen in responding patients suggesting that in the early reports benefits were masked by the non-responders. The impact on quality of life and in particular fatigue following treatment may also be influenced by the side-effects of the treatment given where adverse events may mask the benefits of an improved platelet count.

## 19.7. Improving the Standard of Care

While there is no treatment specifically directed at the fatigue it is important that the patient is thoroughly assessed at presentation both to confirm the diagnosis and to identify any associated conditions that may be contributing to the problem, such as anaemia, an underactive thyroid or associated condition. A decision should also be made as to whether the ITP requires therapy. It can be argued that while the level of platelets and/or the bleeding state may be such that therapy is not required the presence of severe fatigue alone is an indication to initiate treatment. It is therefore important that as part of assessment the patient's views are taken into account and they are part of the decision making strategy. This has been emphasised in a publication for patients produced by the UK ITP Support Association in partnership with the UK ITP Clinical Forum, which emphasises making the right choices in ITP management and care and is a shared decision making toolkit for patients [63].

While fatigue may improve with disease-orientated treatment a proportion of patients with active ITP, irrespective of their platelet response, remain fatigued. Non-pharmacological interventions for fatigue have shown benefit in other disorders; for example, mindfulness-based training, cognitive behavioural therapy (CBT) and supervised exercise programs have all been advocated. Similarly, fatigued cancer patients have also benefited from physical activity programs, energy conservation and psychosocial support [49]. The National Institute for Health and Care Excellence have recently published their guidance on Chronic Fatigue Syndrome (NICE NG2021) much of which is transferable to the patient with ITP and chronic fatigue.

The importance of the advice produced by NICE is that to a great extent the solutions are patient led, with support from a trained healthcare professional, placing much of the emphasis on energy management. While not claiming to be curative it provides coping strategies that include all types of activity, supporting the patients cognitive, physical, emotional and social needs, while taking into account their overall level of activity. It helps the patient use the amount of energy they have while reducing their risk of post-exertional exhaustion and, importantly, not worsening their symptoms by exceeding their limits. It acknowledges that each person has a different energy limit, that may fluctuate, and that they are best placed to judge their own limits. Such an approach can help the healthcare professional recognise when the patient is approaching their limit. This is particularly important for children and adolescents who may find it harder to judge their limits and can overreach them. Such a flexible, tailored approach is designed so that activity is never automatically increased but is maintained or adjusted (upwards after a period of stability or downwards when symptoms are worse) as required. This can be combined with a more holistic approach that gives the patient a 'pick and mix' approach that suits their own particular needs [26].

While it is now clear that fatigue is a major symptom in ITP at presentation and may improve with treatment it has been shown to continue to deteriorate over the first few months following diagnosis [17, 102] but improving by 12 months. It is therefore important to initiate effective treatment as early as possible but also to formally monitor the patient's quality of life and levels of fatigue during the first few months of treatment. Patients want to be involved in their own management plan and they want to have more of a 'partnership' with their ITP care providers. They want to be included in treatment decisions and want to be educated on all available treatment options [51]. First-line therapy is usually initiated with steroids in some form as they are less expensive than most other options, are easier to administer but it is acknowledged that while they often increase the platelet count, relapses are frequent and further lines of treatment are required. The early response seen following steroids is rarely associated with cessation of symptoms and the approach does not recognize the long-term burden steroids cause and the impact of daily living [4]. Newer ITP therapies such as thrombopoietin receptor agonists (TPO-RAs) have been shown to be effective with fewer side effects, and current guidelines suggest that if used earlier in the course of the disease, there may be better clinical outcomes for patients with an increased rate of treatment free remission [26]. It is now accepted that the use of steroids should be restricted [61, 72]. With the increasing recognition of the importance of a guideline-based approach, it is recognised that patients are best managed by clinicians with an up-to-date experience of the condition. A more clinical trial-based approach to treatment should be pursued to explore first line alternates to steroids and more effective early phase treatment that minimises the period of fatigue aiming for long-term response.

## 19.8. Conclusion

We now recognise fatigue as a major component of the symptoms that patients' complain about when initially diagnosed with ITP and this, plus other HRQoL measures are often more important to the patient than the level of their platelet count. Unfortunately this is often the reverse level of priorities for their attending clinician. As fatigue may improve with response to treatment, early and effective therapeutic intervention is important. However, fatigue may worsen in the first few months and not all who have a platelet increment will show improvement in their symptoms. This reflects the complex pathophysiology of the condition and reflects the disordered cytokine milieu associated with active disease, which may persist irrespective of platelet response. It is therefore important that patient reported outcome measures are regularly reviewed, along with the platelet count, during clinical review. The measures that have been developed to assess fatigue and, more generally, HRQoL should be used on a routine basis so the management approach can be guided by the patients' needs. The introduction of non-therapeutic interventions to help energy management should also be considered as an integral component of patient care. While a specific therapeutic approach to fatigue would be valuable a more realistic approach is the early use of clinically effective ITP treatment, with minimal side-effects, that leads to an early and sustained response. The associated reduction in disease activity is the most likely approach that will lead to an improvement in fatigue and quality of life.

## Disclosure

The author has acted as a consultant for Amgen, Angle, Argenx, Grifols, GSK, Novartis, Pfizer and UCB Biosciences; participated in advisory boards and/or as a speaker at medical education events sponsored by Amgen, Argenx, Grifols, GSK, Novartis and Roche; and received research support from Amgen, BMS, GSK, Novartis and Octapharma.

## References

1. Adelman JS, Martin LB (2009) Vertebrate sickness behaviors: adaptive and integrated neuroendocrine immune responses. Integrative and Comparative Biology, 49, 202-214.

2. Arnold DM, Heddle NM, Carruthers J, et al. (2012) A pilot randomized trial of adjuvant rituximab or placebo for non-splenectomized patients with immune thrombocytopenia. Blood, 119, 1356-1362.

3. Barsevick AM, Cleeland CS, Manning DC, et al. (2010) ASCPRO recommendations for the assessment of fatigue as an outcome in clinical trials. Journal of Pain and Symptom Management, 39, 1086-1099.

4. Berti D, Moons P, Dobbels F , et al. (2008) Impact of corticosteroid-related symptoms in patients with immune thrombocytopenic purpura: results of a survey of 985 patients. Clinical Therapeutics, 30, 1540-1552.

5. Blatt J, Weston B, Gold S (2010) Fatigue as marker of thrombocytopenia in childhood idiopathic thrombocytopenic purpura. Pediatric Hematology and Oncology, 27, 65-67.

6. Bussel JB, Cheng G, Saleh MN, et al. (2007) Eltrombopag for the treatment of chronic idiopathic thrombocytopenic purpura. N Engl J Med. 357(22):2237-2247.

7. Bussel J, Kruse A, Kruse C, et al. (2019) The burden of disease and IMPACT of immune thrombocytopenia (ITP) on patients: Results from an ITP survey. Blood. 134 Suppl_1:1076.

8. Castro-Marrero J, Zaragoza M, Lopez-Vilchez I , et al. (2021) Effect of melatonin plus zinc supplementation on fatigue perception in myalgic encephalitis/Chronic Fatigue Syndrome: A Double-Blind, Placebo-Controlled Trial. Antioxidants. 2021030234.

9. Cauch-Dudek K, Abbey S, Stewart DE, Heathcote EJ (1998) Fatigue in primary biliary cirrhosis. Gut, 43, 705-710.

10. Cheng G, Saleh MN, Marcher C, et al. (2011) Eltrombopag for management of chronic immune thrombocytopenia (RAISE): a 6-month, randomised, phase 3 study. Lancet, 377, 393-402.

11. Cines DB, Bussel JB (2005) How I treat idiopathic thrombocytopenic purpura (ITP). Blood, 106, 2244-2251.

12. Cooper N, Kruse A, Kruse C, et al. (2021a) Immune thrombocytopenia (ITP) world impact survey (I-WISh): patient and physician perceptions of diagnosis, signs and symptoms, and treatment. Am J Hematol. 96:188-198.

13. Cooper N, Kruse A, Kruse C, et al. (2021b) Immune thrombocytopenia (ITP) world impact Survey (I-WISh): impact of ITP on health-related quality of life. Am J Hematol. 96(2):199-207.

14. Cuker A (2010) Toxicities of the thrombopoietic growth factors. Seminars in Hematology, 47, 289-298.

15. Del Vecchio GC, Giordano P, Tesse R, et al. (2012) Clinical significance of serum cytokine levels and thrombopoietic markers in childhood idiopathic thrombocytopenic purpura. Blood Transfusion, 10, 194-199.

16. Dittner AJ, Wessely SC, Brown RG (2004) The assessment of fatigue: a practical guide for clinicians and researchers. Journal of Psychosomatic Research, 56, 157-170.

17. Efficace F, Mandelli F, Fazi P, et al. (2016) Health-related quality of life and burden of fatigue in patients with primary immune thrombocytopenia by phase of disease. Am J Hematol. 91(10):995-1001.

18. Emilia G, Morselli M, Luppi M, et al. (2002) Long-term salvage therapy with cyclosporin A in refractory idiopathic thrombocytopenic purpura. Blood, 99, 1482-1485.

19. Fabiola A, Nucera V, Masala IF , et al. (2019) IL-6 involvement in pain, fatigue and mood disorders in rheumatoid arthritis and the effects of the IL-6 inhibitor sarilumab. Pharmacol Res. 149, 104402.

20. Felger JC, Miller AH (2012) Cytokine effects on the basal ganglia and dopamine function: the subcortical source of inflammatory malaise. Frontiers in Neuroendocrinology, 33, 315-327.

21. Fisk JD, Ritvo PG, Ross L, et al. (1994) Measuring the functional impact of fatigue: initial validation of the fatigue impact scale. Clin Infect Dis. 18 Suppl 1:S79-83.

22. Fisk JD, Doble SE (2002) Construction and validation of a fatigue impact scale for daily administration. Quality of Life Research, 263-272.

23. Flores A, Klaassen RJ, Buchanan GR, et al. (2017). Patterns and influences in health-related quality of life in children with immune thrombocytopenia: A study from the Dallas ITP cohort. Pediatr. Blood Cancer; 64(8): doi: 10.1002/pbc.26405.

24. Frederiksen H, Schmidt K (1999) The incidence of idiopathic thrombocytopenic purpura in adults increases with age. Blood, 94, 909-913.

25. George JN, Mathias SD, Go RS , et al. (2009) Improved quality of life for romiplostim-treated patients with chronic immune thrombocytopenic purpura: results from two randomized, placebo-controlled trials. British Journal of Haematology, 144, 409-415.

26. George JN, Buchanan GR. Fatigue in ITP (2019). www.itpsupport.org/download/Fatigue%20in20in %ITP %202019.pdf.

27. Giordano P, Lassandro G, di Melo NA, et al. (2019) A narrative approach to describe QoL in children with chronic ITP. Front Pediatr. 7:163.

28. Goelz N, Bosch AM, Rand ML, et al. (2020). Increased levels of IL-10 and IL-1Ra counterbalance the proinflammatory cytokine pattern in acute pediatric immune thrombocytopenia. Cytokine; 130: 155078.

29. Grace RF, Klassen RJ, Shimano KA, et al. (2020) Fatigues in Children and Adolescents with Immune Thrombocytopenia. British Journal of Haematology. 191(1): 98-106.

30. Grainger JD, Young NL, Blanchette VS, Klaassen RJ. (2013) Quality of life in immune thrombocytopenia following treatment. Arch Dis Child. 98(11):895-897.

31. Grainger JD, Blanchette VS, Grotzinger KM, et al. (2019). Health-related quality of life in children with chronic ITP treated with eltrombopag in the PETIT study. British Journal of Haematology 185(1): 102-106.

32. Gudbrandsdottir S, Birgens HS, Frederiksen H, et al. (2013) Rituximab and dexamethasone vs dexamethasone monotherapy in newly diagnosed patients with primary immune thrombocytopenia. Blood, 121, 1976-1981.

33. Guidry JA, George JN, Vesely SK, et al. (2009) Corticosteroid side effects and risk for bleeding in immune thrombocytopenic purpura: patient and haematologist perspectives. Euro J Haematol. 83; 175-182.

34. Hauber AB, Johnson FR, Grotzinger KM, Ozdemir S (2010) Patients' benefit risk preferences for chronic idiopathic thrombocytopenic purpura therapies. Ann Pharmacother. 44(3):479-488.

35. Haznedaroglu IC, Buyukasik Y, Kosar A , et al. (1999) Selectins and IL-6 during the clinical course of idiopathic thrombocytopenic purpura. Acta Haematol. 101(1); 16-20.

36. Helal AMH, Shahine EM, Hassan MM , et al. (2012) Fatigue in Rheumatoid Arthritis and its relation to Interleukin-6 serum levels. The Egyptian Rheumatologist. 34, 4; 153-157.

37. Hewlett S, Chalder T, Choy E, et al. (2011) Fatigue in rheumatoid arthritis: time for a conceptual model. Rheumatology (Oxford), 50, 1004-1006.

38. Hill QA, Newland AC (2015) Fatigue in immune thrombocytopenia. British Journal of Haematology. 170(2):141-149.

39. Hockenbury MJ, Hinds PS, Barrera P, et al.(2003) Three Instruments to assess Fatigue in Children with cancer. The Child, Parent and Staff Persectives. Journal of Pain and Symptom Management, 25, 4, 319-328.

40. Huyser BA, Parker JC, Thoreson R et al. (1998) Predictors of subjective fatigue among individuals with rheumatoid arthritis. Arthritis and Rheumatism, 41, 2230-2237.

41. Jernas M, Hou Y, Stromberg Celind F , et al. (2015) Altered cytokine levels in pediatric ITP. Platelets. 26: 589-92.

42. Kamath J, Yarbrough GG, Prange Jr AJ, Winokur A (2009) The thyrotropin-releasing hormone (TRH)-immune system homeostatic hypothesis. Pharmacology & Therapeutics, 121, 20-28.

43. Karshikoff B, Sundelin T, Lasselin J (2017) Role of Inflammation in Human Fatigue: relevance of multidimensional assessments and potential neuronal mechanisms. Front. Immunol. 20, 21.

44. Kaser A, Branacher G, Steurer W, et al. (2001) Interleukin-6 stimulates thrombopoiesis through thrombopoietin: role in inflammatory thrombocytosis. Blood. 98 (9); 2720-2725.

45. Kappers-Klunne MC, van't Veer MB (2001) Cyclosporin A for the treatment of patients with chronic idiopathic thrombocytopenic purpura refractory to corticosteroids or splenectomy. Br J Haematol, 114, 121-125.

46. Khelif A, Saleh MN, Salama A, et al. (2019) Changes in health-related quality of life with long-term eltrombopag treatment in adults with persistent/chronic ITP: findings from the EXTEND study. Am J Hematol. 94(2): 200-208.

47. Klaassen RJ, Blanchette VS, Barnard D, et al. (2007) Validity, reliability, and responsiveness of a new measure of health-related quality of life in children with immune thrombocytopenic purpura: the Kids' ITP Tools. Journal of Pediatrics, 150, 510-515.

48. Klaassen RJ, Kinahan JY, Graham JMI, et al. (2019) Patient-Reported Outcome Measures (PROMs) in Pediatric Non-Malignant Hematology: A Systematic Review. Blood. 134, S1; 2180.

49. Koornstra RH, Peters M, Donofrio S,et al. (2014). Management of fatigue in patients with cancer—a practical overview. Cancer Treat Rev. 40(6):791-799.

50. Kruse C, Kruse A, Watson S, et al. (2018) Patients with immune thrombocytopenia (ITP) frequently experience severe fatigue but is it under-recognized by physicians: results from the ITP World Impact Survey (I-WISh). Blood. 132:2273.

51. Kruse C, Kruse A, DiRaimo J. (2021) Immune thrombocytopenia: the patient's perspective. Ann Blood 2021;6:9.

52. Kuter DJ, Mathias SD, Rummel M (2012) Health-related quality of life in non-splenectomized immune thrombocytopenia patients receiving romiplostim or medical standard of care. Am J Hematol, 87, 558-561.

53. Lee TW, Iser JH, Sparrow MP , et al. (2009) Thiopurines, a previously unrecognised cause for fatigue in patients with inflammatory bowel disease. Journal of Crohn's and Colitis, 3, 196-199.

54. Lewis G, Wessely S (1992) The epidemiology of fatigue: more questions than answers. Journal of Epidemiology and Community Health, 46, 92-97.

55. Ma D, Zhu X, Zhao P, et al. (2008) Profile of Th17 cytokines (IL-17, TGFbeta, IL-6) and Th1 cytokine (IFN-gamma) in patients with immune thrombocytopenic purpura. Annals of Hematology, 87, 899-904.

56. Mathias SD, Gao SK, Miller KL, et al. (2008) Impact of chronic Immune Thrombocytopenic Purpura (ITP) on health-related quality of life: a conceptual model starting with the patient perspective. Health Qual Life Outcomes. 6:13.

57. Mathias SD, Bussel JB, George JN, et al. (2007) A disease specific measure of health-related quality of life for use in adults with immune thrombocytopenic purpura: its development and validation. Health and Quality of Life Outcomes, 5, 11.

58. Matzdorff AC, Arnold G, Salama A, et al. (2011). Advances in ITP – Therapy and Quality of Life – A Patient Survey. PLOS ONE, 6 (11) e27350.

59. McDonald V, Newland A, Morgan M, et al. (2021) Patient preferences and experiences regarding thrombopoietin-receptor agonists for immune thrombocytopenia in the United Kingdom and Ireland (TRAPeze UK & IE study). Hematology, 26:1, 799-808.

60. Miller AH, Ancoli-Israel S, Bower JE, et al. (2008) Neuroendocrineimmune mechanisms of behavioral comorbidities in patients with cancer. Journal of Clinical Oncology, 26, 971-982.

61. Neunert C, Terrell DR, Arnold DM, et al. (2019) American Society of Hematology 2019 guidelines for immune thrombocytopenia. Blood Adv. 3(23): 3829-3866.

62. Newland AC, Godeau B, Priego V et al. (2016) Remission and platelet responses with romiplostim in primary immune thrombocytopenia: final results from a phase 2 study. British Journal of Haematology, 172, 262-273.

63. Newland AC, Hill Q, Morgan M, et al. (2021) Making the right choices in ITP management and care; a shared decision making toolkit. https://bit.ly/3INsdKe.

64. Newton JL, Reese JA, Watson SI, et al. (2011) Fatigue in adult patients with primary immune thrombocytopenia. Eur J Haematol. 86(5):420-429.

65. National Institute for Health and Care Excellence. (2021) NICE Guideline [NG206]. Myalgic Encephalitis(or encephalopathy)/Chronic Fatigue Syndrome: diagnosis and management. Available from: https://www.nice.org.uk/guidance/ng206. Accessed December 5, 2021.

66. Nikolaus S, Bode C, Taal E, van de Laar MA (2013) Fatigue and factors related to fatigue in rheumatoid arthritis: a systematic review. Arthritis Care & Research, 65, 1128-1146.

67. Ogawara H, Handa H, Morita K, et al. (2003) High Th1/Th2 ratio in patients with chronic idiopathic thrombocytopenic purpura. European Journal of Haematology, 71, 283-288.

68. Panitsas FP, Theodoropoulou M, Kouraklis A, et al. (2004) Adult chronic idiopathic thrombocytopenic purpura (ITP) is the manifestation of a type-1 polarized immune response. Blood. 103:2645-7.

69. Pardini M, Cordano C, Benassi F , et al. (2011). Amisulpride vs Fluoxetine treatment of Chronic fatigue syndrome. European Neuropsychopharmacology, 21 (3): 282-286.

70. Pedraz-Petrozzi B, Neumann E, Sammer G (2020) Pro-Inflammatory markers in patients with depression: a case controlled study. Scientific Reports. 10, Article number 9494 (open access).

71. Peerschke EI, Andemariam B, Yin W, Bussel JB (2010) Complement activation on platelets correlates with a decrease in circulating immature platelets in patients with immune thrombocytopenic purpura. British Journal of Haematology, 148, 638-645.

72. Provan D, Arnold DM, Bussel JB, et al. (2009) Updated international consensus report on the investigation and management of primary immune thrombocytopenia. Blood Adv. 3(22):3780-3817.

73. Rabin DU, Kuter DJ, Liebman HA, Bussel JB. (2010) What do healthcare providers ask their patients with immune thrombocytopenia? Am J Hematol. 85(8):629-631.

74. Ricci JA, Chee E, Lorandeau AL, Berger J (2007) Fatigue in the U.S. workforce: prevalence and implications for lost productive work time. Journal of Occupational and Environmental Medicine, 49, 1-10.

75. Riemsma RP, Rasker JJ, Taal E, et al. (1998) Fatigue in rheumatoid arthritis: the role of self-efficacy and problematic social support. British Journal of Rheumatology, 37, 1042-1046.

76. Rocha AMC, DeSouza SC, Rocha GA, et al. (2010) IL1RN VNTR and IL2-330 polymorphic genes are independently associated with chronic immune thrombocytopenia. British Journal of Haematology, 150, 679-684.

77. Romanov DV, Volel BA, Petelin DS (2018) Approaches to therapy for depressions in neurology: prospects for the use of agomelatine. Neurology, Neuropsychiatry, Psychosomatics. 10(4): 101-110.

78. Ruggeri M, Tosetto A, Palandri F, et al. (2014) Thrombotic risk in patients with primary immune thrombocytopenia is only mildly increased and explained by personal and treatment-related risk factors. Journal of Thrombosis and Haemostasis, 12, 1266-1273.

79. Sarpatwari A, Watson S, Erqou S, Anderson H, Grainger J, Higgins JP, Newland AC (2010a) Health-related lifestyle in adults and children with primary immune thrombocytopenia (ITP). British Journal of Haematology, 151, 189-191.

80. Sarpatwari A, Bennett D, Logie JW, Shukla A, Beach KJ, Newland AC, Sanderson S, Provan D (2010b) Thromboembolic events among adult patients with primary immune thrombocytopenia in the United Kingdom General Practice Research Database. Haematologica, 95, 1167-1175.

81. Satoh T, Pandey JP, Okazaki Y, et al. (2004) Single nucleotide polymorphisms of the inflammatory cytokine genes in adults with chronic immune thrombocytopenic purpura. British Journal of Haematology, 124, 796-801.

82. Schmeding A, Schneider M (2013) Fatigue, health-related quality of life and other patient reported outcomes in systemic lupus erythematosus. Best Practice & Research. Clinical Rheumatology, 27, 363-375.

83. Schubert C, Hong S, Natarajan L , et al. (2007) The Association between fatigue and inflammatory marker levels in cancer patients: A quantitative review. Brain, Behaviour and Immunity. 21; 413-427.

84. Semple JW, Milev Y, Cosgrave D, et al. (1996) Differences in serum cytokine levels in acute and chronic autoimmune thrombocytopenic purpura: relationship to platelet phenotype and antiplatelet T-cell reactivity. Blood, 87, 4245-4254.

85. Semple JW (2008) ITP three R's: regulation, routing, rituximab. Blood. 112(4); 927-928.

86. Semple JW, Provan D (2012) The immunopathogenesis of immune thrombocytopenia: T cells still take center-stage. Curr Opin Hematol. 19:357-62.

87. Shimano KA, Neunert C, Bussel JB , et al. (2021) Quality of life is an important indication for second-line treatment in children with immune thrombocytopenia. Pediatr Blood Cancer. 68(6):e29023.

88. Signorovitch J, Brainsky A, Grotzinger KM (2011) Validation of the FACIT-fatigue subscale, selected items

from FACT-thrombocytopenia, and the SF-36v2 in patients with chronic immune thrombocytopenia. Quality of Life Research, 20, 1737-1744.

89. Stasi R, Cooper N, del Poeta G , et al. (2008) Analysis of regulatory T-cell changes in patients with idiopathic thrombocytopenic purpura receiving B Cell-depleting therapy with rituximab. Blood. 112(4); 1147-1150.

90. Suvajdzic N, Zivkovic R, Djunic I, et al. (2014) Health-related quality of life in adult patients with chronic immune thrombocytopenia in Serbia. Platelets 2014;25:467-9.

91. Swain MG (2000) Fatigue in chronic disease. Clinical Science (London, England: 1979), 99, 1-8.

92. Swain MG (2006) Fatigue in liver disease: Pathophysiology and clinical management. Can J Gastroenterol Vol 20 No 3; 181-188.

93. Takahashi N, Saitoh T, Gotoh N, et al. (2017) The cytokine polymorphisms affecting Th1/Th2 increase the susceptibility to, and severity of, chronic ITP. BMC Immunol. 18, 26.

94. Trotter P, Hill QA (2018) Immune thrombocytopenia: improving quality of life and patient outcomes. Patient Relat Outcome Meas. 9:369-384.

95. Tsukune Y, Komatsu N. (2016) Management of Adult Chronic Immune Thrombocytopenia in Japan: Patient and Hematologist Perspectives from a Multicenter Cross-sectional Questionnaire Survey. Intern Med. 55(17):2379-2385.

96. Viana R, D'Alessio D, Grant L et al. (2021). Psychometric Evauation of ITP Life Quaity Index (ILQI) in a global survey of patients with Immune Thrombocytopenia. Adv Ther. Doi: 10.1007/s12325-021-01934-0 (online ahead of print).

97. Wada H, Minamikawa K, Ohiwa M , et al. (1991) Elevated plasma interleukin-6 inpatients with idiopathic thrombocytopenic purpura. Rinsho Ketsueki. 32(7); 773-776.

98. Wang RT, Liu XG, Hou Y , et al. (2021) A Physician-Patient survey for primary immune thrombocytopenia: Chinese subgroup analysis of I-WISh International Survey. Zhonghua Xue Ye Xue Za Zhi. 42(5); 369-375: e29023.

99. Wang YM, Jin BZ, Ai F, et al. (2012) The efficacy and safety of melatonin in concurrent chemotherapy or radiotherapy for solid tumors: a meta-analysis of randomized controlled trials. Cancer Chemotherapy and Pharmacology, 69, 1213-1220.

100. Wong RSM, Saleh MN, Khelif A, et al. (2017) Safety and efficacy of long-term treatment of chronic/persistent ITP with eltrombopag: final results of the EXTEND study. Blood. 130(23):2527-2536.

101. Wu KH, Peng CT, Li TC, et al. (2005) Interleukin 4, interleukin 6 and interleukin 10 polymorphisms in children with acute and chronic immune thrombocytopenic purpura. British Journal of Haematology. 128 (6); 849-852.

102. Zhou Z, Yang L, Chen Z, et al. (2007) Health-related quality of life measured by the Short Form 36 in immune thrombocytopenic purpura: a cross-sectional survey in China. European Journal of Haematology, 78, 518-523.

103. Zhao H, Du W, Wang D, et al. (2010). The expression of IFN-gamma, IL-4, Foxp3 and perforin genes are not correlated with DNA methylation status in patients with immune thrombocytopenic purpura. Platelets. 21: 137-43.

104. Zhan Y, Zou S, Hua F, et al. (2014) High-dose dexamethasone modulates serum cytokine profile in patients with primary immune thrombocytopenia. Immunology Letters, 160, 33-38.

105. Zielinski MR, Systrom DM, Rose NR (2019) Fatigue, sleep, and autoimmune and related disorders. Front Immunol. 2019; 10: 1827.

106. Zilber R, Bortz AP, Yacobovich J, et al. (2012) Analysis of health-related quality of life in children with immune thrombocytopenia and their parents using Kids' ITP tools. J Pediatr Hematol Oncol 34:2-5.

107. Zlott DA, Byrne M (2010) Mechanisms by which pharmacologic agents may contribute to fatigue. PM & R: The Journal of Injury, Function, and Rehabilitation, 2, 451-455.

# 20. Guidelines for using ITP management guidelines

Clinical management guidelines are documents formulated by individuals or, more often, panels of experts assembled by professional organizations, societies, agencies, or educational institutions with the aim of offering uniform definitions and overall management recommendations for patients with a disease or group of related conditions. The number of such guidelines has proliferated during the past several decades [1], resulting in their creation for virtually every disease that affects human beings, including immune thrombocytopenia (ITP).

Guidelines come in many forms, although virtually all focus on patient diagnosis and management. Sometimes their scope is broad, whereas in other circumstances it is limited to, for example, patients of a certain age and/or with a specific disease complication. Management guidelines should be based primarily or exclusively on scientific evidence, but in many cases they represent opinions, usually a consensus among the group of appointed experts. Since guideline documents should make recommendations which are evidence based, during their development process the scientific data are ideally rigorously reviewed and their quality assessed in a formal manner by one or more "methodologists" who are experts with training and experience in the process. The strength of each management recommendation derived from the evidence is generally measured by one of a variety of "grading" systems, one of the most highly regarded and frequently used of which is termed GRADE [2]. Strong recommendations for diagnostic tests or treatments should be supported by high quality evidence, such as multiple randomized clinical trials. Yet for many disease-oriented guidelines (including ITP) this is usually not feasible.

Many forms of "management guidelines" in ITP and other conditions are not necessarily constructed in the rigorous fashion described above.

| Reference | Sponsoring society or organization | Patient population described | Method(s) |
|---|---|---|---|
| George, 1996 [3] | American Society of Hematology | Comprehensive* | Evidence-based and expert consensus |
| Neunert, 2011 [4] | American Society of Hematology | Comprehensive* | Evidence-based (GRADE system) |
| Provan, 2010 [5] | International Working Group | Comprehensive* | Evidence-based and expert consensus |
| Rodeghiero, 2009 [6] | International Working Group | Comprehensive terminology and definitions | Evidence-based and expert consensus |
| Provan, 2003 [7] | British Committee for Standards in Haematology General Haematology Task Force | Comprehensive* | Evidence-based |
| Ghanima, 2012 [8] | None | Second line treatment of adults | Opinion of authors |
| Pabinger, 2012 [9] | Austrian Society of Hematology | Primary ITP in adults | Expert consensus |
| De Mattia, 2010 [10] | AIEOP (Italy) | Children with chronic ITP | Evidence-based and expert consensus |
| Sanz, 2012 [11] | Spanish Hematology Societies | Comprehensive* | Expert consensus |

***Table 20.1:*** Diversity of ITP management guidelines. * Comprehensive = most or all adults and children with ITP.

Some are simply individual or multi-authored review articles which do not assess all of the evidence and grade its quality. Other publications labeled as "management guidelines" are, in fact, editorials or review articles which present a specific and potentially biased point of view.

## 20.1. Guidelines for management of ITP

So what is the state of affairs specifically regarding management recommendations in immune thrombocytopenia (ITP)? Not surprisingly, a number of ITP guidelines have been published during the past several decades in peer reviewed hematology journals targeted to clinicians and scientists [3-7]. Some have a rather limited scope focusing on, for example, topics such as chronic refractory ITP, acute ITP during childhood, or treatment of ITP in the elderly [8]. Others emphasize detailed management recommendations regarding specific treatments for ITP (e.g., splenectomy, rituximab, thrombopoietin receptor agonists, etc.) and/or describe treatment strategies recommended for use in a specific country in which clinicians practice [9-11]. Examples of some (but for certain an incomplete listing) of these many types of ITP guidelines are summarized in Table 20.1.

Most hematologists as well as other physicians caring for patients with ITP frequently rely on such guidelines to enhance their clinical decision making. Hematologists are also accustomed to employing guidelines in the many other diseases that they encounter, including thrombotic thrombocytopenic purpura, thromboembolic disease, sickle cell disease, etc. The examples of ITP guidelines published during the past decade or two which are displayed in Table 20.1 highlight their diversity with regard to supporting organization, targeted population of ITP patients, and methods employed. In most instances a literature review was undertaken to identify levels of evidence that were felt to support the strength of the recommendations that were made. Moreover, because of a paucity of good evidence from published studies, most recommendations have included consensus opinions among experts on the guidelines panel. In some cases where a structured literature review was not undertaken, examples of which are the "How I Treat" articles regularly published in *Blood* [8], it is clear that the recommendations are based primarily on the authors' personal experience and their interpretation of the literature.

## 20.2. Pros and cons of guidelines

Disease focused guidelines have many merits, providing important information for physicians to guide their management decisions. Many primary care, emergency department, or hospitalist physicians who may initially encounter bleeding ITP patients benefit greatly from the advice provided in a guidelines document. Moreover, hematology-oncology specialists who care for some ITP patients but whose focus is primarily on oncology may occasionally be asked to consult on or even care for ITP patients, so they also will benefit from guideline recommendations. Even hematologists keen on ITP and familiar with every aspect of this disorder usually find information in guideline documents reassuring, helping them remain up-to-date regarding their knowledge of ITP. So guidelines can be extremely helpful to physicians caring for patients with ITP and their families. It is noteworthy that some guidelines documents have actually incorporated in their writing committees patient advocates and/or representatives of ITP support groups or organizations to assure that the recommendations are appropriately patient-centered [7].

So what are the disadvantages of ITP guidelines? The pitfalls of guidelines and cautions to take when using them have been emphasized repeatedly in the literature [1, 12]. Potential disadvantages of ITP guidelines are similar to those used in other medical conditions. A recent editorial highlighted some of these concerns, including the overreliance of expert opinion and the "marketing" of guidelines documents by organizations or institutions seeking publicity or financial gain [9]. Moreover, certain guidelines documents have been generously supported by industry, resulting in potential conflicts of interest when a specific drug used for ITP patients is strongly recommended for use even though the scientific evidence does not necessarily provide justification [13, 14]. An additional concern is how recommendations made in a guideline might be incorrectly viewed by trial lawyers and juries as the "standard of care" and then used in court proceedings to label physicians whose management strategy differed from the guideline recommendation as being negligent when an adverse outcome occurred. Moreover, guidelines have the potential, especially when the recommendation is strong and evidence compelling, to be used inappropriately by hospital quality assurance committees as performance measures which are then rigidly enforced.

| Pros |
|---|
| • May prove extremely useful to guide physician decision-making<br>• Defines a consensus of acknowledged experts regarding diagnosis and management of patients with an acute or chronic medical condition<br>• Often helpful to patients as source of information about their disease and its treatment<br>• Establishes different opinions and approaches, thus allowing for choice of management options |
| **Cons** |
| • May conflict with a patient's desires and values<br>• Too often based on opinion and bias rather than on strong evidence<br>• Employed inappropriately in legal proceedings and as performance ratings<br>• Used as marketing and public relations tools by industry and professional societies |

***Table 20.2:*** Pros and cons of management guidelines.

## 20.3. Evidence based vs. patient centered management

The "bottom line" for those of us treating ITP patients is to deliver to them the best care possible. Guidelines can be helpful in our decision making about which tests to perform or treatments to give, one option always being observation, watchful waiting, or "active non-intervention" [15]. Evidence based medicine may indeed inform the most highly regarded guidelines published in the best medical journals. However, we must use more than scientific evidence when caring for our patients. The values, beliefs, activity levels, and environment of our ITP patients always come first. We must listen to them and to give them the best possible treatment that is "right" for them. Such patient-centered care often transcends what the guidelines state. This is certainly true in ITP just as it is in many other medical conditions where evidence is often lacking or conflicting. Maybe there should be a self-enforced moratorium on developing additional ITP clinical guidelines in order to reflect awhile on those guidelines already available to us. Let's focus on doing what is "best" for our patients, irrespective of what the latest guidelines recommend.

## References

1. Sniderman AD, Furberg CD. Why guideline – making requires reform. JAMA 2009;301:429-431

2. Guyatt GH, Oxman AD, Vist GE, et al. Grade: an emerging consensus on rating quality of evidence and strength of recommendations. BMJ 2008;336:924-926

3. George JN, Woolf SH, Raskob GE, et al. Idiopathic thrombocytopenic purpura: a practice guideline developed by explicit methods for the American Society of Hematology. Blood 1996;88:3-40

4. Neunert C, Lim W, Crowther M, et al. The American Society of Hematology 2011 evidence-based practice guidelines for immune thrombocytopenia. Blood 2011; 117:4190-4207

5. Provan D, Stasi R, Newland AC, et al. International consensus report on the investigation and management of primary immune thrombocytopenia. Blood 2010;115: 168-186

6. Rodeghiero F, Stasi R, Gernsheimer T, et al. Standardization of terminology, definitions and outcome criteria in immune thrombocytopenic purpura of adults and children: report from an international working group. Blood 2009;113:2386-2393

7. Provan D, Norfolk D, Bolton-Maggs P, et al. for British Committee for Standards in Haematology General Haematology Task Force. Guidelines for the investigation and management of idiopathic thrombocytopenic purpura in adults, children, and in pregnancy. Br J Haematol 2002;120:574-596

8. Ghanima W, Godeau B, Cines DB, Bussell JB. How I treat immune thrombocytopenia: The choice between splenectomy or a medical therapy as a second-line treatment. Blood 2012;120:960-969

9. Pabinger I, Gasti G, Steurer M, et al. Primary immune thrombocytopenia in adults – diagnostic and treatment. Consensus statement of the Austrian Society of Hematology and Oncology (OGHO). Wien Klin Wochenschr 2012;124:111-123

10. De Mattia D, Del Vecchio GC, Russo G, et al. Management of chronic childhood immune thrombocytopenic purpura: AIEOP consensus guidelines. Acta Haematol 2010;123:96-109

11. Sanz MA, Vicente GV, Fernandez A, et al. Guidelines for diagnosis, treatment, and monitoring of primary immune thrombocytopenia. Med Clin (Barc) 2012;17: 261.e1-261,.

12. Shaneyfelt TM, and Centor RM. Reassessment of clinical practice guidelines: Go gently into that good night. JAMA 2009;301:868-869

13. George JN. Management of immune thrombocytopenia – something old, something new. N Engl J Med 2010;363:1959-1961

14. Provan D, Newland AC. Guidelines for immune thrombocytopenia. N Engl J Med 2011;364:4

15. Maguiness SM, and Frieden IJ. Current management of infantile hemangiomas. Semin Cutan Med Surg 2010; 29:106-114

# 21. State of the Art and future Considerations of ITP

Behind immune thrombocytopenia (ITP) lies heterogeneous manifestations and natural histories, an unknown etiology, and a complex pathogenesis, resulting in controversies in the management of patients with ITP. To further develop this field, evidence-based analyses of different heterogeneities are needed and subgroups need to be defined in order to manage the individual patient with ITP.

## 21.1. Heterogeneity of ITP

### Clinical manifestation

Confronted with an individual patient with newly diagnosed ITP it is initially unknown whether it is primary ITP characterized by bleeding and isolated destructive thrombocytopenia in an otherwise healthy person, or secondary ITP due to infection, primary immune deficiency, other autoimmune, oncologic, or drug related disorders, or due to other as-yet unrecognized disorders. The clinical presentation may involve mild, moderate, or (rarely) severe bleeding, and the response to an indicated intervention will be heterogenous, ranging from a spontaneous recovery – frequently observed in children with a post- or para-infectious history – to a long-term chronic disease.

The main concern in a patient with ITP is bleeding [1, 2], which is unpredictable even when platelet counts are extremely low. Other factors contributing to easy bleeding beside platelet count, such as platelet associated antibodies or immune complexes bound to platelets, may be indicators of etiology, i.e., undetected inborn or acquired, qualitative platelet function defects or endothelial vascular component alterations [3]. Existing assessments and bleeding scores are increasingly used and reported in studies, but validation of these proposals needs to be adapted.

The heterogeneity of the natural history of ITP is exemplified in three studies concerning age and gender (☞ Figure 21.1+21.2 with their respective references) and on Table 21.1 concerning reported differences and similarities in children and adults adapted from reference [4]. In children, the rate in the first year of age (infants) is markedly higher in boys, while between the ages of 1 and 16 years, it is higher in girls (☞ Figure 21.1). In almost all adult age groups, the rate of female patients is higher than that of males. The number of patients with ITP is markedly higher after the age of 60 years than in younger age groups [5-9] (☞ Figure 21.2 with references).

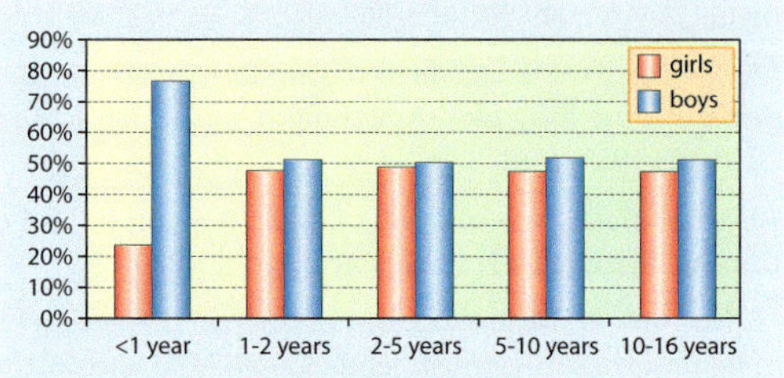


***Figure 21.1:*** Age of girls and boys with newly diagnosed ITP in different age groups. Results from the prospective, intercontinental cooperative ITP study group (n = 2,031), published in J Pediatr 2003;143:605-8.

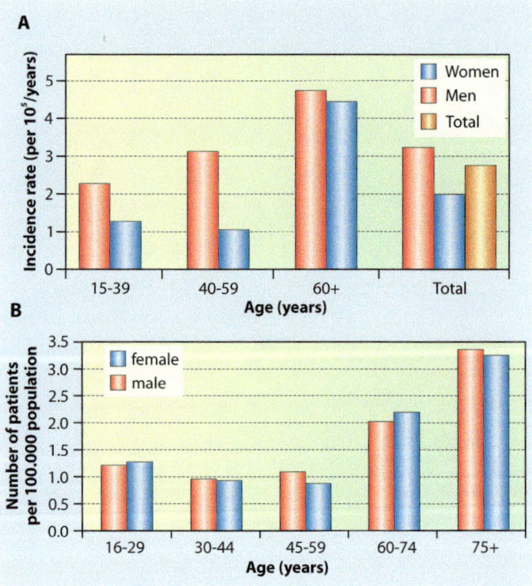


***Figure 21.2:*** Incidence of adults with newly diagnosed ITP from two studies, published in Blood 1999; 94:909-13 (**A**) and Brit J Haematol 2003;122:966-74 (**B**).

### Management

Management of ITP is also heterogeneous. The goal is for the individual to reach a platelet count that allows adequate hemostasis and/or the prevention of bleeding [28]. The decision and recommendation of different management options while

| | Children | Adults | Ref. in Despotovic [4] |
|---|---|---|---|
| Epidemiology | 5-10:100,000 | 3.3-3,7:100,000 | D5 |
| Bleeding at presentation | 90% | 69% | D1 |
| Marked bleeding | 20% | 9.6% | D14 |
| Intracranial hemorrhage (ICH) | 0.5-0.6% | 1.5-1.7% | D6, 17, 19, 28 |
| Comorbidities | 3.5% | >30% | D5, D8 |
| 2 years after diagnosis | 10.7% | 30.7% | D6, Schiff18 |
| Remission rate | 71% | 56% | D6, D10 |
| In chronic ITP | 28% | 30% | D6 |
| Management | | | |
| Observation only | frequent | rare | D5, 6, 12-14, 35, 36 |
| Intravenous immunoglobulins (IVIg) | frequent | optional | D4-6 |
| QoL: Reduction of activities | 23,3% | 9,5% | D58 |
| Similarities (D12, 13, 22-27) | | | |
| Presenting platelet counts | = | = | |
| Bleeding tendency | = | = | |
| Management: Steroids | = | = | |
| QoL: Fatigue | = | = | |

***Table 21.1:*** Reported differences and similarities between children and adults.

avoiding adverse effects caused by specific medications depends on various factors. In patients with mild or no bleeding and platelet counts above 10,000, a period of observation may be an option. If an intervention is indicated, clinicians can decide between three main options:

1) decreasing the autoantibody production by steroids, IVIg, immunosuppressants, or anti-CD20 monoclonal antibody;

2) blocking the rapid clearance of platelets by IVIg and steroids, splenectomy, or the new Syk-inhibitor; or

3) enhancing platelet production by TPO-RAs. The latter may be indicated in combination with one of the other options due to different mechanisms of action, but clinical studies into the use of such a combination are needed in the future.

## Terminology and guidelines

The international working group into standardization, definitions, and outcome criteria in adults and children with ITP published their recommendations in 2009 [11, 29-31]. This group began at an expert meeting of the Intercontinental Cooperative ITP Study group (ICIS) in 2006 in order to get and analyze more results. It is now imperative to build upon these published statements by validating their impact and translating their theory into practice. In addition, prospective registries and studies are required for patients with ongoing ITP to develop recommendations regarding tests for early detection of chronic ITP [32] or the various secondary diseases associated with ITP [33]. Most therapeutic procedures and many published guidelines are not evidence-based; the latter, however, include qualified opinions by experts in the field.

Furthermore, information is still needed regarding the individual quality of life depending on age, activity, anxiety, environmental and social aspects, ethnicity, and other issues.

The evaluation of health-related quality of life instruments (such as surveys, questionnaires, or the Kid's Tool (34-36) is an important future issue in the management of primary ITP. The early attempts at validation [37] and the relationship between platelet count, bleeding severity, and patients' health-related quality of life need to be further clarified. Validation of the Kid's Tool failed to be significant except for some details among children with newly diagnosed ITP and with chronic ITP. New, more simplified concepts of measurement of persistent ITP (3-12 months' duration after diagnosis) or chronic ITP are now a priority. To achieve this, research could focus on factors including the patient's fatigue, depression, and sleep disturbances, and their possible relationship to chronic, subclinical inflammatory disease, disturbed immunity, and patients', children's, and parents' anxiety. In addition, the patient's (and parent's) own perspectives of ITP, gained by information from social media, patient support organizations, and other sources, must be evaluated.

## 21.2. Unknown etiology of ITP

In children, approximately 70% of newly diagnosed ITP occur after or during infectious disorders; cross-reactive antibodies or immune complexes may be causative for early platelet destruction in susceptible individuals. In patients with chronic ITP it is hypothesized that acquired recognition of new self determinants (cryptic epitopes), i.e. triggered by infection [38] and exposed to T-cells [39] lead to autoantibody production by B-cells [40]. This indirectly indicates that the immune tolerance is disturbed in patients with ITP by loss of tolerance.

Molecular genetic studies may direct to the etiology of weak tolerance for self antigens. Furthermore, for many years the trigger of infectious particles is not sufficiently studied in ITP with exception of *H. pylori*, HCV and HIV. Together with molecular genetic studies infectious agents may be the key for research of the etiology in autoimmune disorders.

Infection-related oxidative stress may induce the immune disturbance in ITP. Zhang and colleagues reported differences on gene expression and molecular-oxidative stress in children with chronic ITP [43]. Overexpression of the gene vanin-1 (VNN1) – an oxidative stress sensor – was associated with chronic ITP only. VNN1 plays an important role in oxidative stress response and mediates production of inflammatory cytokines. From this new finding early prognostic estimation of transient or long-term ITP may be possible.

Some attempts of susceptibility by research on polymorphisms are promising [41], but single nucleotide polymorphisms (SNPs) may vary from one ethnic population to the other [42].

## 21.3. Immunomodulation in inflammatory and autoimmune disorders

Since many years the causative factor of platelet destruction in ITP seems to be related to antibodies, immune complexes or autoantibodies. In recent years, the debate of pathophysiology focuses on the disturbed immune response including the whole innate and adaptive immune system [44]. The rapid response and the research of the mechanisms of action of antibody concentrates (IVIg) [45-47] changed the immunosuppressive to the immunomodulatory approach. Later on, the anti-D-immunoglobulin treatment and the translation to monoclonal anti-CD20 antibody (rituximab) treatment [48] and other targeted therapeutics supported the immune pathogenesis of ITP, as well the direct destruction of platelets by cytotoxic T-cells [49]. The switch from one of the compounds of the immune cascade (antibodies) to multiple parts of immune disturbance dominates not only the pathophysiology of ITP, but many other inflammatory and autoimmune disorders [44].

PubMed has indexed over 78'800 publications on IVIg since 1981, of which over 8,000 are focused on the mechanisms (☞ Chapter 2.5., Table 2.3). When the different findings of the mechanisms of action of IVIg were allocated to a schema of the whole immune system it could be recognized that many (if not all) components of the innate and adaptive immune system were involved after IVIg administration (☞ Figure 21.3). The immunomodulatory effects described in thousands of peer-reviewed laboratory, *in vitro* and animal experiments, as well as in clinical reports support, that the immune cascade is disturbed in these conditions and can be synergistically modulated by administration of IVIg [44]. Humbly, however, one has to conclude that IVIg evoked a synergistic interaction in patients with a disturbed immune system, which resulted in a new balance of the complex immune response. Further research has to clarify immune pathophysiologic details.

In many other inflammatory and autoimmune disorders similar pathophysiological mechanisms and immunomodulatory treatment possibilities have been found. The initially triggering event, however, remains unclear. In addition, there are uncertainties, if pathophysiological animal models can be translated to humans. The research in immunopathology will continue. Pathophysiological analogies between infection, autoimmunity, immunodeficiency and oncology may elucidate common mechanisms of action [50].

## 21.4. Platelet stimulation by thrombopoietin receptor agonists (TPO-RA) of megakaryopoiesis

☞ also Chapter 2.6.

A second development is the pathophysiologic influence of autoantibodies to the megakaryocytopoiesis and the therapeutic effect by platelets stimulation, which is somewhat unexpected, because the majority of patients with ITP has normal or slightly elevated serum thrombopoietin levels. McMillan and Chang [51-53] showed, that the pathogenic effects – especially the autoantibodies – affect the megakaryopoiesis as well. The second generation of thrombopoietin receptor agonists (TPO-RA) – romiplostim for subcutaneous, eltrombopag and avatrombopag for oral administration – have the potential to stimulate platelets. The agonists have a high affinity to the thrombopoietin receptor, activate the intracellular cascade, which stimulate the platelet production [54]. They have been clinically evaluated by standardized phase I-III studies and approved by the authorities more than 10 year ago. Thus, the stimulatory effect of megakaryocyte by TPO-RAs may indirectly overcome the autoantibodies-based megakaryocytic suppression by high production of platelets.

It is important to note that each individual patients showed a broad range of different response of platelet increase in all clinical studies. This is the case not only in ITP, but also in patients with platelet production disturbances and in thrombocytopenic patients with cancer and/or under platelet suppressive treatments. As we can see, each patient's plasma had an individually different degree of suppression.

As an example, in a phase III study of eltrombopag, broad ranges of platelet increase over six months of continuous treatment were observed in patients with chronic, refractory ITP (☞ Figure 21.3) [55-57]. After ceasing the drug (post-treatment in Figure 21.3) the majority of patients' platelets counts returned to baseline, while some patients retained higher counts. This is an important new observation. It may be a preliminary confirmation that platelets themselves are not only responsible for coagulation, but have immunological activities, which may support the spontaneous recovery of ITP when the platelets are present in adequate numbers within some months of effective treatment – however, this is still hypothetical.

In the future, clinical studies of TPO-RA in patients with early refractory ITP might be indicated for confirmation of beneficial therapeutic results, activation of platelet and megakaryocytic functions, and other aspects of the response.

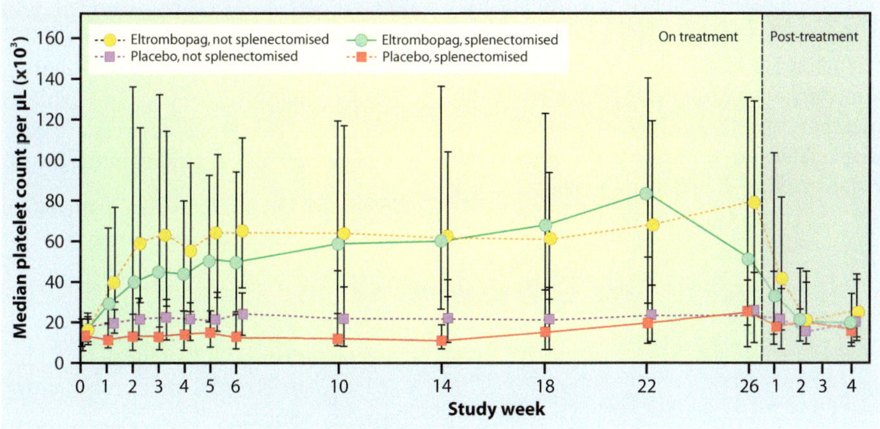


***Figure 21.3:*** Median platelet counts and broad ranges in patients with/without splenectomy during eltrombopag versus placebo treatment through 26 weeks and after ceasing the drugs.

## 21.5. Future progress and the question of adequate management of ITP

Since 1992 guidelines based on extensive reviews and followed by many national or local guidelines have been published [11, 30, 31, 58]. These guidelines and reports are not evidence-based, today; they serve as arguments of adequate management recommendations. As a result of controversies emerging over the large heterogeneities in individuals with ITP, current practice does not always follow these recommendations. Validation programs are now important for guidelines.

Ongoing efforts to define the natural history and management of ITP by expert groups, i.e., to harmonize terminology [29] based on international cooperative ITP studies and registries (www.itpbasel.ch) and updates of international expert groups will facilitate the clinical use of such guidelines.

The Pediatric and Adult Registry on Chronic ITP (PARC-ITP) database aims to define subgroups of ITP based on natural history, genetics, comorbidity, management, treatments, adverse effects and other criteria in collaboration with international scientists and centers. This has promise in the development of algorithms for diagnostic procedures and practical management to steadily improve the care of patients with ITP [59].

Results of subgroups of patients from the above mentioned registries will be helpful for eligibility criteria of patient inclusion and for endpoints in clinical studies and treatment recommendations. The ongoing, long-term Pediatric and Adult Registry on Chronic ITP (PARC-ITP) especially serves to define such subgroups [59] (☞ Figure 21.4). Results from studies with subgroups of patients with ITP concerning risk factors including analyses of qualitative platelet dysfunctions will ameliorate the decision-making in ITP management.

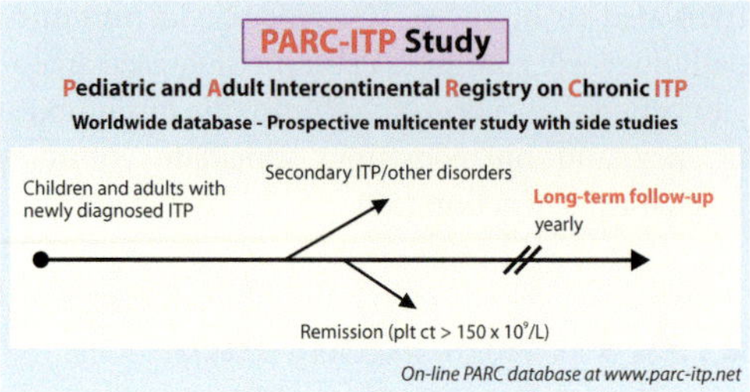


***Figure 21.4:*** Structure of the Pediatric and Adult Registry on Chronic ITP (PARC-ITP).

On the basis of clinical studies platelet counts as a decision measure for treatment endpoint remain important. In clinical practice other factors than platelet counts may be considered for an intervention: the individual pattern of bleeding signs, the health-related quality of life, the cost-benefit factor and others. Continuation of bleeding assessments with validation, correlation of other risk factors [60] and adverse effects of a specific treatment are mandatory. An important decision-making factor of management is the consensus between the individual patient with ITP and the physician.

An important issue of management is the low frequency of severe bleeding which was prospectively confirmed in registries of the Intercontinental Cooperative ITP Study Group (ICIS; ☞ Chapter 2., Table 2.1) and in other population-based studies [61, 62]. However, the individual risk for life-threatening bleeding is still unknown. Most of bleeding risk factors associated with ITP, such as severity of bleeding, individual activities, e.g. sport, the anxiety of parents and patients, as well as the pre- and peri-surgery support remain unstudied. An exception of low severity of bleeding [5] and other frequent complications are elderly patients with ITP over 60 years of age (☞ Table 21.1 and Figure 21.2). This group deserves a special attention of natural history studies in the future.

Confronted with an individual patient, considerations have to be done concerning:

- their stage of disease (newly diagnosed, persistent, chronic, or refractory ITP),
- the individual quality of life depending on age, activity, anxiety, and environmental (familiar) aspects, ethnicity,
- different management options, and therapeutic adverse effects

- evaluation of the patient's and parents' own perspectives; today, patients (and parents) inform themselves regarding ITP mainly by social media, patient support organizations, and other sources.

Algorithms for the practical management are a new development [59] and have to be evaluated in the future: In patients, especially in children, with newly diagnosed or persistent ITP a period of critical observation without further diagnostic analyses, either for a watch and wait phase in patients with no or mild bleeding or with a treatment intervention in patients with risk of bleeding and, mostly, with less than 10,000 platelet counts may be recommended. For treatment intervention in children with newly diagnosed or persistent ITP 1-2 times IVIg, which has a short time to response and a high rate of response, but the longterm stable responses and the remission rates are similar as with steroids [63, 64], which is still the alternative option to IVIg; another possibility starts with high dose steroids (dexamethasone) [65, 66] followed by low dose steroids with a faster response than with low dose steroids only. In an emergency situation a combination of high dose steroid and IVIg, if necessary, in combination with a platelet transfusion is still indicated. A new possibility in patients, who do not satisfactorily respond to the initial treatment, is the recommendation of TPO-RA, since the mechanism of action is different to steroids or IVIg.

As soon as a suspicion of refractory or chronic ITP within the first months after initial diagnosis of ITP emerge, it is recommended to check for second ITP, to exclude a chronic infection and/or to perform analyses for other causes of thrombocytopenia.

In recent analysis of the ICIS PARC ITP Registry with 3,974 children and with a prospective observation time of at least 2 years (59), there were 113 children with confirmed second ITP beside a group of additional children with still not confirmed second ITP (n=110). As shown on the graphic, chronic infections and autoimmune disorders were the frequently diagnosed second ITP beside aplastic anemia, malignancy, immune deficiency and drug related disorder (☞ Figure 21.5).

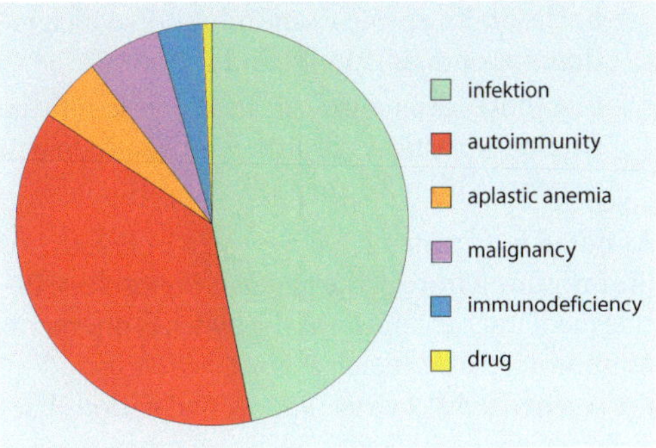


***Figure 21.5:*** Distribution rates of secondary ITP in 113/3,974 children with at least two years ongoing chronic ITP from the prospective PARC ITP Registry (ref.).

If a patient still has primary, chronic and or refractory ITP, the possible therapeutic options currently are:

- Thrombopoietin agonists (TPO-RA, ☞ also Chapters 2.6. and 21.4.) [67-74, 76], which are economically expensive for long-term treatment, and adverse effects such as thromboembolism, deposition of reticulin fibers within the bone marrow need further long-term observation [75]
- Anti-CD20 (rituximab) [78, 79], which have a good response rate, but an unsatisfactory long-term outcome, high risks of adverse effects and is still not evidence-based and approved by authorities for the indication of ITP
- Splenectomy have a good outcome, but has been postponed in favor of newer drugs [80]. The main disadvantage of splenectomy is the life-long, unpredictable risk of severe infections, especially in infants and young children and elderly patients. There may be an unknown number of patients dying after splenectomy [81-83]
- Immunosuppressants as a single drug or in combination with another option are indicated for a limited time period due to adverse effects [84]
- New targeted therapeutics will enlarge the options such as
  - the recently approved Syk-inhibitor (fostamatinib), which inhibits the phagocytosis [85-88]
  - the neonatal FCR antagonists in phase II/III evaluation, which mainly reduce the antibody production [89, 90]

- bortezomib, a proteasome inhibitor, which induces apoptosis [91, 92] and
- low dose decitabine, a therapeutic of the myelodysplastic syndrome, which is studied in patients with refractory ITP [93-94].

As noted in Chapter 2.7. a new area of research is the immune nature of the platelets themselves: Beside mediator of hemostasis the platelets interact as immunoregulatory agent against viruses including the recent Covid19 virus [95, 96] and various bacteria, together with endothelial and other components of the immune e system [97, 98].

In conclusion, decisions reflecting the heterogeneous background of ITP in the management of patients with ITP include:

1) observation with the patient's consent and knowledge of risks, and

2) treatment of patients with bleeding or risk of bleeding with immunomodulatory agents or the recent developed platelet stimulating agents.

For scientists future considerations should focus on studies involving etiology of ITP, including molecular genetic analyses of immune disturbances in the pathogenesis of ITP.

## References

1. Neunert C, Noroozi N, Norman G, Buchanan GR, Goy J, Nazi I, Kelton JG, Arnold DM. Severe bleeding events in adults and children with primary immune thrombocytopenia: a systematic review. J Thromb Haemost. 2015;13:457-464.

2. Mithoowani S, Cervi A, Shah N, Ejaz R, Sirotich E, Barty R, Li N, Nazy I, Arnold DM. Management of major bleeds in patients with immune thrombocytopenia. J Thromb Haemost. 2020;18:1783-1790.

3. Arnold DM, Nazy I, Clare R, Jaffer AM, Aubie B, Li N, Kelton JG. Misdiagnosis of primary immune thrombocytopenia and frequency of bleeding: Lessons from the McMaster ITP Registry. Blood Adv. 2017;1:2414-2420.

4. Despotovic JM, Grimes AB. Pediatric ITP: is it different from adult ITP? Hematology Am Soc Hematol Educ Program. 2018;2018(1):405-411.

5. Cortelazzo S, Finazzi G, Buelli M, et al. High risk of severe bleeding in aged patients with chronic idiopathic thrombocytopenic purpura. Blood. 1991;77:31-33.

6. Grimaldi-Bensouda L, Nordon C, Michel M, Viallard JF, Adoue D, Magy-Bertrand N, Durand JM, Quittet P, Fain O, Bonnotte B, et al. Immune thrombocytopenia in adults: A prospective cohort study of clinical features and predictors of outcome. Haematologica. 2016;101:1039-1045.

7. Kühne T, Buchanan GR, Zimmerman S, Michaels LA, Kohan R, Berchtold W, Imbach PA. Prospective comparative study of 2540 infants and children with newly diagnosed idiopathic thrombocytopenic purpura (ITP) from the Intercontinental Childhood ITP Study Group. J Pediatrics. 2003;143:605-608.

8. Imbach P, Kühne T, Müller D, Berchtold W, Zimmerman S, Elalfy M, Buchanan GR. Childhood ITP: 12 months follow-up data from the prospective registry I of the Intercontinental Childhood ITP Study Group (ICIS). Pediatr Blood Cancer. 2006;46:351-356.

9. Jaime-Pérez JC, Aguilar-Calderón P, Jiménez-Castillo RA, Ramos-Dávila EM, Salazar-Cavazos L, Gómez-Almaguer D. Treatment outcomes and chronicity predictors for primary immune thrombocytopenia: 10-year data from an academic center. Ann Hematol. 2020;99: 2513-2520.

10. Terrell DR, Beebe LA, Vesely SK, Neas BR, Segal JB, George JN. The incidence of immune thrombocytopenic purpura in children and adults: a critical review of published reports. Am J Hematol. 2010;85(3):174-18.

11. Neunert C, Terrell DR, Arnold DM, Buchanan G, Cines DB, Cooper N, Cuker A, Despotovic JM, George JN, Grace RF, et al. American Society of Hematology 2019 guidelines for immune thrombocytopenia. Blood Adv. 2019;3:3829-3866.

12. Kuhne T, Berchtold W, Michaels LA, et al; Intercontinental Cooperative ITP Study Group. Newly diagnosed immune thrombocytopenia in children and adults: a comparative prospective observational registry of the Intercontinental Cooperative Immune Thrombocytopenia Study Group. Haematologica. 2011;96(12):1831-1837.

13. Schifferli A, Holbro A, Chitlur M, et al; Intercontinental Cooperative ITP Study Group (ICIS). A comparative prospective observational study of children and adults with immune thrombocytopenia: 2-year follow-up. Am J Hematol. 2018;93(6):751-759.

14. Saeidi S, Jaseb K, Asnafi AA, et al. Immune thrombocytopenic purpura in children and adults: a comparative retrospective study in Iran. Int J Hematol Oncol Stem Cell Res. 2014;8(3):30-36.

15. Neunert C, Lim W, Crowther M, Cohen A, Solberg L Jr, Crowther MA; American Society of Hematology. The American Society of Hematology 2011 evidence-based practice guideline for immune thrombocytopenia. Blood. 2011;117(16):4190-4207.

16. Kuhne T, Imbach P, Bolton-Maggs PH, Berchtold W, Blanchette V, Buchanan GR; Intercontinental Childhood ITP Study Group. Newly diagnosed idiopathic

thrombocytopenic purpura in childhood: an observational study. Lancet. 2001;358(9299):2122-2125.

17. Neunert C, Noroozi N, Norman G, et al. Severe bleeding events in adults and children with primary immune thrombocytopenia: a systematic review. J Thromb Haemost. 2015;13(3):457-464.

18. Sailer T, Lechner K, Panzer S, Kyrle PA, Pabinger I. The course of severe autoimmune thrombocytopenia in patients not undergoing splenectomy. Haematologica. 2006;91(8):1041-1045.

19. Noergaard M, Jensen AØ, Engebjerg MC, et al. Long-term clinical outcomes of patients with primary chronic immune thrombocytopenia: a Danish population-based cohort study. Blood. 2011;117(13):3514-3520.

20. D Zhou F, Xu Y, Zhang Z, Wu X, Jin R. Severe hemorrhage in Chinese children with immune thrombocytopenia. J Pediatr Hematol Oncol. 2015;37(3):e158-e161.

21. Cuker A, Cines DB, Neunert CE. Controversies in the treatment of immune thrombocytopenia. Curr Opin Hematol. 2016;23(5):479-485.

22. Neunert CE, Buchanan GR, Imbach P, et al; Intercontinental Childhood ITP Study Group Registry II Participants. Severe hemorrhage in children with newly diagnosed immune thrombocytopenic purpura. Blood. 2008;112(10):4003-4008.

23. Neunert CE, Buchanan GR, Imbach P, et al; Intercontinental Cooperative ITP Study Group Registry II Participants. Bleeding manifestations and management of children with persistent and chronic immune thrombocytopenia: data from the Intercontinental Cooperative ITP Study Group (ICIS). Blood. 2013;121(22):4457-4462

24. McMillan R, Bussel JB, George JN, Lalla D, Nichol JL. Self-reported health-related quality of life in adults with chronic immune thrombocytopenic purpura. Am J Hematol. 2008;83(2):150-154.

25. Mathias SD, Gao SK, Miller KL, et al. Impact of chronic immune thrombocytopenic purpura (ITP) on health related quality of life: a conceptual model starting with the patient perspective. Health Qual Life Outcomes. 2008;6:13.

26. Grace R, Despotovic J, Bennett C, et al. Fatigue in pediatric immune thrombocytopenia (ITP): baseline prevalence in patients starting second line therapies in the first ITP Consortium of North America research study (ICON1). Pediatr Blood Cancer. 2016;63:S20.

27. Flores A, Klaassen RJ, Buchanan JR, Neunert CE. Patterns and influences in health-related quality of life in children with immune thrombocytopenia: a study from the Dallas ITP Cohort. Pediatr Blood Cancer. 2017;64 (8):e26405.

28. Hato T, Shimada N, Kurata Y, Kuwana M, Fujimura K, Kashiwagi H, Takafuta T, Murata M, Tomiyama Y. Risk factors for skin, mucosal, and organ bleeding in adults with primary ITP: A nationwide study in Japan. Blood Adv. 2020;4:1648-1655.

29. Rodeghiero F, Stasi R, Gernsheimer T, et al. Standardization of terminology, definitions and outcome criteria in immune throm-bocytopenic purpura of adults and children: report from an international working group. Blood. 2009;113:2386-2393

30. Provan D, Arnold DM, Bussel JB, Chong BH, Cooper N, Gernsheimer T, Ghanima W, Godeau B, González-López TJ, Grainger J, et al. Updated international consensus report on the investigation and management of primary immune thrombocytopenia. Blood Adv. 2019; 3:3780-3817.

31. Matzdorff A, Meyer O, Ostermann H, Kiefel V, Eberl W, Kühne T, Pabinger I, Rummel M. Immune Thrombocytopenia — Current Diagnostics and Therapy: Recommendations of a Joint Working Group of DGHO, ÖGHO, SGH, GPOH, and DGTI. Oncol Res Treat. 2018; 41 (Suppl. 5):1-30.

32. Edslev PW, Rosthøj S, Treutiger I, et al; NOPHO ITP Working Group. A clinical score predicting a brief and uneventful course of newly diagnosed idiopathic thrombocytopenic purpura in children. Br J Haematol 2007; 138:513-516.

33. Cines DB, Bussel JB, Liebman HA, Luning Prak ET. The ITP syndrome: pathogenic and clinical diversity. Blood. 2009;113:6511-21.

34. Snyder CF, Mathias SD, Cella D, et al. Health-related quality of life of immune thrombocytopenic purpura patients: results from a web-based survey. Curr Med Res Opin. 2008;24:2767-2776.

35. Barnard D, Woloski M, Feeny D, et al. Canadian Children's Platelet Study Group. Development of disease-specific health-related quality-of-life instruments for children with immune thrombocytopenic purpura and their parents. J Pediatr Hematol Oncol. 2003;25:56-62.

36. Buchanan GR, Adix L, Klaassen R, et al. Quantitative assessment of drug treatment side effects in children with idiopathic thrombocytopenic purpura (ITP). Blood. 2004;104:3030.

37. Klaassen RJ, Blanchette VS, Barnard D, et al. Validity, reliability, and responsiveness of a new measure of health-related quality of life in children with immune thrombocytopenic purpura: the Kids' ITP Tools. J Pediatr. 2007;150:510-515.

38. Zhou B, Zhao H, Yang RC, Han ZC. Multi-dysfunctional pathophysiology in ITP. Crit Rev Oncol Hematol. 2005;54:107-116.

39. Kuwana M, Kaburaki J, Kitasato H, et al. Immunodominant epitopes on glycoprotein IIb-IIIa recognized by autoreactive T cells in patients with immune thrombocytopenic purpura. Blood. 2001;98:130-139.

40. Semple JW. Immune pathophysiology of autoimmune thrombocytopenic purpura. Blood Rev. 2002;16: 9-12.

41. Foster CB, Zhu S. Erichsen HC, et al. Polymorphisms in inflammatory cytokines and Fcgamma receptors in childhood chronic immune Thrombocytopenic Purpura: a pilot study. Br J Haematol. 2001;113:596-599.

42. Zhao H, Du W, Gu D, et al. DNMT3B 579G>T Promoter Polymorphism and the Risk for Idiopathic Thrombocytopenic Purpura in a Chinese Population. Acta Haematol. 2009;122:31-35.

43. Zhang B, Lo C, Shen L, Sood R, et al. The role of vanin-1 and oxidative stress-related pathways in distinguishing acute and chronic pediatric ITP. Blood. 2011; 117:4569-4579.

44. Imbach P, Lazarus AH, Kühne T. Intravenous immunoglobulins induce potentially synergistic immunomodulations in autoimmune disorders. Vox Sang. 2010; 98:385-394.

45. Imbach P, Barandun S, d'Apuzzo V, et al. High-dose intravenous gammaglobulin for idiopathic thrombocytopenic purpura in childhood. Lancet. 1981;1:1228-1231.

46. Imbach P, Berchtold W, Hirt A, et al. Intravenous immunoglobulin versus oral corticosteroids in acute immune thrombocytopenic purpura in childhood. Lancet. 1985;2:464-468.

47. Lemieux R, Bazin R, Néron S. Therapeutic intravenous immunoglobulins. Mol Immunol. 2005;42:839-848.

48. Arnold DM, Dentali F, Crowther MA, et al. Systematic review: efficacy and safety of rituximab for adults with idiopathic thrombocytopenic purpura. Ann Intern Med. 2007;146:25-33.

49. Olsson B, Andersson PO, JErnas M, et al. T-cell-mediated cytotoxicity toward platelets in chronic idiopathic thrombocytopenic purpura. Nat Med. 2003;9: 1123-1124.

50. Schifferli A, Cavalli F, Godeau B, Liebman HA, Recher M, Imbach P, Kühne T. Understanding Immune Thrombocytopenia: Looking Out of the Box. Front Med (Lausanne). 2021;8:613192.

51. McMillan R, Luiken GA, Levy R, Yelenosky R, Longmire RL. Antibody against megakaryocytes in idiopathic thrombocytopenic purpura. JAMA. 1978;239:2460-24635.

52. Chang M, Nakagawa PA, Williams SA, Schwartz MR, Imfeld KL, Buzby JS, Nugent DJ. Immune thrombocytopenic purpura (ITP) plasma and purified ITP monoclonal autoantibodies inhibit megakaryocytopoiesis in vitro. Blood. 2003;102: 887-895.

53. McMillan R, Wang L, Tomer A, Nichol J, Pistillo J. Suppression of in vitro megakaryocyte production by antiplatelet autoantibodies from adult patients with chronic ITP. Blood. 2004;103:1364-1369.

54. Imbach P, Crowther M. Thrombopoietin-receptor agonists for primary immune thrombocytopenia. N Engl J Med. 2011;365:734-741.

55. Wong RSM, Saleh MN, Khelif A, Salama A, Portella MSO, Burgess P, Bussel JB. Safety and efficacy of long-term treatment of chronic/persistent ITP with eltrombopag: Final results of the EXTEND study. Blood. 2017; 130:2527-2536.

56. González-López TJ, Pascual C, Álvarez-Román MT, Fernández-Fuertes F, Sánchez-González B, Caparrós I, Jarque I, Mingot-Castellano ME, Hernández-Rivas JA, Martín-Salces M, et al. Successful discontinuation of eltrombopag after complete remission in patients with primary immune thrombocytopenia. Am J Hematol. 2015;90:E40-E43.

57. Mishra K, Pramanik S, Jandial A, Sahu KK, Sandal R, Ahuja A, Yanamandra U, Kumar R, Kapoor R, Verma T, et al. Real-world experience of eltrombopag in immune thrombocytopenia. Am J Blood Res. 2020;10:240-251.

58. Eden OB, Lilleyman JS. Guidelines for management of idiopathic thrombocytopenic purpura. The British Paediatric Haematology Group. Arch Dis Child. 1992; 67:1056-1058.

59. Schifferli A, Heiri A, Imbach P, Holzhauer S, Seidel MG, Nugent D, Michel M, Kühne T. Misdiagnosed thrombocytopenia in children and adolescents: analysis of the Pediatric and Adult Registry on Chronic ITP. Blood Adv. 2021;5(6):1617-1626.

60. Neunert CE, Buchanan GR, Blanchette V et al. Relationships among bleeding severity, health-related quality of life, and platelet count in children with immune thrombocytopenic purpura. Pediatr Blood Cancer. 2009;53: 652-4.

61. Kühne T, Imbach P. Management of children and adolescents with primary immune thrombocytopenia: controversies and solutions. Vox Sang. 2013;104(1):55-66.

62. Zeller B, Rajantie J, Hedlund-Treutiger I, et al; NOPHO ITP. Childhood idiopathic thrombocytopenic purpura in the Nordic countries: epidemiology and predictors of chronic disease. Acta Paediatr. 2005;94:178-184.

63. Wang L, Xu L, Hao H, Jansen AJG, Liu G, Li H, Liu X, Zhao Y, Peng J, Hou M. First line treatment of adult pa-

tients with primary immune thrombocytopenia: A real-world study. Platelets. 2020;31:55-61.

64. Zhou Z, Qiao Z, Li H, Luo N, Zhang X, Xue F, Yang R. Different dosages of intravenous immunoglobulin (IVIg) in treating immune thrombocytopenia with long-term follow-up of three years: Results of a prospective study including 167 cases. Autoimmunity. 2016;49:50-57.

65. Mithoowani S, Gregory-Miller K, Goy J, Miller MC, Wang G, Noroozi N, Kelton JG, Arnold DM. High-dose dexamethasone compared with prednisone for previously untreated primary immune thrombocytopenia: A systematic review and meta-analysis. Lancet Haematol. 2016;3:e489-e496.

66. Ma J, Fu L, Chen Z, Gu H, Ma J, Wu R. High-dose dexamethasone as a replacement for traditional prednisone as the first-line treatment in children with previously untreated primary immune thrombocytopenia: A prospective, randomized single-center study. Int J Hematol. 2020;112:773-779.

67. Kuter DJ. Milestones in understanding platelet production: a historical overview. Br J Haematol. 2014;165 (2):248-258.

68. Neunert C, Despotovic J, Haley K, et al; Pediatric ITP Consortium of North America (ICON). Thrombopoietin receptor agonist use in children: data from the Pediatric ITP Consortium of North America ICON2 Study. Pediatr Blood Cancer. 2016;63(8):1407-1413.

69. Roumier M, Le Burel S, Audia S, Chauchet A, Gousseff M, Hamidou M, Liferman F, Moulis G, Lioger B, Galicier L, et al. High dose romiplostim as a rescue therapy for adults with severe bleeding and refractory immune thrombocytopenia. Am J Hematol. 2021;96(2): E43-E46.

70. Kuter DJ, Arnold DM, Rodeghiero F, Janssens A, Selleslag D, Bird R, Newland A, Mayer J, Wang K, Olie R. Safety and efficacy of self-administered romiplostim in patients with immune thrombocytopenia: Results of an integrated database of five clinical trials. Am J Hematol. 2020;95:643 651.

71. Kuter DJ, Newland A, Chong BH, Rodeghiero F, Romero MT, Pabinger I, Chen Y, Wang K, Mehta B, Eisen M. Romiplostim in adult patients with newly diagnosed or persistent immune thrombocytopenia (ITP) for up to 1 year and in those with chronic ITP for more than 1 year: A subgroup analysis of integrated data from completed romiplostim studies. Br J Haematol. 2019; 185:503-513.

72. Yang R, Hou M, Li J. Effect of eltrombopag on platelet response and safety results in Chinese adults with chronic ITP-primary result of a phase III study (abstract). Blood. 2014;124:1464.

73. Wong RSM, Saleh MN, Khelif A, et al. Safety and efficacy of long-term treatment of chronic/persistent ITP with eltrombopag: final results of the EXTEND study. Blood. 2017;130(23):2527-2536.

74. Li Y, Shi Y, He Z, Chen Q, Liu Z, Yu L, Wang C. The efficacy and safety of low-dose rituximab in immune thrombocytopenia: a systematic review and meta-analysis. Platelets. 2019;30:690-697.

75. Janssens A, Rodeghiero F, Anderson D, Chong BH, Boda Z, Pabinger I, Cervinek L, Terrell DR, Wang X, Franklin J. Changes in bone marrow morphology in adults receiving romiplostim for the treatment of thrombocytopenia associated with primary immune thrombocytopenia. Ann Hematol. 2016;95:1077-1087.

76. Jurczak W, Chojnowski K, Mayer J, Krawczyk K, Jamieson BD, Tian W, Allen LF. Phase 3 randomised study of avatrombopag, a novel thrombopoietin receptor agonist for the treatment of chronic immune thrombocytopenia. Br J Haematol. 2018;183:479-490.

77. Doptelet®Prescribtion Information. Available online: www.accessdata.fda.gov/drugsatfda_docs/label/2018/210238s000lbl.pdf (accessed on 8 January 2021).

78. Arnold DM, Vrbensky JR, Karim N, et al. The effect of rituximab on antiplatelet autoantibody levels in patients with immune thrombocytopenia. Br J Haematol. 2017; 178(2):302-307.

79. Patel VL, Mahevas M, Lee SY, et al. Outcomes 5 years after response to rituximab therapy in children and adults with immune thrombocytopenia. Blood. 2012; 119(25):5989-5995.

80. Bhatt NS, Bhatt P, Donda K, et al. Temporal trends of splenectomy in pediatric hospitalizations with immune thrombocytopenia. Pediatr Blood Cancer. 2018;65(7): e27072.

81. Chaturvedi S, Arnold DM, McCrae KR. Splenectomy for immune thrombocytopenia: Down but not out. Blood. 2018;131:1172-1182.

82. Vianelli N, Palandri F, Polverelli N, Stasi R, Joelsson J, Johansson E, Ruggeri M, Zaja F, Cantoni S, Catucci AE, et al. Splenectomy as a curative treatment for immune thrombocytopenia: A retrospective analysis of 233 patients with a minimum follow up of 10 years. Haematologica. 2013;98:875-880.

83. Kwiatkowska A, Radkowiak D, Wysocki M, Torbicz G, Gajewska N, Lasek A, Kulawik J, Budzyñski A, Pêdziwiatr M. Prognostic Factors for Immune Thrombocytopenic Purpura Remission after Laparoscopic Splenectomy: A Cohort Study. Medicina (Kaunas). 2019;55 (4):112.

84. Wang J, Li Y, Wang C, Zhang Y, Gao C, Lang H, Chen X. Efficacy and Safety of the Combination Treatment of Rituximab and Dexamethasone for Adults with Primary

Immune Thrombocytopenia (ITP): A Meta-Analysis. Biomed Res Int. 2018;2018:1316096.

85. Newland A, Lee EJ, McDonald V, Bussel JB. Fostamatinib for persistent/chronic adult immune thrombocytopenia. Immunotherapy. 2018;10:9-25.

86. Bussel J, Arnold DM, Grossbard E, Mayer J, Trelinski J, Homenda W, Hellmann A, Windyga J, Sivcheva L, Khalafallah AA, et al. Fostamatinib for the treatment of adult persistent and chronic immune thrombocytopenia: Results of two phase 3, randomized, placebo-controlled trials. Am J Hematol. 2018;93:921-930.

87. Bussel JB, Arnold DM, Boxer MA, Cooper N, Mayer J, Zayed H, Tong S, Duliege AM. Long-term fostamatinib treatment of adults with immune thrombocytopenia during the phase 3 clinical trial program. Am J Hematol. 2019;94:546-553.

88. Boccia R, Cooper N, Ghanima W, Boxer MA, Hill QA, Sholzberg M, Tarantino MD, Todd LK, Tong S, Bussel JB. Fostamatinib is an effective second-line therapy in patients with immune thrombocytopenia. Br J Haematol. 2020;190:933-938.

89. Robak T, Kazmierczak M, Jarque I, Musteata V, Treliñski J, Cooper N, Kiessling P, Massow U, Woltering F, Snipes R, Ke J, Langdon G, Bussel JB, Jolles S. Phase 2 multiple-dose study of an FcRn inhibitor, rozanolixizumab, in patients with primary immune thrombocytopenia. Blood Adv. 2020;4:4136-4146.

90. Newland AC, Sánchez-González B, Rejtõ L, Egyed M, Romanyuk N, Godar M, Verschueren K, Gandini D, Ulrichts P, Beauchamp J, et al. Phase 2 study of efgartigimod, a novel FcRn antagonist, in adult patients with primary immune thrombocytopenia. Am J Hematol. 2020;95:178-187.

91. Li G, Wang S, Li N, Liu Y, Feng Q, Zuo X, Li X, Hou Y, Shao L, Ma C, et al. Proteasome Inhibition with Bortezomib Induces Apoptosis of Long-Lived Plasma Cells in Steroid-Resistant or Relapsed Immune Thrombocytopaenia. Thromb Haemost. 2018;118:1752-1764.

92. Beckman JD, Rollins-Raval MA, Raval JS, Park YA, Mazepa M, Ma A. Bortezomib for Refractory Immune-Mediated Thrombocytopenia Purpura. Am J Ther. 2018; 25:e270-e272.

93. Ding K, Fu R, Liu H, Nachnani DA, Shao ZH. Effects of decitabine on megakaryocyte maturation in patients with myelodysplastic syndromes. Oncol Lett. 2016;11: 2347-2352.

94. Zhou H, Qin P, Liu Q, Yuan C, Hao Y, Zhang H, Wang Z, Ran X, Chu X, Yu W, et al. A prospective, multicenter study of low dose decitabine in adult patients with refractory immune thrombocytopenia. Am J Hematol. 2019;94:1374-1381.

95. Pavord S, Thachil J, Hunt BJ, Murphy M, Lowe G, Laffan M, Makris M, Newland AC, Provan D, Grainger JD, et al. Practical guidance for the management of adults with immune thrombocytopenia during the COVID-19 pandemic. Br J Haematol. 2020;189:1038-1043.

96. Mahévas M, Moulis G, Andres E, Riviere E, Garzaro M, Crickx E, Guillotin V, Malphettes M, Galicier L, Noel N, et al. Clinical characteristics, management and outcome of COVID-19-associated immune thrombocytopenia: a French multicentre series. Br J Haematol. 2020; 190:e224-e229.

97. Maouia A, Rebetz J, Kapur R, Semple JW. The Immune Nature of Platelets Revisited. Transfus Med Rev. 2020;34(4):209-220.

98. Semple JW, Rebetz J, Maouia A, Kapur R. An update on the pathophysiology of immune thrombocytopenia. Curr Opin Hematol. 2020;27(6):423-429.

# 22. List of abbreviations

| Abbreviation | Meaning of the abbreviation |
|---|---|
| AA | Aplastic anemia |
| ADAMTS | A disintegrin and metalloprotease with thrombospondin-1-like domain |
| ALPS | Autoimmune lymphoproliferative syndrome |
| Anti-D | Intravenous anti-Rh(D) |
| APS | Antiphospholipid syndrome |
| ASH | American Society of Hematology |
| Bregs | Regulatory B cells |
| BSS | Bernard-Soulier syndrome |
| BTK | Bruton tyrosine kinase |
| CDC | Complement dependent toxicity |
| CIDP | Chronic inflammatory demyelinating polyradiculoneuropathy |
| CLL | Chronic lymphocytic leukemia |
| CMP | Common myeloid progenitor |
| CMV | Cytomegalovirus (infection) |
| CR | Complete response |
| CTL | Cytotoxic lymphocyte |
| CVID | Common variable immune deficiency |
| DC | Dendritic cells |
| DDAVP | Desmopressin |
| DMS | Demarcation membrane system |
| EBV | Epstein-Barr virus (infection) |
| EMA | European Medicines Agency |
| FcR | Fc receptor |
| FcRn | Neonatal Fc receptor |
| FDA | Food and Drug Administration |
| GBS | Guillain-Barre syndrome |
| GP | Glykoprotein |
| GPS | Gray platelet syndrome |
| GR | Glucocorticoid receptor |
| GWAS | Genome-wide association studies |
| HCV | Hepatitis C virus (infection) |
| HIV | Human immunodeficiency virus (infection) |
| HRQoL | Health-Related Quality of Life |
| HSC | Hematopoietic stem cell |
| ICH | Intracranial hemorrhage |
| ICIS | Intercontinental Cooperative ITP Study Group |
| IFN | Interferon |
| Ig | Immunoglobulin |
| IL | Interleukin |
| IPF | Immature platelet fraction |
| IQR | Interquartile range |
| IT | Inherited thrombocytopenia |
| ITAM | Immunoreceptor tyrosine-based activation motif |
| ITIM | Immunoreceptor tyrosine-based inhibitory motif |
| ITP | Immune thrombocytopenia |
| IVIg | Intravenous immunoglobulin |
| IWG | International Working Group |
| JBS | Jacobsen syndrome |
| L | Liter |
| MAC | Membrane attack complex |
| mDC | Myeloid dendritic cells |
| MDS | Myelodysplastic syndrome |
| MEP | Megakaryocyte erythroid progenitor |
| MK | Megakaryocyte |
| mTOR | Mammalian Target of Rapamycin |
| PARC-ITP | Pediatric and Adult Registry on Chronic ITP |
| pDC | Plasmacytoid dendritic cells |
| PEG rHu MGDF | Pegylated human recombinant megakaryocyte growth and development factor |
| PGE | Prostaglandin E |
| PRO | Patient reported outcome |
| QoL | Quality of Life |
| R | Response |
| RES | Reticuloendothelial system |
| rhTPO | Recombinant human thrombopoietin |
| SLE | Systemic lupus erythematosus |

| Abbreviation | Meaning of the abbreviation |
|---|---|
| SMOG | Skin (S), visible mucosae (M), and organs (O), with gradation (G) of severity |
| TAR | Thrombocytopenia with absent radii |
| TCPT | Paris-Trousseau thrombocytopenia |
| TE | Thromboembolic event |
| TGF | Transforming growth factor |
| TNF | Tumor necrosis factor |
| TPO | Thrombopoietin |
| TPO-RA | Thrombopoietin receptor agonist |
| TRA | Thrombopoetin receptor agonist |
| Tregs | Regulatory T cells |
| TTP | Thrombotic thrombocytopenic purpura |
| VWF | Von Willebrand factor |
| WAS | Wiskott-Aldrich syndrome |
| XLT | X-linked thrombocytopenia |

***Table 22.1:*** Selection of important abbreviations used in this textbook. Further abbreviations are explained either directly in the text or in table and figure legends.

# Index